The Adult Autism
Assessment Handbook

of related interest

The Little Book of Autism FAQs
How to Talk with Your Child about their Diagnosis & Other Conversations
Davida Hartman
Illustrated by Margaret Ann Suggs
ISBN 978 1 78592 449 1
eISBN 978 1 78450 824 1

The Autism and Neurodiversity Self Advocacy Handbook
Developing the Skills to Determine Your Own Future
Barb Cook and Yenn Purkis
ISBN 978 1 78775 575 8
eISBN 978 1 78775 576 5

Autism and Masking
How and Why People Do It, and the Impact It Can Have
Dr Felicity Sedgewick, Dr Laura Hull and Helen Ellis
ISBN 978 1 78775 579 6
eISBN 978 1 78775 580 2

An Adult with an Autism Diagnosis
A Guide for the Newly Diagnosed
Gillan Drew
ISBN 978 1 78592 246 6
eISBN 978 1 78450 530 1

THE ADULT AUTISM ASSESSMENT HANDBOOK

A Neurodiversity-Affirmative Approach

Davida Hartman, Tara O'Donnell-Killen,
Jessica K. Doyle, Dr Maeve Kavanagh,
Dr Anna Day and Dr Juliana Azevedo

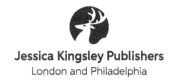

Jessica Kingsley Publishers
London and Philadelphia

First published in Great Britain in 2023 by Jessica Kingsley Publishers
An imprint of Hodder & Stoughton Ltd
An Hachette Company

1

This book was typeset in accordance with accessible principles, but it does contain a high
volume of text and information in order to be fully comprehensive. It is also available as an
eBook, where text can be resized or converted to speech using text-to-speech software.

All pages marked with ✳ can be downloaded at https://library.jkp.com/redeem for personal use with this
programme, but may not be reproduced for any other purposes without the permission of the publisher.

Content warning: This book mentions mental health, anxiety, abuse and trauma.

A CIP catalogue record for this title is available from the British Library and the Library of Congress

ISBN 978 1 83997 166 2
eISBN 978 1 83997 167 9

Printed and bound in Great Britain by TJ Books Ltd

Jessica Kingsley Publishers' policy is to use papers that are natural, renewable and recyclable
products and made from wood grown in sustainable forests. The logging and manufacturing
processes are expected to conform to the environmental regulations of the country of origin.

Jessica Kingsley Publishers
Carmelite House
50 Victoria Embankment
London EC4Y 0DZ

www.jkp.com

This book is dedicated to the Autistic people who have chosen to work with us in The Adult Autism Practice and Thriving Autistic. We are grateful to them for honouring and trusting us with their stories.

It is also dedicated to the wider Autistic community: those who have shared their stories and found connection on social media, the advocates who have borne the brunt of the prejudice against Autistic people as they push for basic human rights and demand that our voices are the ones leading the conversation about us, the Autistics who remain in institutions around the globe, punished by a world that seeks to extinguish that which it does not understand, Autistics who hold multiple marginalized identities and have exponentially greater barriers and prejudices to navigate, Autistic parents who daily navigate outside pressure to force their children to conform to neurotypical societal norms, and the Autistic clinicians, practitioners and researchers who work tirelessly and bare their soul daily, all for the greater good of protecting and promoting the rights and wellbeing of the Autistic community.

Acknowledgements

Thank you to our families and those precious to us: Max, Ely, Juno and Alex, Martina, William and Ríona. Gavin, Oisín, Ray, Lucas, Sam, Aoife, Aideen, Keelin and Hughie. Jim (Dad), Siún, Beth, Fred, Emmet, ET, Thérèse, Astro and Owli. Barry, Ben, Maisie, Vera, Barry, Kieran and Karen. Daisy, Flower, Teddy and Peanut. Celso, Regina, Julia, Mateus, Tatiana, Fabiana and Rodrigo. Thank you to Philomena, Kieron and the entire Adult Autism Practice team. Thank you to Alice, Ann, Claire, Dana, Jasper, Jennie, Nic, Rajita, Teri, Vauna and the entire Thriving Autistic team. Thank you to Shelley Carr for her helpful insights. Thank you to Olatunde Spence and Elaine McGreevy. Thank you to our editor Amy Lankester-Owen and the entire publishing team at Jessica Kingsley Publishers.

Contents

1

Introduction

Who We Are and Why We Are Writing This Book

Our writing team is a mixed group of Autistic, otherwise neurodivergent and neurotypical professionals working together within the wider Adult Autism Practice and Thriving Autistic teams. We are psychologists, an assistant psychologist/ Autistic researcher, friends and colleagues who have come together with the shared purpose of, and passion for, supporting Autistic people to live their best lives, recognizing that for them to do so there are significant societal changes that need to be made in relation to how we understand and assess Autistic neurology. We have all seen first hand in our work the enormous, positive benefits that correct identification of being Autistic brings, as well as the life-changing benefits of having been assessed through a Neuro-Affirmative framework, and we are passionate about sharing this knowledge and learning with our wider colleagues.

The Adult Autism Practice is a private company specializing in remote adult autism assessment (which includes as standard post-assessment support delivered by the team at Thriving Autistic). It is a multidisciplinary team of Autistic, otherwise neurodivergent and neurotypical professionals (psychologists, occupational therapists and speech and language therapists) who work together to provide timely, respectful, collaborative, LGBTQIA+ and Neuro-Affirmative adult autism assessments where strengths are emphasized and passions and differences celebrated. It is part of The Adult Autism Practice's mission to continue to employ and be shaped by Autistic professionals and the Autistic community.

Davida Hartman (one of the authors of this book) founded the Practice in 2020 to fill the huge gap in services that were, and continue to be, present. Tara O'Donnell-Killen and Dr Maeve Kavanagh (also authors of this book) have been involved with the Practice from its inception, and have been vital collaborators, influencing how the Practice has been shaped thus far. As well as comprehensive adult autism assessments, The Adult Autism Practice also provides consultations for clients who are unsure if they want to go ahead with a full assessment but would like to talk it all through with someone. The team is a mix of Irish and UK-based professionals, and because the assessments are remote, they see clients worldwide (apart from Canada and the USA).

Thriving Autistic is a non-profit organization that specializes in support services for Autistic adults. It is the world's first multidisciplinary team of professionals (psychologists, psychotherapists, counsellors, occupational therapists, speech and language therapists, educators and coaches) who are all Autistic or otherwise neurodivergent themselves. Tara O'Donnell-Killen (one of the authors of this book) founded it in 2020, to provide the global Autistic community with Neuro-Affirmative support services, create employment for neurodivergent practitioners and to light the way for all people of conscience to adapt their thinking and practice to a more human-rights based approach to neurodiversity. In 2021 Thriving Autistic became a legal non-profit with the support of another of this book's authors, Jessica K. Doyle, who is also a director at Thriving Autistic. The global Thriving Autistic team provide post-assessment support services for adults from all over the world. They also provide continuing professional development and education to psychologists and therapists, and consultations to private organizations on Neuro-Affirmative best practices.

Starting in early 2022, our next goal as a collaborative Thriving Autistic and Adult Autism Practice team is to start capturing the short- and long-term benefits of Neuro-Affirmative autism assessments (as well as broader Neuro-Affirmative approaches) through research, not only on our clients' experiences, but also how undertaking assessments in this way has revitalized and remotivated our teams. We also aim to publish a Neuro-Affirmative **child** autism assessment handbook, and are in the process of developing a Neuro-Affirmative autism diagnostic assessment tool (as none are currently available).

All the authors of this book were involved in the planning and reviewing of **all** sections of this book, and it was a collaborative and joyful process to write. However, certain sections were led by authors who hold a particular interest or expertise in the area – for example, Tara O'Donnell-Killen led our chapter on post-assessment support (Chapter 13) and Jessica K. Doyle led our chapter on Autistic perception (Chapter 6).

An Introduction to Autism Assessment

▓ **Important note:** The concepts and paradigms in this book are not our 'creations', but the culmination and ongoing journey of a great many Autistic and disability rights advocates.

As of the time of writing (2022), this is the first book specifically on the topic of adult autism assessment, and the Wikipedia page related to autism assessment and diagnosis doesn't even mention adults. As you will learn later, best practice guidelines worldwide to support adult autism assessments are hard to find and outdated in relation to newer ways of understanding and talking about Autistic people. There are also no standardized tests that are validated or appropriate to assess Autistic adults. It has therefore been difficult for clinicians wishing to undertake best practice adult autism assessments to find information on just how to go about them. It is our aim to fill this gap.

Despite its lack of prominence in the literature and best practice guidelines, accurate identification of someone's Autistic neurology is **vitally** important. In 2020, the Royal College of Psychiatrists reported that **most Autistic people are adults, undiagnosed and without an intellectual disability** (Berney 2020). A Swedish study in 2022 found that out of all new patients referred to an adult psychiatric outpatient unit, the estimated prevalence of Autistic people was at least 18.9 per cent, with another 5–10 per cent showing signs of being Autistic but who were 'subthreshold' (Nyrenius et al. 2022). Cassidy et al. (2022) found elevated Autistic traits to be significantly overrepresented in those who died by suicide in England (identifying evidence of possible undiagnosed Autistic people in 41.4 per cent of cases). Statistics like this show the very real-world implications for Autistic people of not correctly understanding their neurology, and the great need for the upskilling of **all** healthcare professionals in this area.

The core goal of this book is for professionals to stop missing Autistic people diagnostically because of outdated views or ignorance. It is also for professionals involved in adult autism assessments to make the vital shift to a Neuro-Affirmative paradigm in their work and assessments so that they can see the quite phenomenal short- and long-term benefits to their clients.

Until relatively recently the term 'Neuro-Affirmative' was new to the majority of us – we only started using it in early 2020 to perfectly conceptualize a slow and then more recently rapidly changing landscape in how Autistic and otherwise neurodivergent people understand and talk about their individual neurology. We were first introduced to the term by Tara O'Donnell-Killen, the inspiration for much of our changes of thinking in this area. Thankfully, the concept is now quickly growing in popularity and awareness, and it feels that we are currently on the crest of a wave in relation to this paradigm shift, arising from a phenomenal amount of work over the years from Autistic (and otherwise neurodivergent) advocates.

We have been working with our adult clients on autism identification, diagnosis and post-assessment support since 2020, and have seen the truly life-changing benefits our clients experience having gone through the process of a collaborative, supportive, therapeutic, respectful, LGBTQIA+ and Neuro-Affirmative assessment. At Thriving Autistic, we hear on a daily basis from many people self-referring to our support service about how devastating and traumatizing the current traditional ways of assessing autism can be for Autistic adults, even when conducted by well-meaning and kind professionals wanting the best for their clients.

Our intention is that this book will be a practical 'how to' guide to adult autism assessments, as well as covering the vital background information that professionals need to know before starting. We have therefore included up-to-date information about Autistic neurology, a history of Autistic people and the neurodiversity movement and paradigm, important areas and possible differential diagnoses that professionals will need to consider alongside their assessment, how to make assessments accessible, how to actually conduct assessments and post-assessment support, and vitally, how to develop self-reflection skills in this area, with Reflection Points throughout.

We have also included helpful resources that clinicians can use in their own assessments as well as a great deal of personal reflections and learning from us, as clinicians, working in this area. We hope that through changing your practices to be more Neuro-Affirmative, you, too, will experience the rich, genuine and moving connections that we have daily with the people who allow us the privilege of taking this part of their journey with them. These have been some of the most profound connections of our clinical experience, reflected in the beautiful words that many Autistic people have shared with us about their experience. This way of working is both life-affirming and joyous.

▦   **Important note:** This is a **rapidly** evolving area as new learning is made every day. In the year that it has taken to write this book, we have had to rewrite and edit whole sections to take into account new learning and new language use. We are almost constantly updating how we work and how we talk about Autistic people. It is very important for professionals to bear this in mind, and to realize that the information in this book is provided with what we understand to be best practice **at this time.** But it is **vital** to continue to keep up to date with Autistic-led research and thinking in this area, and to be constantly updating practice to reflect that.

Our aim is to provide professionals with the critical thinking tools and avenues to continue this journey independently, and we have a wealth of accompanying materials available online to download.

Copies of the appendices found in this book can be downloaded from
https://library.jkp.com/redeem using the code LNFRFAX

Declaration of Privilege

We are aware of our privilege in being part of the writing process of this book. Collectively, we hold many marginalized identities, yet we acknowledge and hold the tension of knowing that we are, for the majority, white people. There are many other amazing Autistic professionals who hold multiple ethnic and gender identities who (in this book) did not have the same opportunity. Our aim has been to include as many perspectives as possible, without speaking for those other identities.

If you are contemplating carrying out an adult autism assessment, it is imperative that the earlier chapters of this book should be read prior to engaging with Chapter 12.

2

Language Guide

Important note: Language evolves over time. The language recommended in this book was the Autistic community (in the global North) consensus at the time of writing. Our sources of information were from the Autistic community themselves (e.g., through Autistic-led research, Autistic advocacy groups and online surveys with Autistic respondents). We recommend professionals keep up to date with evolving language preferences by using these sources of information going forward.

Key Neuro-Affirmative Terminology
(with a Focus on Autistic Neurology)

- Neurodiversity: The broad array of different neurology (brains) in the human population.

- Neurodiverse: Refers to a group of people with a broad array of different neurology (brains), including neurotypical people as well as Autistic people. It does not refer to individual people.

- Neurodivergent: Someone whose brain differs to the perceived neuro-majority, e.g., if they are Autistic or ADHD.

- Autistic: An individual who has an Autistic neurotype.

- Autistic developmental trajectory: Autistic people have a developmental trajectory that is different (not delayed or disordered) as compared to non-autistic people.

- Neurotypical: A term describing the majority neurotype of the population.

- Non-Speaking: Someone who does not use their mouth to speak.

The person may be Non-Speaking at times, or intermittently. They may use other modes of communication and be known as multi-modal communicators.

- Identity-first language: Referring to yourself with your identity before your personhood, e.g., how the Autistic community choose the terminology 'I am Autistic' over 'I have autism'.

- The Autistic community: A community of people who are all Autistic, and of all ages.

- The Autism community: A community of people that also includes non-autistic people (as well as Autistic people), e.g., non-autistic parents, professionals and allies.

Examples of their use:

Neurotypical people can often struggle to understand the lived experience of Autistic and otherwise neurodivergent people.

My family is neurodiverse, it includes Autistic, Dyspraxic as well as neurotypical people.

I am Autistic, which means that I am neurodivergent.

My child is Autistic, and so their development is on an Autistic, not a neurotypical, developmental trajectory. Please don't judge their progress by neurotypical standards.

I like the neurodiversity paradigm that sees value in a wide range of different neurologies, including being neurotypical, Dyspraxic, Dyslexic and Autistic.

I am an Autistic person and I have a different experience of the world because my perception is created differently to how a non-autistic person's perception is created.

I am 10, I like clouds, I am Autistic and a member of the Autistic community. My mum prefers clear skies and she is not Autistic but is a member of the Autism community.

Introduction

Language is one of our most powerful tools to shape how we think and talk about difference and disability. The American Psychological Association has clearly stated that to honour the language preference of any disability group is both a sign of professional awareness and respect, as well as a way of offering solidarity.[1] By using a community's language of choice, and avoiding ableist and damaging language, we can help build more accommodating and understanding societies for Autistic (and otherwise neurodivergent) people to thrive in.

However, changing our language can be difficult. Humans naturally rely on bias to navigate the world, and we have evolved in such a way that we value familiarity and generally dislike change. This can often make it easier to build up evidence for something we have always believed to be true rather than take the sometime difficult steps to reflect and enter the unknown, to examine our bias on what might be underpinning our beliefs, and to try to consider a new perspective.

As professionals working with Autistic people, it is not only our responsibility to diagnose or provide therapeutic support to the best of our ability and knowledge; it is also our responsibility to more broadly support and advocate for the community we serve. As Desmond Tutu so wisely said, **we need to stop fishing people out of the water and instead look to why they are falling in in the first place**. And then, of course, take the steps needed to stop this happening. Part of this advocacy role is counteracting negative stereotypes and listening to the community to whom we entrust our livelihoods. This is not specific to the Autistic community, and is the same across distinct groups and cultures that have the right to decide for themselves how they choose to be spoken about.

You personally may have opinions about the use of certain words or phrasing, but if you are not Autistic, these will need to be put aside out of respect for the community you are serving. The fact is that Autistic people hear and see the language you use about them. And they feel **deeply** hurt and unheard when you do not use their language preferences. It is part of our role as health and caring professionals to keep up to date with respectful language use for a community or population of people. Using outdated, harmful or incorrect terminology is a sign to Autistic people that you do not care about their voice, that you do not personally know or listen to any Autistic people, and ultimately it damages your professional reputation with them. Using the language choices of a community shows that you are a professional who is respectful and inclusive. It reflects good manners and sensitivity.

---

1   See https://apastyle.apa.org/style-grammar-guidelines/bias-free-language/disability

■ **Important note:** Sometimes the language individual people use to describe themselves will differ with wider community preferences. When working with **individual** people, with **them**, always use the language **they choose** to use to describe themselves.

Here are the **current** language preferences for the majority of the Autistic community.

Use 'Autistic Person', Not 'Person with Autism'

If you are new to using identity first-language, for all of the reasons outlined here it can feel uncomfortable for a while. It was for the neurotypical authors of this book, who were using identity-first language for months before it felt natural.

The consensus is clear that the majority of the Autistic community and Autistic-led Autistic organizations prefer the use of identity-first language (i.e., 'Autistic person') over person-first language (i.e., 'person with autism'). Countless research, blogs and opinion polls conducted with and by Autistic people have now shown this to be fact.

Not only do the Autistic community prefer identity-first language over person-first language, they often find person-first language offensive and disrespectful to their neurotype. You would never, for example, say 'a person with woman-ness'. The same principle absolutely applies to Autistic individuals and communities, and hurts every bit as deeply. If not already clear, continuing to use person-first language when you are aware that the Autistic community prefer identity-first language is offensive and disrespectful for reasons we will further outline in this section.

Being Autistic is integral to who someone is. It is intrinsic to how a person develops through a distinct Autistic developmental trajectory, communicates through Autistic communication styles, experiences and interacts with the world through distinctly Autistic perceptual mechanisms, and learns and understands through Autistic cognitive processing. Being Autistic is the neurological foundation from where each Autistic person grows. Being Autistic is not a **part** of a person, or in any way detachable or an impediment to be removed. Being Autistic **is** a naturally occurring neurology.

To get to the point of being a professional supporting an individual's discovery of being Autistic, you have undoubtedly attended a multitude of training courses that framed the Autistic neurotype as an overwhelmingly negative experience and a disorder, and all co-occurring conditions (e.g., epilepsy, intellectual disabilities, obsessive-compulsive disorder (OCD)) and responses to environment (e.g., mental health issues and anxiety) as being a direct consequence of being Autistic. It is likely that within these courses person-first language was used and recommended, either explicitly or implicitly. Unless you are Autistic yourself, outside of your professional life, in the media and in non-autistic-led community groups, person-first language has also likely been the dominant framing.

However, disability and personhood are not mutually exclusive, and it is shameful that we would even need to think to remind ourselves that Autistic people are people. But still this remains an argument for the continued use and promotion of person-first language, even when it is against the community's preferences. The argument follows that person-first language helps the person using that language to remember that the person is a 'person first' and not just their neurology. The analogy of a person with cancer is often cited, explaining that it would be dehumanizing for a doctor to call their patient a 'cancer person', as (language being powerful) this would lead to the doctor unconsciously not seeing the full person that their patient is. But there is a crucial difference here. Cancer, unlike being Autistic, describes a **disease** the person has **acquired**, and is something that needs to be eradicated. It is not the essence of a person's neurology. The 'with' creates a separation between the label and the person, while the 'is' has no separation and illustrates an integral connectedness. So, yes, in this instance the doctors will be treating and hopefully eradicating this thing called cancer. But this is not a fundamental part of that person, the way that being Autistic is.

Jim Sinclair (an Autistic activist who wrote some of the formative Autistic rights essays, including 'Why I dislike "person-first" language' in 1999[2]) has made the important point that the only time we separate a person from their condition is when we see that condition in negative terms or believe it is incompatible with their human side. In his seminal 1993 essay 'Don't mourn for us', he wrote about how it is not possible to separate the experience of being Autistic from the person, that there is no neurotypical child hiding inside an Autistic shell, that autism is not something that can be picked up or put down like a cup, but is instead a construct to describe an Autistic person.

Looking at other identity descriptions that we consider neutral, positive or integral to people (not just a part that can be taken away), we use identity-first language.

---

2   https://autismmythbusters.com/general-public/
     autistic-vs-people-with-autism/jim-sinclair-why-i-dislike-person-first-language

For example, we might describe someone as a woman, Irish or a doctor; we do not say a 'person with womanhood', a 'person with Irishness', or a 'person with doctorhood'. The reason we don't feel uncomfortable framing our language this way is because we do not hold negative connotations towards those identities.

After reading this book you will probably continue to see professionals incorrectly using person-first terminology (we have done so in earlier publications!). You might up to this very moment be using person-first terminology yourself. You may also hear professionals or others incorrectly saying that there is no consensus in the Autistic community regarding language (this is incorrect – while it is not a 100 per cent consensus, it is a clear majority[3]). You may also read a guideline document that recommends using person-first language, or a mix of both (they are also incorrect). Adapting to a new understanding and new language use is challenging and requires conscious and consistent effort, and begins with making the **choice** to do so. For those who take the steps to reflect and examine thoughtfully the feelings that identity-first language bring up in us can reveal a lot, highlighting our ableism, bias for familiarity and unconscious negative attitudes towards Autistic people. It shows just how much being Autistic is categorized in our heads alongside burdens and life-limiting medical conditions.

Important note: Respecting individual preferences when working with people is important. But for books, reports, research papers, policy documents and people whose preference you do not yet know, or who are only at the first impression stage, it is **vital** to choose identity-first language.

Interestingly, it would appear that most Autistic people who prefer person-first language have spoken mostly to professionals (who use outdated language) only, and have not yet linked in with the Autistic community, or are unaware of the neurodiversity movement or paradigm. The first professional to talk to a person about being Autistic will have a lasting impact on their language use going forward.

Many professionals worry that by using identity-first language they will upset or alienate clients or their families (or indeed other professionals). Of course, all of us as clinicians want to be seen as caring and respectful, and it is true that some people around you may not be so up to date with respectful language choices and may query your choice of words. But if this is the case, **be a force for change**. Explain to people **why** you are using identity-first language. Use these situations as a learning opportunity to teach people about the Autistic community and the importance of listening to them. It may be one of the most valuable lessons you impart.

---

3   See, for example, https://autisticnotweird.com/autismsurvey and https://autisticadvocacy.org/about-asan/identity-first-language

Just Call It 'Autism', Not 'Autism Spectrum Disorder', 'ASD', 'Autism Spectrum Condition' or 'ASC'

Using just 'autism' plain and simple is not only easier and shorter; it also shows respect to the Autistic community who fully reject the framing of their natural ways of being as a disorder or a condition (Kenny et al. 2016).

Use 'Disabled Person', Not 'Person with a Disability'

In modern discourse, many disability groups choose identity-first language as a preference – 'disabled person' as opposed to 'person with a disability'. It is interesting to note that it is the disability groups that **embrace** being disabled as part of their cultural and/or personal identity that are more likely to prefer identity-first language. For them, the use of identity-first language is used as an expression of cultural pride and reclamation of a disability that once conferred a negative identity.

This has not always been the case, as previously person-first language (a 'person **with** a disability') was how the majority of disabilities were framed and spoken about in the media and research journals. This has changed over time as disability activists have fought hard for the use of person-first language to combat how they had been dehumanized and abused historically. They sought to be treated and spoken about with the same respect and dignity as those who weren't disabled. Now, paradoxically, it is mostly non-disabled people who advocate for the retention of person-first language.

▨ **Important note:** There are some disability groups who prefer person-first language, for example the intellectual disability community. There are also some disability groups who, while being similarly disabled, live in different countries or regions and disagree with each other as to how they would like to be referred to. Where it is unclear, research preferred language choices by contacting advocacy groups and organizations in the country you are working in. Again, make sure that the organization is led, or at least heavily influenced by (e.g., having a high percentage of disabled people on the board of a charity), the community you are investigating.

Again, the common argument used to promote person-first language in relation to being disabled in general was that it helped the person using that language to remember that the person was a 'person first' and not just 'their disability'. This highlights a misunderstanding of why identity-first language is preferred. Today, it is recognized and understood that identity-first language ('disabled person') is preferred because it acknowledges that it is not that the person 'has' disabilities, but that they are a 'disabled person' because they are **disabled by society** and how it is not designed for, or indeed by, them. Identity-first language acknowledges the role of the environment and the external factors that disable the person. A disabled person is disabled because they are actively disabled by the environment (an external force), rather than focusing on a person 'having' a disability, which incorrectly suggests the disability as being within the person, belonging to the person, an issue with the person, or something that is the sole responsibility of the person to change or to live with.

Working with Parents on Language Use

Although this book has been written specifically for clinicians diagnosing adults, there should be no distinction between how we talk about Autistic adults and how we talk about Autistic children. Parents learn their language from professionals for the most part, and leading by example is vital. Most important in our minds should be the Autistic children we are supporting, and the effect on them of growing up feeling that 'autism' is something that is a small and detachable part of them, that could or should be removed.

At times, however, there is a need to gently introduce these concepts because many parents (who, remember, have quite a high likelihood of being Autistic themselves) also grew up in the same world we did, with all its negative messaging about Autistic people and being taught to 'see the person first', which is shorthand for 'see the neurotypical person first'. If you are also identifying Autistic children, you will meet many parents with a strong preference for their child to be spoken about using person-first language, and this needs to be explored in more depth with them in relation to the foundations of where this comes from (as outlined in this book). The Neuro-Affirmative concepts described within this book need to be introduced with compassion.

But it is also our job as clinicians to educate and support parents to understand that language is powerful, and how parents conceptualize the Autistic experience (and neurodiversity in general) now will have an impact on how their children understand themselves and their community in the future. Educating families helps break ongoing stigma, and ultimately links parents in with an important community that their child (and likely at least one of the parents) belongs to, a community of people who care about their child, and the future of their shared community. The way you, as a professional, frame being Autistic to these families will affect how they go forward in their lives and how they think about themselves. It will affect how these children come to understand themselves, how they value themselves and being Autistic, and how others see and value them and their integral Autistic neurology. As Virginia Satir (an influential American author and psychotherapist) said, **heal the family, heal the world.**

■ **Important note:** Parental priorities are heavily influenced by the professionals they first meet as well as the resources and books they are then provided with post diagnosis. Remember that many parents you meet may actually have already discovered they are Autistic (and have chosen not to disclose to you), and so, when talking about their child being Autistic, you are also talking about them. Respecting the place that parents are at in their journey is vital for trust, but continuing to educate and gently point them towards information that is up to date and respectful is also vital, and will benefit the family as a whole in the long term.

Talk about 'High' or 'Low' Support Needs in Specific Areas, Not 'High' or 'Low Functioning'

Using 'high' or 'low functioning' is an outdated and disrespectful way to talk about people. Instead, talk about a person's individual support needs, and be specific about the areas you are talking about. For example: 'Zavier currently has high support needs in relation to mobility in busy places, and needs and wants a person to accompany him when out in the community. Zavier has low support needs in relation to advocating for his own needs. He prefers to communicate by text or email, and has good IT skills.'

When someone is labelled 'low functioning', what naturally follows are low expectations and segregation. Yet when someone is labelled 'high functioning', what naturally follows is people not believing how high some of this person's support needs may be, for example not believing or understanding that this person may experience burnout, shutdown or is unable to speak at times. Thus they are expected to struggle through difficult situations, often to the detriment of their mental health. Ableism is also inherent in these terms, implying that to be Autistic and to openly show Autistic traits (e.g., stimming) is wrong in itself and means someone is 'lesser' than another. An often-quoted phrase in the Autistic community is 'High functioning doesn't have to do with how disabled someone is. It is to do with how well they pass as neurotypical.'

The experience of being Autistic in a world not designed for you brings different strengths and challenges that are individual to the person within different environments. These are not static and are dependent on context. They change depending on environment, internal states, external influences, energy levels, life events and seasons, moment by moment. For example, one Autistic person without co-occurring conditions may successfully attend work in an office each day, but on returning home, find that the sensory demands of the busy office environment, and the commute home, render them unable to perform self-care tasks such as cooking for themselves or communicating through spoken language. Another Autistic person with co-occurring intellectual disabilities may love the busy environment of working in a kitchen, but find the social chit-chat of sitting down to eat food and hearing people eat to be unbearable, and be exhausted engaging in chit-chat. Another Autistic person might avoid cooking at all costs but love night clubs, busy environments and dancing in crowds, and find being by themselves to be lonely and only be able to sleep with loud music playing.

There are so many different ways of being Autistic that using such black and white terms as 'high' or 'low functioning' is nonsensical and unhelpful. It is like saying just how 'high' or 'low functioning' on the scale of neurotypicality are you? Or where are you on a scale of womanhood? Within the Autistic population the same amount of diversity exists in the neurotypical population. Across both populations there are people with, for example, different skills, preferences, abilities, types of intelligence, sensory systems, values, levels of support required, ways of being independent, things that are considered important to them. Using 'high' and 'low functioning' is like using a blunt axe to pick apart and describe the multitude of layers and depth that make up each individual person. Time and context add even more layers to be considered, as all people change, grow and fluctuate in the levels of support they need depending on their age, health, life stage, environment and personal circumstances.

This is why the concept of a **spectrum** is so helpful when understanding Autistic people (although please do not use 'on the spectrum', as this implies again that someone is separate and 'on top' of something rather than it being part of their being). The spectrum concept allows people to be individuals, who will need support at different times in their lives, which is individual to them (see Chapters 3 and 4).

Other Ableist Language to Avoid

- Talk about 'passions'. Avoid the use of 'special interests', which is deemed as patronizing.

- Refer to 'neurotypical milestones'. When talking about the likelihood of someone being Autistic, use phrases like 'There is evidence to show an increased likelihood that Mary is Autistic' or 'Mary is showing signs that she may be Autistic.' Do not use phrases such as 'at risk for autism' or 'red flags for autism', both of which are medicalized and deficit-based.

- Talk about an Autistic developmental trajectory instead of developmental issues or delay (Leadbitter et al. 2021). If you refer to developmental milestones, clarify that you are referring to 'neurotypical developmental milestones'. For example, 'Mary began using words to communicate at three years old, which does not align with neurotypical developmental milestones, but may be more in keeping with an Autistic developmental trajectory.'

- Avoid talking about 'concerns' in relation specifically to Autistic traits or characteristics, as this implies that these are inherently negative, or even dangerous. This does not mean that you cannot highlight concerns about areas that are causing distress, such as self-harm, intense pain from sensory experiences, loneliness or mental health issues.

- Use 'Non-Speaking' or 'Non-Speaking (at times)' to refer to a person and lowercase 'non-speaking' or 'non-speaking (at times)' to refer to the action instead of 'non-verbal'. 'Verbal' is the equivalent to using 'language', so to say that someone is 'non-verbal' implies that the person does not have any internal language or external vocalizations. Producing words from your mouth is a motor act. Just because someone does not speak does not mean they don't have language. The Non-Speaking community has claimed 'Non-Speaking' as the preferred term, including how it is spelled.

- Talk about speech and language 'differences' instead of speech and language 'difficulties'.

- Talk about Autistic 'characteristics' or 'features' instead of 'symptoms' or 'impairments'.

- Talk about Autistic communication styles or Autistic communication preferences instead of 'social impairment' or 'lacks social skills' (see Chapter 4 for information about the 'double empathy problem').

- Talk about providing 'supports' or 'adaptations' instead of 'treatment'.

- Talk about the co-occurring needs and challenges instead of attributing all difficulties to being Autistic (see Bottema-Beutel et al. 2021).

Further Recommended Reading

Bottema-Beutel, K., Kapp, S. K., Lester, J. N., Sasson, N. J. and Hand, B. N. (2021) Avoiding ableist language: Suggestions for autism researchers. *Autism in Adulthood 3*(1), 18–29. https://doi.org/10.1089/ aut.2020.0014

Kenny, L., Hattersley, C., Molins, B., Buckley, C., Povey, C. and Pellicano, E. (2016) Which terms should be used to describe autism? Perspectives from the UK autism community. *Autism 20*, 442–462. doi:10.1177/1362361315588200.

Please note that a downloadable Neuro-Affirmative language guide is available at https://library.jkp.com/redeem using the code LNFRFAX and see also Appendix 1.

3

A Brief History of Autistic People and the Neurodiversity Movement

Content warning: The chapter contains information about both historical and ongoing abuse of Autistic children and adults, and so may be upsetting for some readers.

Introduction

Since 'autism' was first coined as a term in 1908 by Swiss psychiatrist Eugen Bleuler, Autistic children, adults and their families have been plagued by flawed and damaging myths, assumptions and untruths about them. Many professionals have perpetrated these, and, while possibly well intentioned, have failed to examine their own biases, and so this prejudice has subsequently had a lasting negative impact that continues today.

Thankfully, alongside this, there have been many determined advocates and parent advocates who (at great personal and emotional cost) have helped bring this once considered rare and judged as shameful diagnosis to both a better understanding and increased recognition of prevalence.

Autistic children were initially, and for a very long time, seen as having a childhood psychiatric disorder, a subset of childhood schizophrenia marked by a detachment from reality. Up until recently, any literature (research or otherwise) to do with the Autistic neurology was focused solely on children, with Temple Grandin (the first Autistic advocate to speak openly about being Autistic) even in the 2000s needing to remind conference attendees that she was not 'recovered' from autism, but was, in fact, still, of course, Autistic.

The 1940s, 'Bad Parenting'

In 1943, Leo Kanner, an American child psychiatrist, published a paper describing a group of 11 children who he later said had 'early infantile autism'. These children were described as being intelligent and displaying a desire for aloneness, repetition of actions and vocalizations and an insistence on sameness. He also noted that the children's parents were highly successful and intelligent. Kanner published his 'autistic disturbances of effective contact' in 1943. In this paper, Kanner described autism as a rare childhood disorder, separate from childhood schizophrenia. As the characteristics of childhood schizophrenia include 'normal' development followed by a state of regression, Kanner's description of Autistic children was characterized by a state of self-absorption present from birth.

In 1944, Hans Asperger, a German scientist, worked in the Heilpadagogik clinic under Erwin Lazar, a physician who had an innovative approach to helping children (even by today's standards). Lazar did not see the children as sick or damaged, but instead believed that their 'burden' originated due to neglect from the society that had failed to provide suitable teaching methods for their unique styles of learning (Silberman 2016). Lazar's clinic utilized an approach developed from the 1800s theory of Heilpadagogik ('therapeutic education'), which helped each child find their own potential as opposed to treating psychological issues in isolation. The approach was one of compassion, to foster environments where children could develop the skills to interact in conditions of mutual respect.

During his time at the clinic Asperger examined more than 200 children who displayed the 'Autistic thinking' previously identified by Bleuler. Asperger also identified Autistic thinking in several adolescents and adults and the children's mothers (Silberman 2016). He wrote about a small group of boys who were similarly described to Kanner's group of children, with the exception of not presenting with echolalia, but instead 'talking' like grown-ups, and having additional fine and gross motor difficulties. This group of traits and characteristics was to become known as 'Asperger's syndrome'.

Asperger also recognized the biological aspect to an 'Autistic pathology' (as he described it). He acknowledged that it ran in families and was not uncommon, and warned his colleagues that it was very unlikely that one single gene could be responsible for such an elaborate system of traits, that it was more likely that the 'Autistic pathology' was polygenetic. These Autistic characteristics included social awkwardness, precocious abilities and an obsession with routine and rules. Asperger acknowledged that the Autistic pathology remained present throughout an individual's life and involved a broad spectrum of people, from the most talented and intelligent individuals to the most disabled. His work was published in German in 1944, but was not translated into English until 1981, by Lorna Wing.

In the late 1940s, psychiatrists said they had found the cause of autism – that it was 'cold' parents (particularly mothers) who did not love their children enough. This theory became known as the 'refrigerator mother' theory, which was popularized by Austrian psychologist Bruno Bettelheim. Bettelheim was heavily influenced by Sigmund Freud, who theorized that emotional or behavioural difficulties in children were all caused by the child's upbringing. Bettelheim was also heavily influenced by Kanner's observation that Autistic children had professional, successful parents, who he judged as not being as emotionally present for their children as stay-at-home parents.

Unfortunately, even Kanner, who had initially felt that being Autistic was something a child was born with, adopted this theory, and with continued support from both Kanner and Bettelheim, it was the prevalent theory of how people 'became' Autistic for decades, with the recommended course of action institutionalization for the child and long-term psychoanalysis for the parents, to investigate why they could not correctly nurture and care for their children.

Parents, especially mothers, were stigmatized and shamed, and children were ripped apart from their families to spend the rest of their lives in horrific, dehumanizing conditions in institutions, often in adult psychosis wards where they were beaten and given electroshock therapy in the name of 'treatment' (see Silberman 2016) (in fact, electroshock therapy for Autistic and otherwise disabled people continues today in some states in the USA as well as in other countries).

Much of Bettelheim's work (not just the 'refrigerator mother' theory) has been discredited since his death, but this did not halt decades being lost in relation to a valid and meaningful understanding of Autistic people. Not only did it influence what people thought was the cause of Autistic neurology, but because of the recommendation of institutionalization for Autistic children, it had an enormous impact on what people thought was the natural lifetime developmental progression for an Autistic child. As most **diagnosed** Autistic children were sent to institutions, naturally all of the research data and anecdotal practice-based information about Autistic children and how they develop into Autistic adults was based on how Autistic people appeared after a life of trauma, abuse and institutionalization. Understandably, many of these children (and subsequent adults) presented with trauma responses, such as self-harm, reduced communication and hitting out (Kerns et al. 2022).

The 1960s and 1970s, Genetics and a Spectrum

The idea that to be Autistic is a fate worse than death can be directly linked to the perception of how Autistic adults in these institutions (i.e., wholly inappropriate and abusive environments) presented. While tragically, many Autistic people continue to live long term in inappropriate 'inpatient' units in hospitals to this day, thankfully, in the 1960s and 1970s, a body of research that included studies of twins disproved the 'refrigerator mother' concept and began to show the genetic and biological underpinnings of being Autistic, and over the next two decades it was increasingly recognized that parenting did not cause Autistic children.

In 1964, Bernard Rimland, an American psychologist with an Autistic child who disagreed with the 'refrigerator mother' concept, wrote *Infantile Autism: The Syndrome and Its Implications for a Neural Theory of Behaviour*. Rimland's work had a large hand to play in the move away from blaming parents, and was subsequently highly influential in relation to how Autistic children were understood. However, while positive in relation to moving away from the idea of blaming parents, Rimland believed that autism was caused by environmental pollutants, antibiotics and vaccinations (although he acknowledged that there may also be a genetic component predisposing children). He also supported chelation, Applied Behaviour Analysis (ABA) and the use of aversives.

In the 1970s, Lorna Wing, a British psychiatrist (whose daughter was Autistic and had learning difficulties), with Judith Gould, undertook the first epidemiological study of autism, concluding that there was a statistically higher incidence of autism than previously thought, and established the 'triad of impairments' that subsequently came to define autism. Wing was the first person to introduce the helpful concept of the 'spectrum' and the vast range of presentations shown by Autistic people, highlighting the great variability between Autistic people, and noting that autism should be considered dimensionally, that it occurs in all ages and in people of all intellectual abilities. It was the first time that it was recognized that Autistic people could be of all ages and abilities, including those with lower support needs. Wing also advocated for parents and professionals to work closely together and for individual rights for Autistic people. In the 1980s she brought the work of Hans Asperger to the English-speaking world, which had a significant influence on subsequent framings of autism.

In 1980, 'infantile autism' (described as a pervasive developmental disorder) was listed for the first time in the *Diagnostic and Statistical Manual of Mental Disorders*, Third Edition (DSM-III; APA 1980), and established autism as its own separate diagnosis distinct from schizophrenia. In 1987, the DSM-III-R (Third Edition, Revised) replaced 'infantile autism' with the broader 'autism disorder', and included a checklist of diagnostic criteria, although autism was still, at this time, considered to be very rare, and was largely unknown to the general public.

The 1980s, and Applied Behaviour Analysis

Hugely influential in the history of autism was the development and subsequent proliferation of Applied Behaviour Analysis (ABA) as the 'gold standard treatment' for Autistic children. In 1987, the Norweigan–American psychologist Ivar Løvaas published his first study related to intensive behaviour therapy for Autistic children, which was to become known as 'ABA'.

In an earlier interview with *Psychology Today*, in 1974, in which he advocated for physical punishment, Løvaas said:

> You start pretty much from scratch when you work with an Autistic child. You have a person in the physical sense – they have hair, a nose and a mouth – but they are not people in the psychological sense. One way to look at the job of helping Autistic kids is to see it as a matter of constructing a person. You have the raw materials, but you have to construct the person. (Chance and Løvaas 1974, p.76)

Important note: Don't skim over this quote as a historical note, but instead, truly 'sit' with it for a few minutes, imagining it was you or your child being described in such terms (i.e., as essentially not human). Really engaging with what was done and said as a reality is to begin to understand the impact that history has had in perpetuating trauma on multitudes of Autistic people in the guise of them being less than human. Indeed, Løvaas also published a study at the time claiming to have 'cured' autism, although this has since been totally discredited due to the fact that his method during research was to use aversive techniques with the children in his care.

ABA is based on influential American psychologist B. F. Skinner's behaviourist framework (from the 1920s), in which the only target for 'treatment' is observable behaviour, and the only way to target the behaviour is by a controlled experimental design. 'Treatment' success is defined as the behaviour changing in the way the experiment was designed to do. Feelings, thoughts, distress, environment, sensory discomfort, **whether** the behaviour should be changed, **who** is deciding that the behaviour should be changed and **why** are not relevant factors in Løvaas' traditional behaviourist framework. A seductive aspect of behaviourism is that it often 'works' at a superficial or surface level in changing short-term behaviour, but we need to ask ourselves, to what end, and with what long-term results? Severely neglected newborn babies, for example, **will** stop crying out to be held, but their need for comfort is not diminished; they have just learned that there is simply no point crying for something that will never come.

Despite limited success, Løvaas further developed his programme to target younger children under five and advocated for 40 hours weekly of therapy (this regimen continues to be recommended today, despite being at odds with a large body of research in relation to how children this age learn best). It is also an entire working week (for an adult) on top of school and the regular business of being a child. How can any child fulfil the job description of being a child subjected to so many hours of direct intervention? Again, despite limited success, the media quickly began reporting about Autistic children 'transformed' into 'apparently normal children' from their engagement with ABA. In the absence of any other well-publicized programme offering hope, worried parents began flocking to ABA to help 'cure' their child, while being Autistic was described to them as 'a fate worse than death'.

While ABA has since grown to become a powerful, multi-billion-dollar industry in the USA and worldwide, it has subsequently been widely denounced and rejected by the Autistic community as harmful and traumatic, denying the validity of Autistic experience, and fundamentally seeking to change Autistic people into something they can never be, or even want to be. It is wholly counter to developing a positive Autistic identity.

The centring from the early days of autism awareness of a behaviourist framework as the 'go-to treatment' for Autistic children has had a dehumanizing impact that still reverberates today in relation to how professionals even begin to understand and support Autistic children. For example, if a neurotypical child experiences a traumatic event and is, for example, speaking less, hitting themselves or running away, the professionals around that child would hopefully know not to implement a behaviour plan with rewards or aversives to shape the behaviour. They should instead try to understand **why** the child is behaving this way, and help provide connection, empathy, consistency, a safer environment, appropriate child-centred therapy and education to the people around the child in relation to the trauma.

The Autistic experience has always been described and framed as observable, undesirable behaviours that need to be ameliorated, and it is part of the legacy of ABA that it is typically the **behaviour** of the Autistic child and how to shape it that is paramount, instead of efforts first being made to empathize and understand **why** the child may be behaving that way, and then changing the environment around them.

The 1980s and 1990s, Self-Advocating and the Internet

Alongside the growth of ABA in 1980s and 1990s, Autistic adults began attending parent conferences about autism and speaking out about their own experiences, often at great emotional cost to themselves. Temple Grandin also began writing books and speaking publicly during this time. This meant that for the first time, parents and professionals were hearing information from Autistic people directly (Autistic people who had **not** spent their lives in institutions), about how they viewed and experienced the world. As well as helping to reduce shame and prejudice, listening to these Autistic adults was revelatory for worried parents, and gave them hope that the diagnosis was not as life-limiting as they had been led to believe. It also helped them to understand for the first time **why** their children experienced the world as they did, and thus helped improve the lives of a great many children and their families.

In the late 1980s only a very small group of people knew what autism was, and even then, it was a very limited conceptualization. Then, in 1989, the film *Rainman* was released to popular acclaim and with an enormous impact on public awareness of autism as it included an Autistic savant with a photographic memory (a character who, while sympathetic and intelligent, was ultimately there to teach the protagonist life lessons before being dispatched back to an institution). Because of its popularity, bolstered by an Oscar for Dustin Hoffman in the title role, after *Rainman* was released many people (which, of course, included parents) knew at least one way that Autistic people could present (although it was such a stereotyped and limited portrayal that it perpetuated myths about what it was to be Autistic).

The growth of the internet in the 1990s allowed new communities across the world to connect, communicate and organize. This included the Autistic community, for whom the medium of the internet may have been particularly suitable given the reduced need to mask or camouflage when communicating, as well as it being less demanding, with less burden of auditory processing, and allowing thinking time, which led to a significant increase in advocacy and activism.

In 1992, Jim Sinclair, with Donna Williams and Kathy Grant (influential Autistic activists) co-founded Autism Network International, which, among other projects, published newsletters 'by and for Autistic people'. In 1993 Sinclair's seminal paper, 'Don't mourn for us', provided a powerful new framing of Autistic identity:

> It is not possible to separate the autism from the person. Therefore, when parents say, 'I wish my child did not have autism,' what they're really saying is, 'I wish the Autistic child I have did not exist and I had a different (non-autistic) child instead.' Read that

again. This is what we hear when you mourn over our existence. This is what we hear when you pray for a cure. This is what we know, when you tell us of your fondest hopes and dreams for us: that your greatest wish is that one day we will cease to be, and strangers you can love will move in behind our faces. (Sinclair 1993)

This was the start of the growth of a strong Autistic advocacy and neurodiversity movement.

The 1990s and 2000s, and the Neurodiversity Movement

In 1996, Autreat was established, the first retreat and conference specifically for Autistic people, which inspired other similar retreats globally. Also in 1996, an email list called 'Independent Living on the Autism Spectrum' was established by Martijn Dekker, an Autistic computer programmer from the Netherlands. What is significant for the development of the concept of 'neurodiversity' was that the list described autism's 'cousin conditions', for example Dyslexia and attention-deficit hyperactivity disorder (ADHD). In 1998 Judith Singer, an Australian Disability and Public Housing activist, first coined the term 'neurodiversity' in her Sociology honours thesis. She spoke about the liberatory, activist aspects of the concept, and the potential for it doing for the neurodivergent person what feminism and LGBTQIA+ rights have done for those groups. The American writer Harvey Blume was the first to publish 'neurodiversity' as a concept in 1997.

With increased access to information about disability activism, the young adults who had been diagnosed as Autistic in the 1990s began looking at the disability rights community and recognizing themselves. Thus, for the first time, a bridge began to grow between the growing Autistic community and the disability rights community. The 1990s and 2000s continued to see the growth of an increasing number of advocacy groups, including the Autism National Committee (AutCom), the Autistic Self Advocacy Network (ASAN), Autistic Women, the Academic Autistic Spectrum Partnership in Research and Education (AASPIRE) and the Non-Binary Network.

An example of activism during this time was Autistic advocate Michelle Dawson challenging the use of ABA in the Supreme Court of Canada. The Auton trial was heard in 2004, and centred on the medical necessity of funding ABA treatment with both parents bringing the case and the British Columbian government taking a deeply pathologizing view of autism. Dawson successfully applied to intervene in the Auton trial to posit an alternative perspective, asserting that the denial of the humanity of Autistic people was the very foundation of ABA therapy.[1]

---

1   See www.lawandthesenses.org

The Court judged that the government was not mandated to fund ABA therapy as 'medically necessary' as there was no right for **all** necessary services to be funded, and acknowledged Dawson's argument when highlighting the 'emergent and controversial nature' of ABA. In her own *Auton vs British Columbia* statement, Dawson wrote that despite being faced with such a negative view of being Autistic during the court case, there had been consideration of an alternative perspective: 'Briefly, the sun broke through and we and our allies celebrated, unnoticed'.

Alongside this growth of activism in the 1990s came the broadening of the diagnostic criteria for autism, and in 1994, 'Asperger's syndrome' was added to the Fourth Edition of the DSM, expanding 'autism' to include people with less care needs. Also at this time, more statistically reliable tests to assess autism became more widely accessible, with an assessment no longer only accessible to those with a connection to a tiny group of experts (and while statistically reliable, these tests did not capture the full breadth of the Autistic experience). These factors, alongside the *Rainman* effect, meant that diagnostic rates of autism began to soar (and have continued to soar since).

Unfortunately, what should have been seen as positive (i.e., that children were being correctly identified and so could finally begin to be understood and supported appropriately) was framed by some organizations and charities as an 'epidemic' to be scourged. They've released prominent, and in our opinion, frightening and damaging media campaigns in which autism was described as 'taking over your child'. This understandably terrified many families, and in our view, that of much of the Autistic and autism community. While it also brought in a lot of money for the charities and for research, much of this went (and continues to go) towards searching for a cause rather than for a greater understanding or the provision of better supports.

Controversy

Andrew Wakefield, a now disgraced UK doctor, then came along to blame the increase in autism diagnoses on vaccines, a simple, seductive and wrong claim, with tsunamic consequences. In 1998 he published a case series suggesting that the measles, mumps and rubella (MMR) vaccine could cause behaviour regression and pervasive developmental disorder in children. This spread rapidly worldwide, and MMR vaccinations immediately began to drop. Although **multiple** studies were quickly published refuting Wakefield's study, the link between autism and vaccines was set in people's minds. His papers have since been retracted, and he has been held guilty of ethical violations, scientific misrepresentation and deliberate fraud, which appears to have taken place for financial gain (Rao and Andrade 2011).

Over the years, a great amount of wasted resources and funding has gone into refuting Wakefield's tiny paper that could have been put to much better use for the Autistic community. Like the 'refrigerator mother' theory, here, again, was another false theory that made a lot of noise while being another impediment to the development of a true understanding of autism for decades. Broadening out from autism, Wakefield's publications can also be seen as the source of exceptionally serious long-term worldwide health implications, including measles outbreaks in the UK and the USA attributed to the non-vaccination of children, the low uptake of vaccines during the COVID-19 pandemic and the current culture war related to vaccines in the USA (Luterman 2020; Rao and Andrade 2011).

What is worrying (and worth bearing in mind when analysing research publications in general) is that it wasn't academic vigilance that highlighted these issues with Wakefield's study, but rather, journalistic investigation. Throughout the 2000s, the Autistic community continued to grow in confidence and numbers, speaking out about what they wanted and needed, namely control over their own lives and an end to the focus on cure and pathologization of their ways of being. What had previously been acceptable began to be unacceptable.

An early example of this was when in 2007 the NYU Child Study Center released advertisements in the form of ransom notes (echoing many previous publicly unchallenged campaigns from Autism Speaks), saying 'We have your son. We will make sure he will not be able to care for himself or interact socially as long as he lives. This is only the beginning.' It was signed 'Autism'. Another said, 'We have your son. We are destroying his ability for social interaction and driving him into a life of complete isolation. It's up to you now', and was signed 'Asperger Syndrome'. The ad campaign was quite rightly accused of using some of the oldest and most offensive stereotypes to frighten parents, and of including untruths and heavily biased ableism.

While during previous Autism Speaks campaigns the Autistic community did not have a voice, now Autistic advocates were mobilized. Spearheaded by Ari Ne'eman (author, PhD candidate in Health Policy at Harvard University and an American disability rights activist who co-founded ASAN), Autistic advocates sparked a huge protest, much to the surprise of the NYU Child Study Center. Ne'eman (with the support of the majority of American disability rights organizations) undertook a highly successful letter-writing campaign that was picked up in many major media outlets in the USA, including the *New York Times*. This was the first and most public time that a major organization needed to reckon with a community that was not looking for a cure or scaremongering, but societal changes. The ads were pulled within three weeks.

The 2000s to Today, Steps Forward and Back

In 2013, the Fifth Edition of the DSM folded all subcategories of autism into one umbrella diagnosis of 'autism spectrum disorder', with 'Asperger's syndrome' no longer seen as a separate diagnosis.

In 2019, Greta Thunberg, Autistic Swedish climate activist, was named *Time* magazine's Person of the Year. Thunberg has, from the start, spoken openly about being Autistic (Asperger syndrome specifically), saying that instead of a hindrance, it has helped her see things from outside the box, and has therefore been **key** to her ideas and success as an activist. Thunberg's high profile has had an enormous positive impact on the general public's perceptions of Autistic people, and has also helped greatly increase awareness of the presence of Autistic girls and women.

In 2020, the Centers for Disease Control and Prevention (CDC) reported that the rates of autism diagnosis were, at that time, one in 54 children in the USA.

Today, the Autistic and neurodivergent community is a thriving culture and community. Alongside an increased openness of Autistic adults to talk about being Autistic, more and more prominent public figures, such as Sir Anthony Hopkins (actor), Wentworth Miller (actor) and Melanie Sykes (presenter) are also openly talking about being Autistic. With reduced societal stigma, more and more parents of Autistic children are recognizing that they themselves are Autistic, and are accessing a diagnosis as well as joining their voices with autism activism. Companies are finally beginning to see that this is something they must address in relation to hiring, disability and equality, with training in Neuro-Affirmative practices fast becoming a booming business.

There has also been an overdue explosion of public Autistic activism, openly Autistic professionals and therapists, Autistic-led and co-produced research, and new Autistic-led organizations and charities.

By the time we came to write this book, a phenomenal amount of research funding had been pumped into searching for the genetic and other 'causes' of autism, with the most recent large-scale studies involving thousands of children indicating that autism is predominantly inherited, with gene-sequencing studies implicating over a hundred different genes (Satterstrom et al. 2020). Despite disproportionate attention from the media and a scared general public in relation to environmental causes (e.g., factors such as the mother's weight or nutritional intake), these studies indicate that environment **does not** have a significant impact. The Autistic community is extremely frustrated with this ongoing focus on 'cause', with the implication of future wide-scale eugenics should a cause be found. (The high rates of Down syndrome pregnancies being terminated mean this fear is not unfounded; see, for example, de Graaf, Buckley and Skotko 2020.)

In a striking example of the emerging power of the Autistic community to shape their future, Spectrum 10K, a large-scale UK-based research project that claimed to be investigating the genetic and environmental factors that contribute to autism and related physical and mental health conditions (although the methodology suggested a possible subdivision of the Autistic community, which is in direct opposition to Autistic-identified research priorities; ASAN 2022; Bascom and Perry 2022), has been put on hold after outcry from the Autistic community. Advocates highlighted a lack of meaningful engagement and co-production with the Autistic community, that the aims of the study and its research area was at odds with community priorities, and queried whether the ultimate goal of the project was cure, that is, eugenics. What the community needs and wants now and going forward are high-quality trials of clinical and community supports that aim to minimize barriers, improve quality of life and nurture individual differences.

Given the history of treatment of Autistic people by the neurotypical-perceived majority, the Autistic community is justifiably angry about being continually spoken over by neurotypical professionals when it comes to matters pertaining to them. In 2021 electric shock therapy was still being given to Autistic people in the Judge Rotenberg Educational Center in the USA, despite continued outcry from the community and the United Nations calling it torture (Human Rights Council 2018). ABA continues to be dominant despite being opposed by **all** Autistic advocacy groups. Many current proponents of ABA claim that 'their ABA' isn't like Løvaas', but the principles remain the same, even if the current delivery may look somewhat different. Fundamentally it is about denying the validity of the Autistic experience. Research on Autistic people continues to be largely ableist and with no real Autistic engagement, and researchers continue to know little about the lives of Autistic adults, women, the intersectionality of minority communities within the Autistic community and the effects of related conditions such as epilepsy.

Compliance-Based Behaviour Therapy

We have provided training (and have spoken) to many professionals who trained and are working within compliance-based behavioural frameworks such as positive behaviour support or ABA. A few themes tend to emerge.

First, it is often our experience that those with a background in ABA, who are excited about the concept of the Neuro-Affirmative model, can see the value of a human rights approach. There is a clear struggle to reconcile their training background and the positive impact they believe they are making with the overwhelmingly negative reception of their modality by the Autistic adult community. They often question us as to the legitimacy of Autistic people's objections, purporting that 'new' ABA is different and there is much of value in their training. On each occasion, when we unpack this argument with an open curiosity, it becomes evident that the 'parts' of ABA they assert are helpful and respectful turn out to be simply good practice from a different modality (e.g., breaking a task down into manageable chunks). It would appear that this good practice has been packaged and 'sold' to them as an ABA strategy exclusively.

Another factor that often raises its head is a misunderstanding of the Autistic developmental trajectory and neuro-normative therapy goals. Goals must be set by the person themself. Goals of compliance or 'fitting in', 'masking' or suppressing natural Autistic expression such as stimming are harmful to Autistic people's mental health, and a potential risk factor for mental health difficulties throughout life.

In the USA in particular we often hear from practitioners that undertaking ABA is the only way to get insurance billing and therefore to access mental health supports, because insurance companies won't fund other therapies. So practitioners tell us that that they are not actually utilizing compliance therapy; they simply bill it as such.

There can also be a confirmation bias when considering ABA with children. Therapists believe the child can have only achieved progress with a desired goal because of ABA, without considering the fact of the Autistic developmental trajectory and the likelihood of the child achieving the goal naturally, or with the support of another therapeutic method (e.g., occupational therapy).

We have two main concerns for the ABA community:

1. Those trained in ABA and who have invested time working in the field must hold the tension that their work has been harmful if they are to adapt. This is an incredibly difficult thing to ask most humans to do. It takes a great deal of self-awareness and openness to listen to the community you believed you were serving and to hear the harm caused.

2. There are many wonderful, well-intentioned ABA-trained therapists and practitioners who, when introduced to and excited by the

human rights-based neurodiversity movement, do not know where to go with their training. They are left at a loss as to how to move forward. This is a conversation in our opinion that needs to happen within the behaviourist community. ABA associations and leadership organizations must listen to and engage with the communities they purport to serve and humbly change course. Up until recently it has been far too easy to dismiss Autistic adults' grievances as a small group of unhappy people, but the issue is clearly much wider. Autistic adults have the support of a growing group of professionals such as the authors of this book, a mix of neurodivergent and neurotypical psychologists, the respected Therapist Neurodiversity Collective and the entire team at Thriving Autistic, along with many more organizations now recognizing the persistent harm and trauma caused by the ABA community in refusing to engage with Autistic voices.

Important note: The history of Autistic people is full of trauma and pain. The conceptualization of the Autistic experience has been problematic from the start, with endorsed 'therapeutic' approaches leading to dehumanizing treatment and trauma. This is not history, however. These models continue to pervade Autistic experience despite tireless work and advocacy by the Autistic community and their allies. When undertaking assessments, clinicians need to remember this history and the damage it has inflicted, and strive to do more to change their lens so that history does not continue to repeat itself.

Common Criticisms of the Neurodiversity Movement

Concerns regarding the neurodiversity movement come from within as well as outside it. For example, there are valid concerns by Autistic advocates that a growing number of clinicians and companies are aligning themselves with the movement by branding themselves as Neuro-Affirmative or 'embracing neurodiversity' when they are not. Often in these cases they may use the language and branding of the neurodiversity movement and talk about strengths as a sales and marketing pitch, but under the surface their systemic processes and thinking are still very much the same as they were before and rooted within the medical paradigm. This has been termed 'neurodiversity lite' (Neumeier 2018).

Traditionally, throughout history, when any previously powerless group comes together and starts asserting itself, it is common for the dominant majority group to find it difficult to change their thinking and language about the minority group.

The majority group also traditionally resist giving up power, and the status quo and equal rights need to be hard fought for. There are parallels and similarities here to other movements such as the LGBTQIA+ and feminist rights movements.

Here are some of the most common criticisms that have been levelled at the neurodiversity movement and paradigm:

Criticism 1: The neurodiversity paradigm claims that autism is not a disability, but just a different way of looking at the world. It sanitizes the Autistic experience and people with high care needs, and presents it as just a 'different' way of being that comes with no difficulties.

Embracing neurodiversity and acknowledging the very real challenges that living with a different neurotype can bring are not mutually exclusive. Autistic advocates and neurodiversity proponents are crying out for support, funding and accommodations, and so this criticism is a profound misunderstanding of the movement.

The neurodiversity movement started within, and continues to be part of, the broader disability rights movement. From the very start it has advocated and fought for a broad range of supports and equal opportunities for Autistic people. Most neurodivergent and Autistic advocates identify as disabled and share the ideals and goals of the wider disability movement. Many of the original proponents of the neurodiversity movement had a range of other disabilities and high support needs in addition to being Autistic.

The neurodiversity movement is fighting for **everyone**'s support needs to be met, and for funding for this. It is fighting for equal rights and an equal voice and position in society for **everyone**, including those with high support needs and those who are Non-Speaking. As an example, there has been a strong focus within the movement on the rights of Non-Speaking Autistics to have equal access to communication, for example with the provision and use of augmentative and alternative communication (AAC) devices in the same way that physically disabled people have rights to access wheelchairs.

While within the neurodiversity paradigm being Autistic is clearly not looked at as a disease or a disorder, and it is not something that needs or wants to be cured, it is still understood for the most part that being Autistic is disabling within the context of the social model of disability. Under this model it is society that disables individuals by being designed for the perceived majority, and not including adequate and appropriate supports for all who need them.

Important note: Remember that many people are talking about neurodiversity publicly. As with any complex topic that involves a lot of people, there will be diverging opinions and different understandings and interpretations of what the neurodiversity movement and paradigm are all about (both within and outside of the Autistic and neurodivergent community). Before accepting a criticism as true, it is important to do some further research into the topic rather than listening to individual people on social media, for example.

Criticism 2: The neurodiversity movement is only relevant for a small subsection of 'high functioning' people.

Note: The use of 'high functioning' here is only used for illustrative purposes as we do not use this stigmatizing terminology. It is used here as a common example of a criticism.

A large part of the issue here is the misunderstanding that Autistic and otherwise neurodivergent advocates all have 'low support needs' and are only speaking to and advocating for people like themselves. There is an assumption that if someone has spoken out articulately, or they have a job or a family, that they couldn't possibly have high support needs. But this is not the case. Many Autistic people who are, for example, professionals, parents and in happy relationships still identify as being disabled and still struggle greatly in other areas of their lives. This is because their needs fluctuate and change over time depending on context and resources. So someone could enjoy communicating verbally early in the day, but later in the day rely on AAC to communicate. Many people have high support needs in one area but need less in another.

In fact, within the Autistic community there is a huge resistance to the division of Autistic people based on their support needs, and a strong desire to support and protect **all** members equally. Huge efforts continue to be made within the community for **all** members to have their views and opinions documented and counted in relation to their collective future. Another big part of the issue here is the misunderstanding that has already been addressed, that the movement focuses on strengths and sanitizes disability. The neurodiversity movement aims for equal rights and prominence for **all** Autistic and otherwise neurodivergent people, and always has.

Neurodiversity is about disability rights, and the neurodiversity movement is the bridge between the worlds of Autistic and otherwise neurodivergent people and disability activism. Disability activism was never about advocating only for those who are less visibly disabled; disability activism's remit is to bring **everyone** along.

It is interesting to note that as a group, people with higher support needs are more generally ignored; their wishes for how their care is managed is discounted as them not knowing what's best for themselves. But when individuals with lower support needs talk about what is needed for their community, they are faced with the criticism that they do not speak for the whole of the Autistic community. So this begs the question – what will it take for the neurotypical majority to listen to the Autistic community?

Criticism 3: The Autistic community and the neurodiversity movement is against all therapy and research.

In relation to research, the Autistic community (including many Autistic researchers) very much welcomes and values research into many areas related to them. This includes research into Autistic wellbeing, the Autistic developmental trajectory and ageing, including areas that can cause distress and that have traditionally been under-researched (e.g., sleep and the provision of appropriate communication supports). The Autistic community also wants research that meaningfully involves Autistic people from the start, and supports community priorities in relation to research. This should be a basic standard when it comes to research with any minority group.

In relation to therapy, again, the Autistic community welcomes support that respects Autistic identity and community priority goals (i.e., quality of life). Autistic parents recognize that children may need to be supported in learning skills. They don't want compliance training, neurotypical social skills training or ABA, but there are many other respectful supports they absolutely do need and want. This includes increasing sensory self-awareness, adapted mental health therapies to foster Autistic wellbeing and individualized personal assistant support, for example, with phone calls, consistent meals and managing life admin such as paperwork. A huge part of the neurodiversity movement and what Autistic advocates are fighting for is **increased** supports, such as speech and language and occupational therapy.

> For an in-depth exploration of the history of Autistic people and the neurodiversity movement, we recommend *NeuroTribes* by Steve Silberman (2016).

4

Understanding Autistic People

Ableism and Why It Is the Core Issue in Need of Addressing

'Ableism' refers to the practices, behaviours, social prejudices and beliefs that discriminate against disabled people in the same way that racism refers to the practices and beliefs that discriminate against people based on their race. To be ableist is to believe that neurotypical abilities are superior to all others in the same way that to be racist is to believe that one race is superior to others. Ableism is a word that has not **yet** entered our common lexicon, unlike other forms of oppression.

In the Western world, ableism may be one of the last socially acceptable forms of discrimination. The medical model of disability, and all classification systems arising from this model (e.g., the DSM-5-TR (Fifth Edition, Text Revision) and ICD-11 (*International Classification of Diseases*, 11th Edition)) are inherently ableist, as each item included is a judgement of how Autistic people are 'less than' neurotypical people. Common and obvious examples of ableism include the use of slurs such as 'retarded', buildings being inaccessible for wheelchair users and companies not hiring people because of their disability.

Like racism, classism and sexism, ableism can be seen in our attitudes and system structures. It can be unintentional (e.g., the focus of media stories related to disability being on pity or 'supercrip' hero stories), covert (e.g., having inaccessibly complicated job application forms) or overt (e.g., not providing wheelchair access to buildings). Equal rights for disabled people (including those who are Autistic and otherwise neurodivergent) is a basic standard that needs to be upheld, and disabled people should not be made to feel grateful for having these supports 'bestowed' on them by the majority group.

Confronting all of these 'isms' is an uncomfortable and ongoing process for both individuals and societies grappling with changes in power and money structures and confronting past wrongs. In the future, we will look back at how we perceived and treated disabled people with the same incredulity and horror we do now at the racist and sexist norms of the past, and wonder how we ever felt they were acceptable.

Important note: As caring professionals, recognizing and reflecting on ableism within ourselves is perhaps particularly uncomfortable as most of us have likely chosen our career path in large part to ease others' suffering, not contribute to it. In order to grow and learn it is important to be able to sit with this discomfort before moving on to more helpful, non-ableist ways of working. It involves unlearning a lot of what we were taught in training and our workplaces, and learning new, better information and ways of thinking and acting. It involves saying to ourselves that we were doing the best we could with what we knew at the time, but now we know better. And then putting effort into implementing this learning into real changes in our lives and working practices.

Ableism and Autistic People

For many professionals (including the authors of this book) it would not be too dramatic to call it revelatory to realize just how deeply ableist our textbooks, diagnostic manuals, beliefs and working practices in relation to autism diagnosis and support are. Once seen, it is impossible to unsee, and soon you will find yourself wincing with shame at the inherently ableist terminology, practices and recommendations that many recommended not too long ago.

Our diagnostic manuals use terms like 'symptoms' (the language of disease), 'disturbances', 'restricted, fixated interests', 'deficits in developing, maintaining and understanding relationships' and 'failure of normal back-and-forth conversation'. Our diagnostic criteria are based on the Autistic person failing as a neurotypical person. The vast majority of the 'interventions' provided to Autistic people (with the word 'intervention' itself being fundamentally ableist in this context) are also ableist. Even environmental and cultural design is biased towards neurotypical people.

The Autistic community has been fighting for equal rights and societal accommodations since the 1980s. Outside of this community, however, the dominant narratives around Autistic people continue to be largely ableist. Here are some examples of ableism against Autistic people:

- Judging certain interests as 'childish' or 'immature'.

- Framing Autistic ways of being as undesirable.

- Expecting Autistic people to have savant or special abilities.

- The assumption that spoken language is the superior form of communication.

- The assumption that everyone should enjoy and be able to engage in social chit-chat.

- The assumption that eye contact when communicating is necessary or superior.

- The assumption that people learn best when their bodies are still.

- Perceiving stimming as negative in any way.

- The belief that to publicly show big emotions is 'wrong' or socially unacceptable.

- Telling someone they should not let their autism define them.

- Telling someone they are doing really well despite being Autistic.

- Celebrating and praising Autistic people for masking their authentic Autistic selves.

- Neurotypical people having the power to decide how Autistic people should be spoken about, assessed, supported and researched.

- Teaching neurotypical social skills as the 'gold standard' way of being.

- The assumption that any treatment or therapy should target Autistic ways of being, and that a 'return to normalcy' and behaving like (or at least passing for) a neurotypical person is the ultimate goal.

- Seeing anxiety, meltdowns or significant mental health issues as inherently a part of the Autistic experience, instead of looking at how growing up and living in a society built for neurotypical people has contributed.

To understand ableism and how it is a crucial part of our shared history, it is important to develop critical thinking skills. In examining if a belief or practice is ableist against Autistic people, ask yourself, why do I have this belief? Why is this thing 'wrong'? What am I basing this on? Would I think the same about gender or race? Is this the respectful and ethical thing to be thinking? Is my thinking biased in any way? Do I need to learn more about this? What do the Autistic community think about this topic? Who is the author? What do they have to gain? How would I feel about it if I was Autistic?

A helpful thought experiment to see if a belief or practice is ableist against Autistic people is to replace it with race, gender or sexuality. Take, for example, something often heard in mainstream education, that there cannot be too many Autistic children included in the mainstream classroom because it would be too distracting for the other children and too much work for the teacher to manage. Sounds relatively reasonable? Now replace it with race or gender, and it is clear how unacceptable either of these justifications are.

Another example is the often-cited reason for providing neurotypical social skills training, that the Autistic person requested it because they want to fit in and want to avoid being bullied or ostracized. Again, this sounds reasonable, but if you do the thought experiment and change it to a gay person coming to you for support, telling you that that they hate being gay because it has 'caused them to be lonely and isolated', and they want to learn either not be gay any more or not to show any outward signs of being gay. No caring professional working within an ethical framework is going to go along with this request from their client, knowing that it would be profoundly damaging and unhelpful in the long term, as well as giving the implicit and explicit message that they agree that being gay is the issue. To do so would be to imply that it is the client's sexuality that was 'causing' the bullying rather than the reality that the blame lies with the perpetrators and a deeply homophobic society. Instead, as a professional you would support your client to embrace their identity, reframe their history, process their trauma, and link them in with LGBTQIA+ community and advocacy groups. You would also likely support and advocate for societal changes in this area in order to greater help your clients. This same process and understanding is what is needed for your Autistic clients.

Another example of ableism and how it relates to the Autistic experience is how Autistic community members and organizations are often ignored or challenged when they speak out about matters pertaining to them. A core motto of the Autistic and wider disability community is 'Nothing About Us Without Us' and yet journalists, authors, researchers and organizations continually write about and research Autistic people's experience with zero engagement from the Autistic community. This is akin to supporting a woman's rights organization that is entirely run by men, whose policies directly contravene what most women say they want and need, or writing about the menopause (for example) and not interviewing a single woman. Or it is akin to having a group of only white panelists on a talk show discussing what it means to grow up Black in the USA. Real, full representation should be a matter of course, not outside of the norm.

The Medical, Social and Biopsychosocial Models of Disability

The medical model of disability

The medical model of disability places all 'problems' related to being disabled as being **within** the person. It asks us, as professionals, to examine what is 'wrong' with that person, how **they** are impaired, and what **they** need to do to change themselves to fit in with the dominant group. According to this model, all ways of functioning that deviate from the 'typical' brain are unhealthy, abnormal or wrong in some way. A natural progression from seeing someone as disabled purely because of an internal impairment (i.e., within-person factors) is to believe that the way to solve the issue is to try to change the person, medically or otherwise.

Through the medical model of disability lens, the Autistic experience is viewed as a pathology, a disorder, a collection of impairments and something to be prevented, intervened with, treated or cured. It posits the misguided and incorrect idea that there was at one stage a perfect brain, until at some stage, something, somehow, went wrong, and the thing that went wrong was autism. Any behaviours or traits arising from this 'impairment' are therefore looked on as problems to be remediated. Current autism diagnostic assessments are based on this medical model of disability and involve professionals looking for evidence of these 'impairments' in the same way that a doctor may look for evidence of a disease in a patient. This applies to all 'disorders' currently outlined in the DSM-5-TR and ICD-11, both fully couched within the medical model of disability.

Because within the medical model of disability Autistic ways of being (e.g., a preference for focusing on one topic in conversation, stimming, eye contact differences and other social communication differences) are looked at as 'impairments', they are then inevitably framed as also being the **source** of the challenges faced by Autistic people and therefore impediments to social or professional success. It then follows that these natural Autistic ways of being are inappropriately targeted for intervention (e.g., through harmful compliance-based programmes to suppress Autistic ways of being) rather than supporting the child or adult in the areas they want help in and which would actually improve their quality of life (e.g., help with poor sleep or increasing sensory self-awareness and adapting environments to suit their sensory perception).

There are, of course, some medical issues (e.g., epilepsy and chronic pain) that cause suffering for many Autistic people, and for these a medical model view, with its focus on cure and intervention, is what is needed to be helpful and improve Autistic lives.

The social model of disability

In contrast to the medical model, the social model of disability views being disabled as being caused by how societal systems and environments are organized and who organizes them rather than by within-person factors. Instead of viewing the person as needing to be fixed, it looks to the wider social contexts and environments in which disabled people live. It centres disabled people as human beings with legitimate needs and rights instead of as problems or burdens on society. It is important to bear in mind that practices to improve access and equal rights for disabled people benefit **all** members of society, not just those who are disabled.

Most of us **should** have learned about the social model of disability at some point in our professional training, and our thinking may have advanced as far as seeing how, for example, wheelchair users are disabled by their environment. It is also clear to most of us how, for these more visible disabilities, structures can be put in place to reduce this inequality (e.g., ramps and wheelchair-accessible toilets). But it is very new to think of this framing in relation to Autistic people.

The social model of disability does not pathologize natural Autistic ways of being. Because it views what is causing the person to be disabled as being outside of that person, its focus is on societal changes, removing barriers and ensuring future design is rooted in the universal design model to ensure **all** members of society have equal access. Shifting to the mindset of being flexible and responsive (and not just doing things as they always have been done) is vital.

Examples of universal design that ensure equal access opportunities to Autistic people in society include balanced, adaptable environments. This means a reduction in uncertain and overloading sensory stimuli such as background noise, unpredictable sensory stimuli, open-plan areas with poor acoustics, travelling sound and visual noise. It also means increases in soothing uplifting stimuli such as soft, non-fluorescent lightening, black-out curtains and moveable furniture to make spaces adaptable and partitioned. All of these should be adaptable depending on the circumstances. Other examples include designing areas of natural light and 'green design' with nature elements, for example inside plants. Universal design also includes clear, jargon-free communication in multiple formats when governments or businesses provide public information. It involves information and interaction options being available for a diversity of communication needs such as a reduced reliance on phone calls to access healthcare for those who struggle with audio communication, but also keeping the phone option for those who struggle with text communication. It includes society-wide education on and acceptance of Autistic ways of being (e.g., the normalization of stimming across environments, including professional workplaces).

The biopsychosocial model of disability

The biopsychosocial model of disability attempts to account for both the medical and social models of disability. 'Bio' refers to physiological aspects, 'psycho' refers to what is going on for that person psychologically – their thoughts, feelings, emotions, beliefs and behaviours – and 'social' refers to the external social, environmental and cultural factors affecting a person.

There are many health professionals, in particular psychiatrists, who work from a biopsychosocial model and who bring this model to their work with Autistic children and adults. There are some ways in which a biopsychosocial model may be helpful to understanding the Autistic experience – for example it allows for the incorporation of theories such as the double empathy theory. It is certainly part of a mindful and respectful journey to becoming more Neuro-Affirmative.

In practice, however, it is our experience that even for professionals who may use this model with other clients, when it comes to Autistic clients the emphasis is placed on the 'bio' aspect, and when examined closely it is a medical model view that is actually being used, with neurotypical standards and neurotypical developmental trajectories as the baseline. This is still counter to a Neuro-Affirmative way of conceptualizing Autistic people.

Is Being Autistic Disabling?

As a starting point, it is not up to anyone to decide for someone else if they are disabled or not. Whether a person feels that their experiences and differences are disabling to them or not, and how they want to frame their life experiences, is that person's story to tell.

Autism is a broad spectrum and Autistic people experience being Autistic in different ways to each other. Also, the way in which disability is understood as a concept can vary between people, cultures and countries.

Most Autistic people agree that they are disabled by a society that actively excludes them, and does not support, understand or adapt to them. There is an important point and distinction to be understood here. What they believe is that it is not that **being Autistic** is disabling. Being Autistic is not the 'problem'. It is the wider societal structures, attitudes and beliefs that are the disabling agents. This view is very firmly within the social model of disability.

There are also Autistic people whose views on being Autistic bridge the traditional

medical and social models of disability. This group of people may feel that for
the **main** they are disabled by the world around them, but also, even when
environmental accommodations exist. Examples include hyperacusis (the mental
overwhelm and physical pain of auditory sensitivity) or interoceptive differences
such as under- or over-recognition of basic functions (e.g., hunger, thirst and bodily
functions) having a significantly negative impact on their lives, and that it **is** these
issues that are disabling and not the environment.

Possibly the best way to frame the answer to this question, then, is that being
Autistic **can** be disabling. This allows room for people who identify and recognize
challenges in their lives (whether they frame these in relation to either or both the
medical and social models of disability) while also making room for people who
do not relate to a disability model of any kind. A framing of 'being Autistic **can** be
disabling' also includes many Autistic people's experience of disabling situations as
a waxing and waning phenomenon in different contexts and environments over the
course of their lives.

Morality, Empathy and Compassion

▦ **Important note:** It is vital that everyone understands that Autistic people
do not lack morality, do not lack empathy and do not lack compassion. To
suggest Autistic people **do** lack any of these is completely unfounded, and
perpetuating such myths causes immense harm and suffering to the Autistic
community. All professionals working with Autistic people need to educate
themselves on how empathy and compassion are experienced and expressed in
the Autistic experience in order to fully support and work with Autistic people.
Understanding both of these separate concepts, how they are similar and
different to each other, and how they relate to Autistic people, will greatly help
the autism assessment process for both you as a professional and the people
coming to you for their assessment.

What is morality?

Morality is such a large concept that it is not within the remit of this book to
fully define it. However, dictionary definitions of morality include 'conformity to
ideals of right human conduct' (Merriam-Webster n.d.), 'a set of personal or social
standards for good or bad behaviour and character' and 'the quality of being right,
honest, or acceptable' (Cambridge Academic n.d.). Morality is also often used as
an umbrella term for a sense of care for others, level of empathy, compassion, love
and concern, along with many other things depending on what is considered right

and acceptable to differing cultural personal and social standards (Decety and Cowell 2014).

While much research uses the constructs of empathy (encompassing compassion) and morality interchangeably (de Waal 2010), there is solid evolutionary, cognitive and biological evidence that these are distinct constructs, that empathy can introduce partiality and interrupt moral decision-making, and that these distinct constructs should be kept separate to reduce risk of furthering misconceptions (Decety and Cowell 2014).

What is empathy?

There is no clear definition of empathy and there are probably as many definitions of empathy as people working in the area (de Vignemont and Singer 2006), although the differences are subtle and hard to disentangle. The most typical definition is that empathy is the active process of experiencing the world as you think another person experiences the world (Bloom 2017).

In its simplest form, empathy can be split into two distinct types:

- **Affective empathy**, which means feeling what another person feels, a shared or vicarious state of being, for example suffering when another person is suffering (Nicolaidis et al. 2019).

- **Cognitive empathy**, which means comprehending what another person is feeling without actually feeling what they are feeling for yourself. You need to have concern for the other's feeling to understand them (Bloom 2017).

These two types of empathy are discrete, and it is possible to have high levels of one and low levels of the other (Nicolaidis et al. 2019).

When empathy is referred to in relation to the Autistic experience, it is often hard to know whether the general term of 'empathy' refers to affective or cognitive empathy, a combination of both, or indeed compassion or a general sense of morality.

Some researchers and clinical practitioners think that empathy is a key element in what makes us human, or in what makes us moral (Hoffman 2010), but empathy is not an estimate of morality. It is influenced by in-group and out-group norms and our impression and judgement about others (Decety and Cowell 2014). Studies of neurotypical people have shown that humans feel more empathy for someone suffering because of outside forces than because of something internal. For example, humans tend to feel more empathy for a person who gets cancer later in life than for a person who is born disabled (Bloom 2017).

Empathy can be an exhausting and draining experience, and Autistic people describe an experience of hyper-pronounced empathy, often termed 'hyper-empathy'.

What is hyper-empathy?

Hyper-empathy is a commonly described experience in the Autistic community. Yenn Purkis describes hyper-empathy as when a person experiences the emotions of others near them almost as if by osmosis (Purkis 2022).

Hyper-empathy involves being highly attuned to feeling others' emotions, often processing them as your own and experiencing them intensely. Autistic people may experience hyper-empathy that is not only more intense, but also more all-encompassing than the neurotypical experience (Fletcher-Watson and Bird 2020). It can be overwhelming, painful, and at times paralysing to be so attuned to the emotions of others, particularly when those around Autistic people may not understand their experience. Despite this, research to date has largely ignored the Autistic experience of hyper-empathy. Assessing clinicians needs to be aware that this experience of hyper-empathy is common for Autistic people.

What is compassion?

Compassion is when you show care and concern for another without matching their feeling to another person's feelings. Compassion can often be confused with affective empathy, but while affective empathy is feeling what another feels, compassion is a more distanced state from others' direct feelings, with the focus being on concern for others, and a desire to find a way to support them to thrive (Bloom 2017).

Compassion also differs from cognitive empathy. Cognitive empathy is when you 'cognitively' or intellectually understand how someone is feeling. It does not involve showing concern or care for another's feelings the way compassion does.

Unlike affective empathy, which is biased toward familiarity and short-sighted motivating actions with instant results in the here and now, but with little concern for its future impacts (Bloom 2017), compassion can be applied to the more general, including non-human, experience. We get a powerful sense of Autistic morality driven by compassion through the work of Greta Thunberg (climate activist) and Dara McAnulty (author and naturalist). Among the Autistic community, there is immense morality and actions of compassion and concern and rational action to create a society where we respect our planet, a place where all life can thrive, where human short-term pleasure is not put above the long-term consequences of manmade destruction.

This is an important aspect for professionals to be aware of when engaging in autism assessment, for example when exploring a client's history and reframing the dynamics of human and non-human relationships, including trauma related to the loss of pets, and the differing ways in which Autistic individuals are motivated by rational compassion to show care for others, driven by an intense sense of social justice and equal concern for non-human life as much as for human life. For example, an Autistic person may respond to another person's distress through compassion by talking to them about how they are feeling, and then doing a deep dive into research on that topic to compile information for the distressed person that might help alleviate their distress or help support them to find a solution.

What is the double empathy problem?

The double empathy problem is a vital theory originally developed by Dr Damian Milton, which all professionals working with Autistic people should be very familiar with. It is a concept that has been hugely influential on our clinical work.

The double empathy problem highlights how any difficulty in interaction between Autistic and neurotypical people comes from the interaction space created between the two groups, rather than judging the issue as being solely with the Autistic person. Problems occur when there is a mismatch between what neurotypical and Autistic people see as important in terms of social expectations, communication styles, life experiences and perception of the world and values (Milton 2017).

As an example of the double empathy problem in action, traditionally the narrative in relation to Autistic people is that Autistic people have 'issues' and 'problems' making friends or in social interactions generally (i.e., the issue is with the Autistic person). However, research exploring the experience of Autistic adults found a key role in social relationships with other Autistic people in quality of life, and that Autistic adults found they were understood better by other Autistic people and felt a stronger sense of belonging (Crompton et al. 2020a). In research that compared interaction through storytelling between Autistic people, neurotypical people and a mix of both, results showed that Autistic people shared the story with other Autistic people as well as neurotypical people shared the story with other neurotypical people, but in the mixed group there was decreased ability to relay the story, and participants reported feeling less connection in communication with each other (Crompton et al. 2020b).

Autistic experience is not familiar to neurotypicals and neurotypical experience is not familiar to Autistic individuals, and so both sides have difficulty engaging empathy for each other and understanding unfamiliar experiences. Challenges for each group to understand and connect with each other arise because of this difference. The social communication issues Autistic people experience when trying to connect with neurotypical people are also the issues experienced by neurotypical people trying to connect with Autistic people. This makes it a double problem, equally experienced by two diverse groups of people, which is known as the 'double empathy problem' (Milton 2012).

Reflection Point

Humans are more likely to be empathetic towards their own group at the expense of an out-group. This, of course, affects health professionals as well as the general public, whereby if you are a neurotypical professional, you may (without ongoing reflective work) show more concern towards the distress of a neurotypical person, as you have familiarity with their experiences. Conversely, it is possible that if you are an Autistic professional, you may (without ongoing reflective work) show more concern towards the distress of Autistic people. Becoming aware of this involves vital ongoing reflection and learning, and will improve both the therapeutic nature of your assessments as well as their outcomes.

Important differences between empathy and compassion

Despite evidence of distinct differences between empathy and compassion, resulting in important consequences, many researchers continue to use affective empathy and compassion interchangeably and without clarity between which of these they are studying.

Affective empathy is biased towards what is familiar (Bloom 2017). Humans have evolved to naturally show more empathy for the similar, such as people who have (for example) similar life experiences, cultural experiences, belong to the same race, the same neurotype, have a similar perception, have similar beliefs, similar home life, similar carers and similar values.

Taking this all into account, Autistic people experience a significantly different reality to neurotypical people, and therefore naturally find it hard to have empathy for each other's unknown experiences. The double empathy problem shows that this is bidirectional, with both neurotypical and Autistic people struggling to experience empathy for each other's unfamiliar experiences. A person might not ever know that there is something to feel empathy for if they have no experience of it, and even with experience, they are likely to find this an extremely difficult if not impossible task if they cannot imagine that experience. Therefore, empathy is most often reserved for things we have some level of familiarity with (Bloom 2017).

Compassion, on the other hand, does **not** require a person to have a similar experience to another person's to show concern for the person feeling it. A person can feel compassion for something or someone else's experience even if they have no notion of what that experience is like, and compassion is not affected by bias and not limited to familiarity, unlike empathy (Nicolaidis et al. 2019). For example, a neurotypical person can feel compassion and provide support for an Autistic person experiencing distress and sensory overload in an environment that the Autistic person perceives as unpredictable and volatile, even if the neurotypical person perceives the same environment as calm and pleasant. The neurotypical person can show concern and provide support through compassion for the Autistic person without actually feeling the distress and pain of sensory overload that the Autistic person experiences being in that environment:

> Despite using the term 'empathy' myself, in the 'double empathy problem' theory, I do have some difficulty with what the concept is really referring to. It seems to mean different things to different people in different contexts. The basic dictionary definition would describe it as the ability to understand and share the feelings of others. Though a full understanding of what it means to be someone else is impossible. What empathy is and how it is theorized are open to much debate. I once saw a prominent academic describe a developing theory of mind in a young girl. She was projecting emotions into a toy doll. I had to point out that dolls do not have minds and so the question was on projecting her learned emotions and constructs. I find categories about cognitive and affective empathy of little use. I would prefer a distinction made about compassion and empathy (Dr Damian Milton, quoted in Nicolaidis et al. 2019, pp.4–11).

Discussion on empathy, compassion and morality

For many years, Autistic people have experienced prejudice due to the myth that they lack empathy, which continues to be incorrectly understood by the public as an all-encompassing measure of morality including care, love, kindness, fairness and compassion. However, it has been proven that Autistic people feel empathy and often experience hyper-empathy, and they also experience a separately intense sense of compassion.

Yet the remnants of this 'Autistic lack of empathy' myth remain, regardless of the evidence. These prejudicial misconceptions continue to cause stigmatization, exclusion and suffering to the Autistic community. While research, and indeed wider society, describes Autistic people in terms of 'lacking' empathy, this does not chime with the lived experience of many Autistic people. It is not that Autistic people have a **lack** of empathy, but rather a **different** experience and expression of it. Understanding this (and just how flawed much of the public understanding about Autistic people's morality is) is vital for professionals undertaking assessments to understand.

The research in relation to empathy and the Autistic experience is confusing, with many inconsistences, misinterpretations, biased reasoning and limitations in findings. One such issue with the empathy research to date is the limitation of current measures, many of which involve a collection of items that describe empathy but that also include items related to but different from empathy. An example of one such measure is Baron-Cohen and Wheelwright's (2004) Empathy Quotient, which consists of 40 empathy items and 20 control items. Some items do capture empathy, such as 'I find it easy to put myself in other people's shoes' (although this is unclear and may be taken literally, leading to confusion), while others capture compassion more than empathy, such as 'It upsets me to see an animal in pain.'

▦ **Important note:** Taking a spotlight view on empathy as the ultimate measure of morality has so far led to a focus on neurotypical ways of being at the expense of Autistic ways of being, and, on a larger scale, a focus on humans as the most important life on Earth at a devastating cost to other ways of being and different life on Earth. Perhaps it would make more sense to remove empathy from its pedestal and focus more on Autistic experiences of compassion and empathy separately? Taking this focus of both as important driving forces for morality allows us to consider both the present and the future, and to take a step back to act rationally in productive ways to create a world that is accessible to everyone, and where all of life can thrive.

Reflection Point

While how both empathy and compassion are conceptualized and operationalized may not always be clear-cut, particularly in relation to how an individual clinician or Autistic person makes sense of both the compassion and empathy constructs personally, it is crucial to consider how we are conceptualizing both in order to be able to incorporate this element properly in our assessment work. Non-autistic clinicians must direct a particularly effortful lens to this.

Non-autistic expectations of how Autistic morality is both expressed and experienced can and will restrict the clinician's ability to explore these constructs with Autistic people, as they do not have the lived experience of Autistic ways of experiencing empathy and compassion. This is particularly important given so many Autistic people will bring with them a lifetime of being told that they have no empathy, which is often understood as no morality, compassion or concern for others. Careful consideration of this, and paying respect and attention to Autistic expression and experience of morality through both compassion and empathy, can support a shift in this narrative away from 'deficits' in Autistic morality towards differences in how both compassion and empathy are expressed.

Current Diagnostic Criteria for Autism

The current diagnostic criteria for autism are firmly deficit-based and within the medical model of disability. In the two diagnostic manuals currently in use, namely, the *Diagnostic and Statistical Manual of Mental Disorders*, Fifth Edition, Text Revision (DSM-5-TR) and the *International Classification of Diseases*, 11th Revision (ICD-11), being Autistic is framed as a disorder, with the language of disorder and disease used throughout.

Although these manuals provide the parameters for what clinicians (including ourselves) currently need to stay within in relation to exploring an Autistic identity, a healthy dose of scepticism and questioning for these classification manuals **in general** (as well as the current Autistic criteria) is needed. For example, it is important for professionals to remember that these classification schemes are based on a current professional consensus of clusters of observed behaviours, not objective biological data or fact – indeed, up until as recently as 1973, 'homosexuality' was included as a disorder in the DSM.

Although Autistic criteria in both the ICD and DSM classifications are problematic and ableist in their framing and language use, when looked at as broad areas in which the Autistic experience differs from the neurotypical experience, these criteria **are** helpful once the judgements within them are removed. As you will see later in this book, the areas within the criteria are the basis of how we, as a team, identify (collaboratively with our clients) whether a person is Autistic or not.

In both the DSM-5-TR and ICD-11, 'autism spectrum disorder' is used as an umbrella term to encompass a wide variety of presentations. Diagnosis is based on a highly subjective set of observed behaviour, and does not take into account the internal feelings or lived experience of the individual being assessed. In both, the 'autism diagnosis' is centred on, and characterized by, persistent challenges with social communication and social interaction coupled with restricted or repetitive patterns of behaviour, interests or activities. Sensory difficulties are also highlighted. All current diagnostic criteria are described using judgement-based terms such as 'restricted', 'difficulties', 'challenges' and 'abnormalities', and are based on how the person has failed to present neurotypically.

▓ **Important note:** While it is important for clinicians to be familiar with the DSM-5-TR and ICD-11 criteria, we do not support the language use and framing of Autistic people within these criteria or within a Neuro-Affirmative assessment process.

Support levels in the DSM-5-TR

The DSM-5-TR also outlines three levels of required support for those diagnosed as 'Autistic': level 1, meaning that they 'require support', level 2, that they 'require substantial support', and level 3, that they 'require very substantial support'.

While superficially it is positive that the DSM-5-TR acknowledges that Autistic people require various levels of support and focuses on support needs rather than ability, these levels are ultimately unhelpful as they do not recognize that sometimes people may require substantial support in one area of their life and no support in other areas. They also do not take into account that the amount of support required in any individual area can vary depending on the day or situation. The DSM-5 and DSM-5-TR model are improvements from the linear 'high' versus 'low functioning' view that the DSM-IV imposed, but there is still room for it to improve to describe the spectrum nature of the diagnosis, and people continue to be categorized in unhelpful ways. These levels are particularly unhelpful to support parents of recently diagnosed children to understand the Autistic experience in any kind of meaningful way, and those of us involved in diagnosis do not use them in our child or adult work.

▓ **Important note:** We don't specifically recommend the use of either the DSM-5-TR or the ICD-11, and services will vary depending on which criteria they use. When using either, it is vital that it is looked at through a critical lens and adapted to be Neuro-Affirmative.

Flipping the narrative

The diagnostic criteria outlined above clearly describe autism through a narrative of deficit. Basing assessments, and wider clinical work, on this framing of the Autistic experience means that implicit messages of deficit are easily given to Autistic people during their discovery of being Autistic and their interactions with services. Given these criteria focus on 'impairment' and 'deficit', assessments embedded in such an approach can leave Autistic people with a sense of being judged as deficient, of being different in a negative way, instead of being different in a joyfully Autistic way.

Conceptualizations of 'deficit' are, of course, defined by the (perceived) predominant neurotype. It is the perceived neuro-majority who drive diagnostic criteria. These arise within the context of the privilege, attitudes and neuro-majority of those who develop them. Their privilege is such that they are not exposed to the experience of having the Self judged as deficient, as occupying a role in the world that is defined in terms of failing to match up to an arbitrary gold standard. And it is arbitrary. Were Autistic people afforded the power of being the perceived neuro-majority, it could be them developing diagnostic criteria for 'neurotypical spectrum disorder'. In general, it is always those in the majority who get to determine what is judged as a deficit or not.

What might these criteria look like? Below we offer an experiential exercise for neurotypical clinicians. If you are a neurotypical clinician reading this, we invite you to attend curiously and thoughtfully to the discomfort that may arise as you see yourself described in terms of 'deficit'. Can you sit with this? Can you hold on to this discomfort and use it to drive a shift in your clinical practice, to support you in catching those moments when it is so easy to be pulled back into deficit-based practice? We encourage you to embrace any discomfort, to treasure and nourish it. Discomfort is where the learning is. It offers the potential to feel, more viscerally, why deficit-based approaches do not merit our attention.

> **Important note:** This is not how Autistic people see or want to see neurotypical people. This is purely a thought exercise, with language use reflecting current diagnostic criteria.

Proposed criteria for neurotypical spectrum disorder

Criteria A: Persistent deficits in social communication and interaction underpin how an individual navigates the social world and interacts with others. Deficits occur in:

- Social-emotional reciprocity: Atypical social approach and response, e.g., over-focus on sharing emotions, deficits in understanding emotions or communication styles of other neurotypes; inability to tolerate silences; inability to discuss meaningful topics; over-reliance on 'small talk'.

- Non-verbal social communication, e.g., over-reliance and over-focus on eye contact (including atypical use of level of eye contact to gauge interest in conversation); insistence on use of overly animated facial expressions.

- Reciprocal relationships: Deficits in developing, maintaining and understanding relationships across neurotypes, over-adjusting behaviour to different contexts, over-focus or reliance on peers; impaired ability to understand Autistic social norms.

Criteria B: Unpredictable behaviours and diversity of interests:

- Rigid adherence to avoiding routines or rituals, despite their practical benefit, e.g., insistence on taking a different route home 'just because'; different meals each mealtime; finding lack of change or inconsistency particularly challenging, which can disrupt preferred chaotic and unplanned schedule.

- May have multiple but superficial interests.

- These behaviours can present in different ways from individual to individual, and are overly flexible, unpredictable and inefficient.

- Marked lack of response to sensory input **or** lack of interest in sensory input (e.g., unaware of small changes in environment, unaware of potential for pleasure from engaging with sensory objects).

These features may present in varying ways for people with neurotypical spectrum disorder. All individuals with neurotypicalism have difficulties in social interaction and social communication, such as insistence on eye contact and an inability to 'read' and respond appropriately to the emotional cues of others from a different neurotype.

What Does Neurotypical Spectrum Disorder Look Like?

Social communication and interaction:

- Over-focus on reciprocity.

- Over-focus on eye contact.

- Deficits in social skills and behaviour including the ability to 'read' others' behaviours and expressions, i.e., those with neurotypical spectrum disorder have pronounced deficits in Autistic theory of mind.

- Over-reliance on making inferences when drawing conclusions.

- May have personal space difficulties (being unaware or intolerant of others' need for space).

- May have difficulties understanding others or norms of social interaction (e.g., sitting in silence together joyfully, turn-taking in information dumping).

- May have too much variation in tone and pitch when speaking.

- May find friendships or making friends difficult outside of their neurotype.

- May have too much (perhaps superficial) interest in others (e.g., spreading gossip).

- May show a 'sheep mindset'.

- May have over-reliance on gestures and displaying facial expressions.

Unpredictable patterns of behaviour, interests and activities:

- May prefer little or no routine.

- May have difficulties in thinking or understanding – difficulties communicating without reliance on sarcasm, metaphors or figures of speech.

- May display marked lack of repetitive movements **or** insistence on denying pencil taps, hair twiddling, etc. are repetitive movements.

- May play in a way that over-relies on others, relies on externalizing scenarios rather than using rich, inner experience.

- May have multiple but superficial interests, or pursue interests valued only by peers.

Should neurotypical spectrum disorder be called a disorder, a condition or a difference? Neurotypical advocates argue that neurotypicalism is a difference (not a disorder), and so strongly oppose any suggestion of cures. While many neurotypical individuals feel that removing that part of them would change them as a person, multiple views exist across the whole community, for example Autistic parents of children with neurotypicalism. We return to neurodiversity as a concept in all neurologies, and neurotypes, including neurotypical, should be respected and not judged.

Reflection Points

- How does it feel being described in a deficit-focused way? Does this feel comfortable?

- Do you recognize yourself in such limited criteria, or are there aspects of neurotypical experience that they do not capture?

- How can you use your reflections to support your clinical work with Autistic people?

- Are you embracing any discomfort, and cherishing it? This will help guide you forward in shifting your lens. Celebrate it gently.

What Does It Mean to Be Autistic?

#autism is dynamic quality in action, picking out notes in a song, losing oneself in an activity, deeply held passionate interests, battling services or just trying to understand a form, nature's answer to overconformity, a description of development, a culture, your best pals... (Damian Milton, @milton_damian)[1]

---

1   Tweet used with permission.

Autism is: Experiencing the world deeply, passionately and viscerally, having the ability to be totally immersed and centred on one experience that I gain intense sensory joy from. I can't imagine not having such an intense experience of the world: sensory experience can be a source of pain but also one of great joy. When I hear or play music, I become the music. I am all the notes, the emotion, the movement, the vibration. Anywhere and everywhere.

Autism opens up the beauty of the world. I would hate not to be so finely tuned to the beauty around me. The unpleasant sensory side is more than counterbalanced by attending to the beauty. I see the beauty in the light, will be mesmerized by simplicity. That is my still point. (Anonymous)

The Richness of Autistic Relationships and Communication: an Autistic Perspective

Many Autistic people have a strong preference for meaningful conversations, involving sharing of interests and passions. It is usually accepted, and indeed most likely expected, that either Autistic communication partner will monologue or 'info dump' about an interest or issue. From a neurotypical and deficit-based perspective such as that reflected in diagnostic criteria, this communication style reflects a 'failure' to hold a back-and-forth conversation. What this perspective misses is the sheer joy of talking in depth about a beloved interest with someone who understands that such extensive sharing can both lead to rich friendships or relationships and reflect the connection that already exists. Put simply, telling someone in depth about a specific passion can be in effect saying 'I care deeply about this topic, and I want to share my passion with you. I care about you.' When Autistic children or adults talk at length about a passion, remember this. You might feel bored, disconnected, find yourself checking out of the conversation or be focused on noting the 'deficits' in the person's communication style. Instead, witness their passion and knowledge and appreciate their choosing to share with you. Look beyond the surface. Remember that there are many ways in which to communicate and many ways in which to develop profound connection.

One such profound connection can be found when Autistic people 'vibe' with each other. This is the experience of a deep connection with someone that is both meaningful and powerful. It may come from a sense of simply 'getting each other', by communicating in a similar way, understanding each other's humour, sharing interests in detail, gifs, stims, music, etc., and finding that the Self is somehow reflected in the Other. Vibing travels far beyond merely enjoying each other's company. It creates a flow experience together, where both communication partners experience connection, understanding and sharing of one's essence. It is not so much about being **on** the same 'wavelength' as **being** that wavelength together. The wavelength finds itself without effortful attention being needed. To vibe deeply with someone is to find moments of freedom.

Not being able to bear witness to the depth of Autistic connection in relationships does not mean it is not there. Remember this.

Being Autistic is a genetically based, for the most part, inherited, neurotype. It is one of a great many possible different neurotypes (including being neurotypical) that have their own profile affecting how people perceive, understand, communicate and experience the world. Autistic people also experience a distinct Autistic developmental trajectory and a different, divergent (not disordered or 'wrong') developmental pathway because of being Autistic.

Individually, Autistic people are, of course, very different to each other, as there is as much diversity within the Autistic community as within the neurotypical community, or any other neurotype. Common ways of experiencing the world that many Autistic people **share** include differences to the majority in relation to sensory perception; using sensory information from the environment to understand and learn about the world; a preference for honesty and clarity in communications; a preference for predictability and control; self-expressive body language; a passionate enjoyment of interests and hobbies; and a strong ability to hyperfocus at times.

Autistic people can also experience emotions intensely, and some can find it difficult to name these emotions (this is termed 'alexithymia'). They often also struggle to relate to neurotypical people in the same way that neurotypical people struggle to relate to them.

Although the majority of the Autistic community do not like the term 'on the spectrum', the concept of the Autistic experience being conceptually like a broad spectrum is helpful to understand the variation and individuality within the Autistic population. Instead of a linear scale, a spectrum allows for Autistic people to experience their Autistic self in different ways, at different times and in different situations.

Being Autistic is not something that can be 'switched off' or 'cured'. It is not that a person has a neurotypical brain except for the 'autism bit'. There is no 'autism bit'.

Being Autistic permeates everything about that person, who moves through the world and experiences it as an Autistic person.

Being Autistic is also to be part of a thriving culture, community and identity. Being Autistic is to be part of a minority group. Over time, the Autistic community has grown and developed, and this shared experience not only encompasses how Autistic people perceive and understand the world because of neurology, but also the shared of experiences of a lifetime of prejudice, pathologization of their core ways of being, discrimination and stereotyping. Autistic people (diagnosed and undiagnosed) are part of the fabric of our society, and it is likely that many clinicians reading this book are themselves Autistic without realizing it.

Autistic people do not have a 'look'. If you are not Autistic, even you have spent your entire professional careers diagnosing Autistic children and adults (as many of the non-autistic authors in this book have) and think you can 'spot' Autistic people easily (as many of the non-autistic authors in this book previously thought), you cannot. In our experience, non-autistic clinicians can at times rely on a 'gut' feeling about whether someone is Autistic or not based on previous experience. This is something that the non-autistic authors have had to de-learn, as a reliance on someone's own personal story is going to be the most important factor here. There are a great many Autistic people who, because of growing up in a neurotypical world, mask their true selves (whether this is conscious or unconscious), and so you will not be able to tell from their observable behaviours if they are Autistic or not. If clinicians assess with only one 'look' in mind, they will miss the vast diversity of the Autistic experience.

When the negative framing and deficit judgement-based language is taken out, the current diagnostic criteria within various classification systems **do** provide helpful areas for clinicians looking to understand and identify with their clients the areas in which most Autistic people experience differences to neurotypical people.

Being Autistic can co-occur with other neurodivergencies (e.g., intellectual disability), and many Autistic people can also present with mental health issues. Unfortunately, diagnostic overshadowing can often occur where the challenges arising from these co-occurring conditions have been mistakenly all lumped together as Autistic 'issues', which has led to a skewed understanding of how Autistic people can present in services. On the other hand, for a great many people being Autistic is not even considered a possibility, despite many clear indications that it should be.

How we discuss and frame the Autistic experience is constantly evolving and changing as more high-quality, Autistic-led and co-produced research is published, and as clinicians it is important we keep up with these changes.

Why Is It So Important for Autistic People to Recognize That They are Autistic?

If you are reading this book, it is likely that you already see the value in someone's Autistic identity being discovered, and you may have already experienced first hand its positive value for your clients or indeed yourself. Unfortunately, however, there is a feeling among many non-autistic professionals (typically those with little experience or knowledge of the adult Autistic community) that there may be no need for being Autistic to be identified at all, particularly when (to them) the person's Autistic traits are not 'obvious' to observers.

Many Autistic adults have told us about how when they first started their journey of attempting to access an autism diagnosis they were told by sometimes multiple, well-meaning professionals that they 'don't see the autism', and that there was no need to pursue such a 'serious' diagnosis or lifelong 'label'. While unhelpful in relation to not being able to see under the surface of someone who has likely spent their lives masking their Autistic traits, this framing of autism reveals just how negative and pathology-based the Autistic experience is in the mind of many professionals.

We all go through our lives with a myriad of labels (e.g., woman, man, doctor, gay, left-handed, Irish), which can be positive, negative or neutral depending on a range of different factors, and ideally, we do not deny or 'hide' these labels from ourselves or others. They are a part of who we are. For a professional to say that it would be a negative thing to be 'labelled' Autistic, and therefore something to be avoided, shows how negative being Autistic is for them, with this message also being passed on loud and clear to their client. Paying attention to the assumptions and biases like this that we bring to our work is vital.

Let's also look at the term 'giving a label', which, along with the problematic power imbalance, implies that some kind of burdensome **thing** has been **given** to the person by you, as a professional. But people are not 'given' an Autistic neurotype in the same way that they are not 'given' their sexuality, gender, hair colour or nationality. The person is Autistic, whether a diagnosis is confirmed or not, and they are always going to be Autistic. They are not choosing to be Autistic, and they can't choose to stop being Autistic. It is as much an integral part of them as their gender. But without an accurate identification, they are lost without this vital understanding of themselves. In addition, all too often if this 'label' is not given, others assign other labels (e.g., 'borderline personality disorder' or OCD), which do not capture their true experience.

Many Autistic adults have documented unhappy and confusing childhoods, followed by the relief and joy that came with a late autism diagnosis and the benefits that this provided, including a sense of belonging, connection, self-acceptance, friends and a community that understands and embraces them. Some typical comments from Autistic adults include:

> I wish I had been diagnosed as a child. If I had known why all that stuff was going on in my head it would have helped me to feel like less of a weirdo.

> For years I saw myself as broken and spent my whole life trying to fix myself. Getting a diagnosis was the best thing I ever did. Now I can get the right kind of support.

> I spent my whole life not knowing the reason why I was weird, odd, rejected, outcast and not coping. I wish I had known earlier why I was different, then perhaps I would have been able to cope better and had access to help. It would have helped me know that the reason for my difference was a wiring difference and not because there is something wrong with me, or it was my fault.

> As soon as I read the description I knew it was me. It was a huge relief. My life made sense. It explained so much. I didn't know other people don't struggle with the things that I do.

> To be honest I don't care if it's a diagnosis or a label. I am just relieved that I am simply Autistic and not a bad, lazy, broken failure.

Being accurately identified as Autistic gives people a 'user manual' and a start to learning their own authentic ways to move through this world. It is the start of a journey of learning about themselves and their neurology, their sensory, perceptual and cognitive processes. It helps them understand **why** they may have felt like a failure time and time again, because they were being expected to be someone they weren't, a square peg being forced repeatedly into a round hole.

It may also be helpful for professionals to look at this in relation to the LGBTQIA+ community, and how positive it is for people in this community who previously masked as cisgender to begin to embrace and understand their sexuality and identity and to start living their authentic lives.

Most importantly, the Autistic community, through advocacy, research and other publications, has spoken out time and time again about how helpful their autism diagnosis was for them, and is advocating for more timely and accessible assessments to make this happen. There is also a growing body of research to support just how positive an impact the diagnosis can be on a wide range of factors in an individual's life. We hope in the future to undertake research that points to the further positive impact of Neuro-Affirmative diagnostic assessments in particular.

Self-Identification

There are currently increasingly large numbers of Autistic people who choose to identify as Autistic although they have not been through an official assessment process. Within the Autistic community, self-identification is fully accepted as valid. For example, to access community-led support or social groups, if someone says they are Autistic, they are Autistic. Many Autistic people say that you don't need to go to a doctor to be told you are gay, so why would you need to be told you are Autistic? Others **want** to go through an assessment process but encounter some of the many barriers explained below. It is a healthcare systems issue that we do not have appropriate pathways to respectful, timely, free, adult autism assessments for the people who need or want them.

It is important for professionals to self-reflect on the feelings and thoughts self-identification may bring up in them, and to also be aware of the many reasons someone may be self-identifying. The fact is that it is currently exceptionally difficult for the majority of adults to access an autism assessment and subsequent diagnosis. Although research has shown that Autistic people present equally across races (Maenner et al. 2021), the further someone is from being white, male, middle class and cisgendered, the harder it is for them to access an autism diagnosis.

Barriers that women experience include outdated views of how autism presents and the current 4:1 male to female ratio statistic, which is not borne out in clinical practice. In The Adult Autism Practice, the majority of people coming to the assessment are women, and anecdotally it would appear that more and more women are accessing a diagnosis worldwide. It is looking increasingly likely that in the future it will be recognized that autism is far more prevalent in women than previously thought, with possibly an even gender split.

Reasons for people self-identifying include the high cost of private assessments, long wait times or lack of services, inaccessible application procedures, a lack of awareness among professionals of how Autistic people present and related professional gatekeeping (e.g., not putting someone forward for an assessment due to good eye contact even when they want an assessment). The requirement for family members to be involved, although the person is an adult and may have fractured relationships with their parents or wider family members, is a huge barrier for many, as is the expectation that a person undergo lengthy verbal interviews in unknown situations when spoken communication is very difficult for them.

Distrust of professionals is also enormous and understandable for many Autistic people, who, alongside knowing the dark history of the treatment of Autistic people in the past by professionals, have been given multiple inappropriate diagnoses (e.g., 'borderline personality disorder') and subsequent treatment pathways. These people have often, over the course of their lives, experienced multiple traumatic experiences within mental and other health services where their neurology was not understood or accommodated.

In online supportive communities, people who have been through traditional autism assessments share their stories about how they were treated, and how their assessments were daunting, difficult, infantilizing and adversarial. Assessments are already a daunting process, where you are expected to open yourself up completely to strangers. The idea that you would do this to strangers who may put you through an outdated and oftentimes traumatizing assessment process, with no real understanding of the Autistic experience, and then ultimately not believe you when you share your life experiences, is understandably too much for many. Or even when they do believe you, they may treat your natural, core ways of being as a pathology, and provide written documentation of all the ways you have failed to be 'normal' throughout your life.

Learning Through Practice

In The Adult Autism Practice, many people come to us for an assessment who are already self-identifying as Autistic, or are fairly confident that they are, but just want to talk it through with a professional. Many are accessing an official diagnosis because of work or college (i.e., to access reasonable accommodations), and many just want to talk it though so that a second person validates what they think is true. The vast majority of the people coming to us have put extensive research into whether they might be Autistic. This is something that has been mulled over, questioned, analysed and processed over a number of years. It is not something that has been decided on a whim or with little thought. We have been struck by the deep levels of self-awareness coming from our clients (completely at odds with traditional ideas of Autistic people lacking insight). The vast majority of people coming to us who are either already identifying, or are close to identifying, ultimately meet the criteria for autism.

We find that having an in-depth consultation, where we discuss the **likelihood** of them being Autistic, is enough for many (we would, of course, not officially diagnose after this one session). This is something to bear in mind for under-resourced services with long wait lists.

5

Theories of Autistic Neurology

Introduction

Since the first conceptualization of the Autistic experience in the 1940s, many different theories and models have been proposed to explain it, some of the most prominent of which we will discuss in this chapter. Some of the theories are holistic, for example van de Cruys et al.'s (2014) predictive coding model of Autistic perception, and their attempt to understand the Autistic neurology, and not just one aspect of it. These holistic theories can be useful in building self-awareness for Autistic people and in increasing understanding of the development of the foundations of Autistic people's experience as they support a person in taking a broader and more comprehensive view of themselves. However, most theories are not holistic; they are domain-specific, and typically only focus on one element of Autistic people's experience rather than considering **all** aspects of it and how they interact with each other.

It could be argued that only when professionals fully understand the theories and mechanisms that create Autistic people's experience will this help non-autistic professionals to start to truly understand what Autistic people experience in different contexts. Too often, however, these theories stray away from simply **objectively describing** Autistic experience and instead make a **subjective judgement**, most often arrived at due to biased comparisons to neurotypical experience.

If instead we remove these judgements and replace them with neutral observations and descriptors of different rather than deficient mechanisms of a neurotype, we can see how many of the theories of Autistic neurology can be critically reframed through a Neuro-Affirmative lens and become useful in understanding the different mechanisms underlying Autistic experience. We can also then more clearly see how some of these theories can be vital in assisting society to design and adapt environments that are inclusive of **all** people and neurotypes, including Autistic people, as it is largely the environment and societal design (not something that is inherent within a person) that leads to most challenges.

While medical, neurological and neuropsychological models **can at times** be unhelpful and reductionist, they can, however, also be helpful in understanding the anatomical, chemical, cognitive, perceptual and developmental factors involved in the Autistic experience, and how these relate to and can potentially improve or refine access to the right help, therapies, medications and supports.

Here are examples of some helpful aspects of a few of the models explained later in this chapter:

- Neural and perceptual models can be useful when they stick to factually describing rather than making a judgement about Autistic people's experience and the ways in which perceptual mechanisms, brain structures and connectivity are developed.

- Exploring differences in structure development and cortical neuromodulators, such as the role of excitation and inhibition neurotransmitters in the Autistic brain, can be useful to understanding how certain medication such as antipsychotics can work differently in an Autistic person's system (Haker, Schneebeli and Stephan 2016).

- Theories of altered connectivity or structural difference can help us understand how Autistic people's cognition may be different.

- Exploring reduction in synaptic pruning or difference in the development of minicolumns may help us begin to understand why there is a higher increase of synaesthetes within the Autistic population compared to the neurotypical population (see more on this later in this chapter) (Ward et al. 2017), and why Autistic people experience elevated levels of intense sensory experiences. These explorations can shed light on how cognitive therapies such as cognitive behaviour therapy (CBT) can have barriers when they are not adapted to be inclusive of formats of thought that are not in words, or how mediums of therapy such as art or music can be beneficial in exploring Autistic people's experience and expression.

- Neutrally exploring Autistic brain development can help us learn more about the process of a distinct Autistic developmental trajectory, and how learning and play and growth progress within the Autistic person's development.

- A predictive coding model of Autistic perception (van de Cruys et al. 2014) can be useful in understanding the role of context and how a situation can be adapted, in particular in highlighting and identifying the barriers of living in a world that has primarily been designed not just for neurotypical individuals, but often also actively excluding Autistic people.

A Brief Overview of Some of the Theories of Autistic Neurology

Broadly speaking, theories of Autistic people's experience can be categorized across three different levels of explanation: perceptual and neural, cognitive processing and action, and interaction. However, many of the models and theories overlap across these three.

We now briefly explore some of the theories of Autistic neurology (including theory of mind, the double empathy problem and monotropism), that aim to explain either the entire Autistic experience or certain Autistic features, and briefly look at their strengths and limitations in terms of working within a Neuro-Affirmative conceptual framework.

Theory of mind and the double empathy problem

Theory of mind (also known as 'cognitive empathy' or 'mind reading') is the ability to be able to make sense of what somebody might be thinking or feeling based on their tone of voice and body language. The theory of mind of Autistic cognition suggests that Autistic people find it difficult to tell what somebody else might be thinking or feeling (Happé and Frith 1996).

Damian Milton's double empathy problem (2012) shows that this is, in fact, a bi-directional problem that occurs when **two groups** who are different and have different views of what is important and salient information, and differing ways of communicating and expressing themselves, have difficulties understanding **each other**. Therefore, it is not that one group has a reduced theory of mind, but that **both groups** struggle to understand experiences that are different from their own (Milton 2012, 2017).

Research has shown that Autistic people go to greater lengths to try to understand the neurotypical experience than neurotypical people will go to understand the Autistic experience (Davis and Crompton 2021). This means, in fact, that the theory of mind problem, or the effort that goes into figuring out the theory of mind issue, often lies with neurotypical people rather than Autistic people.

Important note: Studies have shown that Autistic people show as strong a theory of mind with other Autistic people as neurotypical people do with other neurotypical people (Crompton et al. 2020b).

Monotropism

Monotropism[1] is a theory of Autistic experience developed by a group of Autistic scholars – Dinah Murray, Wenn Lawson and Mike Lesser. It is a cognitive theory of Autistic attention. Monotropism is highly popular and resonates with many of the experiences of those in the Autistic community. It posits that **all** humans have limited resources when it comes to attention, and so the different neurotypes need different mechanisms to deal with this limited attention ability. Monotropism proposes how Autistic people manage their flow of attention to tunnel towards select interests (Murray, Lesser and Lawson 2005), whereas neurotypical people often allocate their attention to many different things in the environment as well as the immediate task around them. So, for example, if hypothetically there are 10 attention points available, an estimate of 5 of those points would be directed at the primary task they are doing, while the other 5 would be allocated to different environmental cues, such as other people in their environment, planning what's for dinner, unrelated mind-wandering ideas, emotional states and basic needs such as hunger and energy levels (Autistamatic 2022), whereas monotropism suggests that **Autistic** people have a monotropic mind that allocates much more attention to the primary task, and, in the example above, Autistic people will only allocate about 1 or 2 of the attention points to other information unrelated to the primary task (Autistamatic 2022).

Engaging with such intensity to one primary task generates an intense energy tunnel towards the primary task, often termed a 'flow state', which can be immensely enjoyable and all-consuming. Monotropism therefore highlights the strong hyperfocus abilities experienced by many Autistic people, who experience the immense joy, playfulness, wonder, curiosity and energy of being engulfed by an interest, delving into the deepest layer of exploration, becoming proficient experts in specialized areas and understanding subjects at an intense level.

However, monotropism also highlights the flip side of this strength, which is, finding it difficult to redirect attention when needed. Autistic people often explain how pulling from their 'flow state' can take tremendous effort, and may even be painful. This intense allocation to the primary tasks means that Autistic people are less likely to recognize that they may need rest, food or water to restore energy.

---

1   See https://monotropism.org for a monotropism repository.

Autistic people can also find it challenging to respond to other tasks, such as daily tasks, responding to others and remembering to eat because they are forgotten to the primary task (Murray 2018). The theory of monotropism shows how switching tasks is easier for neurotypical people as attention is distributed in a way that is fleeting and therefore easier to move from, while in the Autistic brain, attention is allocated to a task with such intensity that it is difficult to switch attention from that deeply immersed state (Murray et al. 2005).

A downloadable deep dive into Autistic perception is available at https://uk.jkp.com/catalogue/book/9781839971662

Executive functioning

Executive ('dys')functioning is a cognitive theory of the Autistic experience (Ozonoff 1997), although 'executive function' itself is a broad term that refers to internal control processes, such as planning, transitioning, sustained attention, focus and memory that enable bodily, cognitive and emotional self-control (Chown 2017; Corbett et al. 2009).

Research has shown that some (but not all) Autistic people can experience difficulties in areas of executive functioning (Demetriou et al. 2018; Hoofs et al. 2018), and executive functioning is not a unitary construct; it can be understood as having separable but related cognitive mechanisms (Snyder, Miyake and Hankin 2015). However, the research findings are inconsistent.

Chown (2017) pointed to several limitations from these studies, including that many do not control for co-occurring intellectual disability or co-occurring neurodivergences such as ADHD. The research has primarily explored only the experience of Autistic children, not adults, and these studies do not often factor in the different developmental trajectories of Autistic children and the possibility of a distinct Autistic executive functioning development trajectory (Chown 2017). In addition, laboratory-based tasks frequently involve illogical or arbitrary tasks. When tasks instead involve rational rules, such as the tubes task, which test for gravity bias (several tubes lead into several different cups, and children see the experimenter drop a ball into one tube; the task is to follow the route of the ball into a cup and to search in the correct cup for the ball; see Hood 1995), Autistic children show no difference in results to their neurotypical peers (Bíró and Russell 2001).

Neural theories and models of Autistic neurology – the minicolumns theory

There is a range of neural theories of Autistic people's experience including those related to differences in connectivity, structure and development of Autistic neurology. It is not possible within this section to review all of these theories, so instead we will look at one prominent theory that links to how we can understand Autistic people's perception, cognition, processing and interaction starting from a distinct Autistic neural development. The Autistic minicolumns theory (Casanova et al. 2006), as research into brain difference between Autistic individuals and neurotypical individuals, has found differences in minicolumns between the two groups.

Minicolumns are located in the neocortex and are thought to be one of the smallest parts of the brain that are capable of processing information (Bogdashina 2016). A minicolumn is a vertical column consisting of glutamatergic (excitatory) and GABAergic (inhibitory) neurons that process thalamus input (Bogdashina 2016). We perceive the world in part from information our senses register from the environment (Friston 2010). This sensory stimulus then takes the journey from the world into our senses, and proceeds to the thalamus (in all cases but in the olfactory (smell) sense, which skips the thalamus). From the thalamus, the information is sent to different parts of the brain where it then travels through the minicolumns located in the different parts of the brain. Studies into minicolumns have found that larger minicolumns are capable of processing information faster, but this leads to overgeneralized processing at the expense of losing details and categorization ability, while smaller minicolumns have found to be capable of processing more information, but a longer processing time is required (Lorincz 2018).

In neurotypical people, the development of minicolumns is different to what is seen in Autistic people. Neurotypical people's minicolumns grow to be bigger as they develop, and more of their minicolumns are pruned. By adulthood they then have far fewer minicolumns than in infancy. In addition, in neurotypical people's brains, information moves through the centre of the minicolumns and doesn't overflow into any neighbouring minicolumns (or stay within the minicolumns for a long period of time) as the minicolumns are surrounded by inhibitory fibres (Casanova et al. 2006).

The study of minicolumns in Autistic people has found that minicolumns in Autistic brains are smaller, and that as Autistic people develop, there is less pruning of minicolumns as compared to the rate of pruning seen in neurotypical development. Autistic minicolumns are thought to stay small and remain numerous in quantity.

It has also been found that for Autistic people, information flows through the minicolumns but the tunnel has holes in it, which can result in information overflowing into neighbouring minicolumns. This means that the information often stays flooded around the minicolumn for longer, which can lead to an amplifying effect. Due to this flooding, the inhibitory fibres around the minicolumns are thought to be less effective in containing the information within individual minicolumns (Casanova et al. 2006).

Importantly, the amplifying effect caused by the flooding through and around the tunnel of the minicolumns also connects to how Autistic people show less habituation to sensory information (Ward 2019). It has been suggested that because there is no overflow in the minicolumns of neurotypical individuals, put simply, it's as if the information passes through and is then gone, meaning that the sensory feeling doesn't 'stay' around for long, and neurotypical people can habituate to it more easily. However, for Autistic people, because the information overflows to neighbouring minicolumns, and because the inhibitory fibres work differently, an intense feeling is created that lasts longer (Casanova et al. 2006). This suggests a mechanism for why the ability to habituate is reduced for Autistic people (Casanova et al. 2006).

The minicolumns theory helps shed some light on how Autistic people experience sensory information at a neural level and the experience of sensory overload, and why Autistic people experience such intense sensory overload, and why it stays with them for longer and is experienced as intense for longer.

Synaesthesia

Synaesthesia is a perceptual experience that is involuntary and automatic and triggered by something, and creates the expertise of an alternative perceptual reality, which is considered beneficial (Eagleman 2014). Synaesthesia = syn (joining) + aesthesia (feeling). It is the experience of a joining of senses, when an individual has a sensory experience that triggers another unrelated sensory experience to happen simultaneously (Eagleman 2014).

Synaesthesia can take many forms and can trigger multiple sensory experiences simultaneously. Common experiences of synaesthesia include for numbers, letters, days of the week or musical notes to be experienced in colours. For example, when someone thinks of Thursday, it triggers the internal experience of purple. Synaesthesia experiences are, however, unique to each individual. For example, seeing the colour blue might taste like vinegar to one person but cardboard to another (Ward 2020). Synaesthesia is thought to run in families – at least 3 per cent of the neurotypical population are thought to have synaesthesia and the rates are thought to be even higher in the Autistic population (Ward 2020).

Research findings related to minicolumns may also help explain the mixing of senses and higher rates of synaesthesia experienced in the Autistic population than in the neurotypical population, with similar brain structures and connectivity observed (Ward et al. 2018).

Similarities between synaesthetes (people who have synaesthesia) and Autistic people include a skill set that falls into a spiky profile, superior memory and a preference for categorization, order and routine and more susceptibility to sensory overload (Ward et al. 2017). Research has also shown that a large number of identified synaesthetes have close relatives who are also Autistic or otherwise neurodivergent (van Leeuwen et al. 2020).

Maurer, Gibson and Spector (2013) write that one idea is that **all** babies have synaesthesia, but that this disappears to a large extent as the neurotypical brain develops, synaptic pruning occurs and minicolumns change. However, this is hard to test as we cannot ask infants how they perceive the world (Ward 2020). In **all** babies, the sensory experience is thought to be more intense (and minicolumns are also more numerous and smaller in size), similar to how they are thought to remain in Autistic people's brains. But as a neurotypical brain develops, the minicolumns become larger and the number are pruned, and for most adults the synaesthesia experiences disappear (Maurer et al. 2013). Therefore, it is thought that what pruned minicolumns in neurotypical brains **may** do is differentiate between the senses and this makes them distinct, while for Autistic individuals (as well as for synaesthetes and infants) the content overflow can lead to a mix of senses across minicolumns, and a more intense, magnifying effect (Bogdashina 2016).

Predictive coding models of Autistic perception

These models propose that perception is created through a process called 'predictive coding', which describes how we combine sensory information from the environment with predictions based on past experience and beliefs we hold about the world to create our perception (for more information on this, see Chapter 6).

Here are three separate theories of Autistic perception, each of which proposes different ways that Autistic perception is created through predictive coding:

- The precision of Autistic predictions is stronger and Autistic people incorporate more sensory information into building a more complex and detailed model of the world based on precise predictions (van de Cruys et al. 2014).

- The precision of Autistic predictions is weaker, and predictions are broader and sensory information outweighs predictions in creating perception (Pellicano and Burr 2012).

- The weighing of predictions and sensory information is unbalanced and not adaptive to different environments, leading to Autistic individuals being 'mildly surprised' at everything (Lawson, Rees and Friston 2014).

Enhanced perceptual theory

Enhanced perceptual theory (Mottron and Burack 2001) suggests that Autistic people have a stronger ability to pick up on the details of a scene compared to non-autistic people. Evidence for this theory comes from laboratory experiments in controlled environments that show Autistic people are less susceptible to optical illusions and more likely to notice small detail changes to a scene compared to neurotypical people (Happé 1996). However, while Autistic people prefer to perceive in detail, this is now thought to be a choice rather than a default, and not at the expense of the bigger picture (Mottron et al. 2006).

The enhanced perceptual theory is an example of how **context** can have an influence on perception. It needs to be considered that the environment in these experiments was a laboratory setting, which is not reflective of neurotypically designed naturalistic environments (as most manmade environments consist of). A laboratory setting is most often calm and controlled. Participants know exactly what's going to happen there, and with ethics procedures ensuring informed consent they have been provided with a great deal of information prior to arriving. This means that there is considerably reduced unpredictability for participants.

Current research suggests that in unpredictable and new situations Autistic people's processing time can be slower because they are aware of increased environmental surprises (Sapey-Triomphe 2017). It therefore makes sense that in a highly controlled environment, such as a laboratory setting, Autistic people would show enhanced abilities, because the environment is designed to be accessible for them. This is not to say that Autistic people don't have enhanced abilities either in a naturalistic world or in a controlled environment. What Autistic perception models do is demonstrate the effect that uncertainty in different contexts has on how Autistic people experience and interact in the world. When high amounts of uncertainty are perceived in busy, neurotypically designed environments, this can create barriers to Autistic people engaging in tasks such as planning, involving several steps or attention switching with multiple competing cues.

Autistic inertia

Autistic inertia is a relatively new theory of Autistic experience that explains the phenomenon that when Autistic people stop doing a task, it is very hard for them to restart. Conversely, it can also occur when an Autistic person has started a task and has difficulty stopping. Generally, inertia is said to come about from an overload of stress, work, sensory overwhelm or lack of sleep.

When it comes to taking action and interacting in the world (Buckle et al. 2021), the theory of Autistic inertia explains the difficulty Autistic people may experience in acting on intentions. Actions such as taking a break to eat food, going to the bathroom to do self-care or transitioning to tasks outside of conscious control can be problematic when the Autistic person is hyperfocused on their interests.

Research has highlighted that Autistic inertia effects Autistic people in several ways, such as through internal experience, which describes the tendency to maintain in activity or in inactivity (Buckle et al. 2021) – for example, intending to take action, but experiencing inability to move, beginning a task even when motivation is high, the lack of conscious control, and confusion and frustration at not being able to do something, leading to fatigue, overload and stress.

Buckle et al.'s research (2021) found that factors that impacted the experience of inertia included helpful factors, such as working in an environment where others were also working, and appropriate environment design, such as working in a space set up like an office. In contrast, it also highlighted unhelpful factors such as movement or noise (which was experienced as stressful and distracting). Another factor identified that the influence of others influenced inertia, which could be experienced as both a positive and a negative influence. For example, some people found prompting from others or an urgent deadline to be useful in pulling them from an inactive state of inertia. Others, however, found influence from other people to be a source of stress.

Participants also explained how inertia affected many aspects of their lives, everything from activities they wanted to do to essential basic activities. Overall, inertia was described as leading to a decrease in productivity and an inability to maintain productivity in multiple spheres, for example only being able to be productive and find challenge in enjoyable leisure activities or hobbies. Inertia also affected people at the beginning of relationships and in maintaining them (Buckle et al. 2021).

While the current information base in relation to Autistic inertia is based on one preliminary and small study, and it needs further investigation, there is still interest in it within the Autistic community.

6

Autistic Perception

If you are a non-autistic clinician, it is vital to spend some time considering and understanding the importance of sensory perception from an Autistic perspective so that you can gain further insight into Autistic people's experiences. For the non-autistic clinicians within our team, the learning we have gained from listening to Autistic colleagues communicate about their experience of sensory perception has been profound and has changed everything about how we understand perception and processing within an Autistic brain.

> A downloadable deep dive into Autistic perception is available at https://uk.jkp.com/catalogue/book/9781839971662

Having a better understanding of the relationship between sensory perception and how an Autistic person's brain is primed to notice and process surprise within their environment has fundamentally changed how we understand this experience and how it relates to real-world experiences of overwhelm in response to, for example, a broken light in a room ruining a person's day, or how a busy environment can be exhausting for a person because of how many surprises there are in that setting. As a clinician, being able to communicate with people during an assessment about how we understand their reactions to surprise or uncertainty in their environment, and also the need that they have for predictability in their life, has a profound impact on how people understand themselves. It provides a framework for understanding the perceptual and cognitive processes that underlie these experiences and in supporting a person to let go of shame, self-berating, guilt and stress in relation to these experiences.

Reflection Point

Spend time learning about perception and how it happens for all humans. Learn about Autistic sensory perception and how there are differences in terms of how

Autistic brains perceive the world. Think about how uncertainty and surprise are experienced when a person's brain processes information in a more detailed way. Understand how overwhelm, meltdowns and shutdowns relate to sensory perception. Reflect on how we cannot remove all uncertainty in the world, but we can do so much to reduce unnecessary uncertainty. Work to accommodate people's needs in relation to sensory perception. Consider how this changes your approach to engaging with Autistic people and your responsibilities within how you serve the Autistic community.

Introduction

Perception is so much more than understanding the senses; it is how humans experience everything, from birth to life to death. Perception is how we create reality, everything we do, feel and think, our high and our lows and all in between. Perception is how we understand the world. Where we go in the world starts from a seed that grows in the soil of our particular perceptual mechanisms that relate to our neurotype, which, on a larger scale, reflects our humanity and our part in life. The human brain is so much more than a computer that passively takes in information from the environment and passively processes and categorizes it to understand the world. It is so much more than our eight senses. Each of us creates our own reality of life from our individual internal and external experience. How we think effects to some extent what we experience. How the Autistic perceptual mechanism works is critical to understanding the Autistic experience. Each Autistic individual, similar to each neurotypical individual, has their own experiences and their unique reality, but each neurotype has its own perceptual mechanism, which has a large effect on how that individually unique reality grows.

This chapter will explain how perception is created for all humans, and then looks at the specific differences seen in the Autistic compared to the neurotypical perceptual mechanism. We will see how context, environmental design, cultural design and societal expectations play a critical role in whether different perceptual mechanisms become strengths or challenges, and how our thinking and human aversion to too much uncertainty can block our learning and the different ways that our beautiful brains adapt context to thrive.

Understanding Autistic perception is vital in the context of autism assessment. If we can begin to understand the foundation from which each Autistic person grows, we can set up and adapt services to make sure that the design of our environment facilitates each person to thrive rather than blocks them in engagement. We can foster and support the growth of authentic development when we understand the foundation from which that self begins. It is much more than understanding 'the senses'. To understand the foundation we need to embrace the detail that makes up the full picture, step away from the general and be engulfed and open to learn something that may be new to many of us.

In The Adult Autism Practice and Thriving Autistic, we place a strong emphasis on exploring with clients their sensory perception and sensory patterns of processing. We highlight that understanding their sensory system supports them to fully understanding their authentic self. The sensory profile (Brown et al. 2001) is a useful tool that can be used with the client and psychologist to explore the client's individual sensory system and the ways they react to sensory stimuli, from the sensory stimuli they crave, what they don't notice, what they are sensitive to and what they avoid.

A referral to an occupational therapist is recommended to further explore the client's sensory profile and how they can adapt the world to suit them. The emphasis should never be on trying to change the Autistic perceptual mechanism to suit the environment, because apart from this not being possible or wanted, it can be dangerous, distressing and have a severe impact on the client's physical and mental health. For example, exposure-based approaches that aim to alter Autistic sensory perception do not work, are invaliding and do not respect Autistic perceptual mechanisms as an equally valid way of experiencing the world, and are harmful and thus unethical.

The Eight Senses

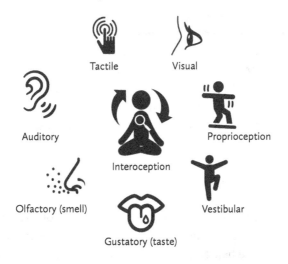

Tactile   Visual

Auditory

Proprioception

Interoception

Olfactory (smell)   Vestibular

Gustatory (taste)

Humans, to a substantial extent, perceive life through their senses:

- **Auditory:** Responsible for hearing and detecting sounds, sound frequency, sound loudness and interpreting language.

- **Tactile:** Helps us process touch sensations from the body and detect light touch, deep pressure, texture, temperature, vibration and pain.

- **Olfactory (smell):** Responsible for processing smells and detecting different odours, discriminating between odours, determining the importance of odours and signalling to the brain about their significance.

- **Gustatory (taste):** Responsible for our sense of taste, detecting safe and harmful foods, and signalling when we need hydration.

- **Visual:** Responsible for seeing and detecting objects, shapes, colours, orientation and motion.

- **Proprioception:** Responsible for sensing position, location, orientation and movement of the body's muscles and joints, detecting where our body parts are in space relative to other parts, and how much effort we use to move our body parts.

- **Vestibular:** Senses our balance and orientation in space. It informs us about the movement, rotation and position of our head relative to gravity. It influences our posture, head and eye movement and breathing.

- **Interoception:** Responsible for detecting and interpreting internal senses that inform us about our physiology and what our internal organs are feeling. It reports what is going on inside our bodies and is the messenger between all the other senses and what is going on physiologically and emotionally. It detects hunger, thirst, tiredness, nausea, heart rate and breathing, and is the foundation of identifying emotions and other bodily sensations. It is intertwined with alexithymia (identifying our own emotions) and how our emotions are represented in our sense and bodily sensations.

Sensory Processing Systems

Before exploring how humans create perception, and the role our expectations about the world play in creating all our diverse perceptions of reality, we first need to consider ways that the human sensory processing system works in registering and reacting to sensory information.

We all have our own unique sensory profile (Brown et al. 2001) made up of our own sensory preferences and patterns of responses and individual ways we experience and react to sensory information that influences how we create perception. How we experience sensory information can have a huge influence on how we feel. The three least known internal senses – proprioception, vestibular and interoception – can have a significant effect on how we feel. What alerts one person may exhaust another – for example, different sensory input can be experienced as alerting, helping us to feel more energized and able to concentrate. For some, going for a run or swimming in the sea can help them feel focused and alert, while sitting in a rocking chair, weight training at the gym or floating in warm water can help others feel relaxed. Other sensory input can have a combined effect to help someone feel more alert and focused but also calm and more grounded, for example, the strong smell of morning coffee, heavy work in the garden, dancing or using a swing.

Autistic sensory processing systems

Autistic people tend to have more diverse sensory profiles to neurotypical people, and in general experience more extremes of what is termed 'under'-responsivity and 'over'-responsivity to sensory stimuli (Ward 2019).

'Over'-responsivity to sensory stimuli, also called 'hypersensitivity', is when someone has an increased response to sensory information, and registers and reacts to sensory information more than most people (Brown, Tse and Fortune 2019). **'Under'-responsivity** to sensory stimuli, also called 'hyposensitivity', is when someone has reduced responses to sensory information, and registers or reacts to sensory information less than most people (Brown et al. 2019).

Sensory seeking or craving is when someone responds much more to a certain sensory stimulus that they find immensely enjoyable and like to experience over and over again. It can also be when someone craves certain sensory stimuli to use as a barrier to protect against other unpleasant sensory stimuli or as a tool to help them engage more and self-regulate (Dunn 2001). They may need a more intense level of this stimulus, and may need to experience it at a higher frequency.

Here are some examples of the many ways in which Autistic individuals can experience hypersensitivity, hyposensitivity and sensory seeking or using sensory stimulus to self-regulate in each sense. However, it is important to note that Autistic people have so many diverse sensory profiles, and what is experienced in a certain way for one person could be experienced in the complete opposite way for another.

Auditory hypersensitivity

- May have hyperacusis – an increased auditory capacity compared to neurotypical people. Hearing 'invisible' sounds that are more likely to be ignored and invisible to neurotypical people can be heard loudly by Autistic people, e.g., the buzz of electricity, the noise of a light bulb that needs to be changed, high-pitched sounds such as the sound of bats, the sound of a horn that is miles away, pen clicks from people in rooms that are on different floors, the noises of fridges in a store, the buzz of a computer fan over a video call, each little droplet of rain falling onto gravel, individual notes of music in a song.

- May experience misophonia – the experience of intense anger and disgust in response to sounds other people make, such as slurping and chewing noises from eating, breathing or swallowing sounds. The noise of rubbing fingers together or cracking knuckles, for example, can be experienced as agitating.

- What is considered a reasonable volume to neurotypicals can be extremely loud to Autistic people, for example, the sound of music playing in stores or the volume of a crowd of people chatting. These noises can be highly distracting, overwhelming, painful or immensely soothing for Autistic people, depending on their sensory profile.

Auditory hyposensitivity

- May not be aware of the volume.

- May shout or whisper when talking, and not be aware of volume of voice.

- May be hyposensitive, hearing sounds that are close sounding far away and muffled.

Auditory seeking/self-regulation

- May like to listen to the same song or line from an audio clip or may play a song repeatedly because they enjoy it like it's the first time every time, or find the familiarity of it soothing.

- May find it is easier to communicate with other people on the phone or through sending voice messages.

- Might like to work while listening to music or with the radio on in the background.

- May find that different music genres can have a significant influence on how they are feeling – they may listen to sombre music in order support them to process a sad emotion or energetic music to help them wake up in the morning.

During their assessment, some Autistic people might find using sounds or music helpful to explain their thoughts, or they may like to make stimming noises or use echolalia to remain self-regulated in sessions. Practitioners need to be actively welcoming and validating of these expressions in sessions. They should also be aware of background sounds that could be distracting or painful for Autistic clients in sessions.

Tactile hypersensitivity

- May experience light touches to be painful or akin to electric shocks.

- May recoil if someone tries to shake their hand, pat their shoulder or give them a hug.

- Clothes shopping may be a nightmare because different textured clothes feel scratchy and itchy.

- May cut the tags off their clothes or wear their socks inside out as the clothes tags or seams of socks feel painful, rubbing against their skin or feet throughout the day.

- May be very aware of temperature and overheat easily or feel the cold intensely.

- May be hypersensitive to pain or find uncomfortable sensations unbearable.

- Wetness or stickiness can feel unbearable, and things like wearing makeup or the experience of kissing and sharing saliva may be intolerable.

Tactile hyposensitivity

- May bump into things or other people without noticing.

- May have something on their face or hands, such as toothpaste, without noticing.

- May not be aware of another person touching them.

- May not feel the cold or the heat or have reduced sensitivity to pain.

Tactile seeking/self-regulation

- May crave certain textures that they seek out to enjoy feeling the pleasant texture over and over again.

- May hug a teddy bear, pet or animal, or find the purring vibration of a cat to be splendidly soothing.

- May engage in skin picking or hair pulling when stressed.

- May love the feeling of being squeezed or getting deep bear hugs.

- May like to bang their hand against surfaces or stamp their feet over and over to feel more alert or energized.

In an assessment setting an Autistic person might feel more comfortable if they can pace or rhythmically drum on a surface while talking or listening. Practitioners should consider the furnishing of an assessment space, and ensure that there are lots of soft non-scratching fabrics. For an online assessment, don't expect clients to be in a formal setting or present in a formal manner, but accept that they may be in their pyjamas, under a blanket, lying in bed, outside on the grass or have their pets with them.

Olfactory hypersensitivity

- May be able to smell foods or scents many others cannot.

- May perceive far away smells as being very close.

- May be hyperaware of the smell of perfume, washing detergent, cleaning products and cologne, and feel nauseous from such scents.

- Subtle scents to others may be experienced as overpowering and bring on headaches or migraines.

- May be very aware of own smell and over-wash.

- May experience flashbacks at times when smells connect to memories. This can be experienced as wonderful but may also be retraumatizing when smells are connected to past traumas.

Olfactory hyposensitivity

- May be 'nose blind' and unable to smell things that others can.

- May use lots of deodorant or perfume without realizing.

- May temporarily lose their ability to smell when overloaded.

- May be able to smell something but may not be able to locate where the smell is coming from.

- May not be able to tell what their body smells like and not be aware of when they need to wash.

Olfactory seeking/self-regulation

- May love certain smells so much that they can get lost in the joy of them and their entire mood can lift when they smell it, such as the smell of soil after it has rained or freshly cut grass.

- May carry essential oil or scent balls with them to smell when they are feeling distressed in order to self-soothe.

- In an assessment, some clients may enquire beforehand about smells that are likely to be in the environment so they can prepare or let others know of their smell sensitivity.

Practitioners should be aware of smells in the assessment space, and not wear overpowering perfume or light scented candles or diffusers before the session. Check any smell sensitivity with clients. Be aware of any lingering food smells, and ensure the space is aired out frequently.

Gustatory hypersensitivity

- May find mixing of tastes or strong tastes makes them gag.

- May prefer to eat plain food and use the same crockery and cutlery as different utensils make food taste different and can significantly alter the eating experience.

- May prefer to avoid new foods for fear of having a negative reaction.

- May separate different food textures and avoid mixed food as each texture and taste mixed together is too much and is uncomfortable to consume.

- May experience food that is considered mildly spicy to others as painful or with a long-lasting overpowering heat and frightening sensation of not being able to breathe.

- Might have a fear of the dentist and dread the feeling of someone poking around in their mouth. The taste and feeling of dentistry tools may be too much.

Gustatory hyposensitivity

- Might drink hot beverages too fast without noticing that their tongue is becoming burnt.

- May find it hard to taste anything and use copious amounts of salt or sauces to try get taste from food, or eat lots of textured or fizzy food to try to make up for the lack of taste.

Gustatory seeking/self-regulation

- May crave the taste of sour, sweet or spicy food and eat it in huge quantities until their mouth is raw or they have acid reflux in their stomach or become agitated.

- Might bite their nails and skin or chew on their hair.

In an assessment, clients might find it helpful to chew on something to focus or stay present.

Visual hypersensitivity

- May be bothered by clutter and messy or crowded environments.

- May find busy visual background information, such as views from windows, views while walking or other people moving, distracting.

- Eye contact may be experienced as too intense and overwhelming, or they may love to stare and get lost in another's eyes.

- May find bright colours such as clothes or environmental designs too visually intense.

- May be aware of flickering lights or dying light bulbs that others aren't detecting. Might find daytime too bright and prefer to do more during the night when it is dark.

- May find strong colours or bright florescent light unbearable.

- May find high-paced TV or action movies disorientating.

- May be an expert in spotting changes or putting together jigsaws.

Visual hyposensitivity

- May often lose things or put things down for a minute and then not be able to find them again among other items.

- May get headaches or have sleep disruptions from looking at too-bright screens for too long but without noticing.

- May experience outlines and perceive only pieces of the visual environment, and at times find it hard to see the whole picture.

- May find it hard to follow moving items.

- May find writing horizontally or without lines difficult.

- May find it hard to distinguish different colours or spelling errors in text.

Visual seeking/self-regulation

- May seek out dark environments such as a sensory room, with calming optic lights.

- May love to exercise in the night, looking up at the stars.

- May seek out and get lost looking at shadows flickering across the ground or tree branches blowing in the fields.

- May wear sunglasses or close their eyes in order to block out visuals and concentrate on what someone is saying.

A busy bus full of people, a waiting area with bright fluorescent lights or a space full of people may be experienced in pieces, with each flicker of the light and each moving limb experienced as unconnected parts leading to overload and experienced as overwhelming, with too much visual noise. This could mean that by the time the client gets into the practice, they may be too exhausted to properly proceed with the assessment. The option for clients to connect online or allow them to wait in a car or area of their choice rather than in a waiting room can help.

Practitioners should also be aware of the visual design of the assessment space and keep it clutter-free, but do include some pops of natural elements, such as plants, warm colours and adjustable lighting. Be aware of background stimulus or things happening outside the window.

Proprioception hypersensitivity

- May be very aware of their body position and find it hard to keep their posture when standing still.

- May find queuing or waiting in line difficult.

- May be hyperaware of changes to the weather – 'heavy' thundering weather can cause extreme fatigue, headaches and decreases in mood.

Proprioception hyposensitivity

- May not notice the force they are using – for example, they may break pencil nibs regularly or bang doors when closing or sit down heavily onto seats.

- Might have bruises but not know where they got them from.

- Might invade other people's personal space without realizing.

- Might find sports like running difficult and painful due to pressing too hard into the ground when they run, and causing injury without realizing.

- Might find it hard to do tasks that involve small fine motor skills, such as tying shoelaces or doing up buttons, or gross motor skills, such as putting on clothes or reaching for objects to be difficult.

- May shake or bounce their legs while sitting without noticing.

Proprioception seeking/self-regulation

- May love and seek proprioceptive activities such as lifting weights, floating on water or dancing.

- May relax by lying under a weighted blanket or wearing lots of tight layers.

In assessments, some may find going for a walk or moving around to be useful as the movement allows them to better express themselves; this proprioceptive input provides self-regulatory input. Others may need to pace while in the assessment space, or may prefer to sit on the ground with their back against a wall rather than sit on a chair. Offering clients the option to use Bluetooth or other free-moving headphones where they can walk freely and talk during an assessment can be very useful.

Vestibular hypersensitivity

- May be intensely aware of movement, and find moving fast or taking transport to be disorientating.

- May experience vertigo.

- May feel dizzy using a lift or escalator, or find heights terrifying.

- May find that being on a swing that can spin in a circle makes them feel nauseous, but if it only goes back and forth, providing linear vestibular input, it might feel incredibly calming and energizing. Others may experience this the other way around.

- May find going for walks with other people in places with lots of new views and unfamiliar landscape too exhausting and overloading. This may be because visual distractions and new surfaces make it too exhausting to talk to others or keep physical balance when moving. They may prefer to walk in a familiar place or walk small laps repeatedly.

Vestibular hyposensitivity

- May always be moving and find it hard to stay still.

- May shake their head or rock their body without noticing.

- May be able to spin in circles without ever getting dizzy.

Vestibular seeking/self-regulation

- May love heights or walking on uneven surfaces.

- May enjoy gymnastics or martial arts sports.

- May enjoy taking risks or be a thrill seeker – may crave the feeling of driving fast, skydiving or moving quickly.

In an assessment some may find sitting in a rocking chair or a swing seat to be soothing and grounding, and it may aid them in interaction.

Interoception hypersensitivity

- May be hyperaware of body sensations such as hunger or thirst, which can result in over-eating or over-drinking. Being hyperaware of their bladder can mean a person experiences repeated urinary tract infections from using the toilet often, even if their bladder is only slightly full.

- May be hypersensitive to pain or uncomfortable sensations such as tickling, which may be felt as pain.

- May be extra-cautious about being ill and have hyperawareness of psychosomatic symptoms such as stomach pains, which may indicate anxiety.

Interoception hyposensitivity

- Might find it difficult to notice and understand body signals, which can make it difficult to work out physically, such as recognizing hunger, fullness or thirst, the need to use the toilet, and identifying tiredness.

- May find it difficult to notice or understand emotional states or identify the build-up of distress.

- May be hyposensitive (reduced sensitivity) to pain and not realize when injured or ill, or find it hard to pinpoint signs of illness.

- May not realize they are dehydrated until they have a headache.

- May get upset but not know why.

- May have trouble recognizing psychosomatic symptoms such as stomach pains that are connected to anxiety.

Interoception seeking/self-regulation

- May enjoy fasting because they crave the feeling of hunger or thirst.

- May engage in high-energy exercise because they crave the feeling of their heart beating fast or fast breathing.

- May exercise a lot to keep getting the feeling of 'the burn' of their muscles.

In an assessment it is important for psychologists to be aware of interoception differences, particularly for clients who experience atypical eating or drinking habits. Explore interoception collaboratively with the client to see if this may make sense for the client as to why they may be experiencing such issues. However, psychologists should also be mindful that Autistic people may not be aware of this difference themselves, and the experience needs to be fully explored.

A Focus on Interoception

Interoceptive differences mean that many Autistic people find it challenging to recognize body signals intuitively. Not recognizing signs of thirst and hunger can mean going without fluids and adequate nutrition for long periods, with concomitant 'knock-on' effects of dehydration and low energy. These can, in turn, impact on mood, sensory sensitivity and increase the likelihood of overwhelm, meltdown or shutdown. This is a key area to examine during assessment as many Autistic people have described a 'light bulb' moment, realizing that interoceptive differences underpin issues with eating and drinking. It can equally be a 'light bulb' moment for neurotypical clinicians, or those without interoceptive differences, to realize that others do not intuitively recognize such signs of hunger and thirst.

Interoception involves **noticing** a body signal or sensation (e.g., butterflies in the stomach) and then **connecting** it to a meaning (e.g., feeling nervous). We can then do something to help us **regulate** (e.g., stimming, getting sleep, drinking water, etc.). Too often, (neurotypical) clinicians assume that because many of them can intuitively recognize body signals and the linked emotion, so can their Autistic clients. We know this is not the case for many Autistic people. Too often the starting part in therapy or other mental health support is on identifying a regulatory strategy (e.g., 'When you feel anxious, try X, Y or Z'), with an implicit message being given that if someone is unable to implement this, that they are 'not trying' or are 'wanting someone else to do the work'. Instead, the first piece needs to be exploring whether the person **can** identify body signals, and then link it to an emotion. Experiencing intense feelings or sensations within our bodies, but not understanding what they mean, can:

- Be frustrating, distressing and overwhelming.

- Make it hard to communicate what is going on for the person.

- Make it very difficult to know how to self-regulate.

Clinicians need to remember that recognizing body signals in a way that is different from how neurotypical people recognize body signals can be challenging when the world is designed in a way that does not consider that way, and having a different sense of body signals in a mismatched environment can make it challenging to respond to emotions, let alone identify and respond to them. Put simply, Autistic people need to know **what** they need help with **before** working out what might help.

Fluctuation in sensory processing systems

A person can experience 'under'-responsivity in one sense, but simultaneously experience 'over'-responsivity in another of their senses – they may be hypersensitive to auditory and hear everything, but be unaware of their body in space and bump into things. Their brain might feel empty, but they may taste every flavour. They might have hyposensitive vision in the morning where they only see outlines, or lights that once seemed bright the night before now seem dull.

Understanding hyposensitivity can show us how dysregulation doesn't always result from too much stimulus but can also come from when there is too little stimulus. Stimming can help regulate when somebody is feeling hypersensitive as well as when they are feeling hyposensitive, helping to arouse the nervous system and self-regulation. While stimming can be used to reduce the effects of too much sensory stimuli, it is also about keeping uncertainty in moderation and maintaining balance when there are not enough sensory stimuli.

There can be fluctuations between hypersensitivity and hyposensitivity (Bogdashina 2016). Autistic people's sensory profiles are not stagnant but can change depending on many factors (e.g., context, internal states, cognitive load, energy levels, etc.). On one day an Autistic person might experience 'under'-responsivity to sound, sounds might sound muffled and far away, or they may shout when talking without realizing, and then the next day they might react to sounds that were invisible to them the previous day and find it uncomfortable to hear people eating or that they need to wear ear plugs because the world now feels too loud. Or something might be experienced as too bright sometimes but dim and dull at other times. Donna Williams explains her experience of fluctuation between hyposensitivity and hypersensitivity as like being on a seesaw without any control (Williams 1996).

Sensory Processing and Communication Styles

Some Autistic people may experience visual or text-processing challenges in interactions and find text-based communication inaccessible. For others, words may all merge or letters may seem disconnected. It may be that reading doesn't lead to understanding, or text feels flat and dull and hard to connect with concepts. For some it may feel as if not enough sensory stimuli are available to engage with text content in a meaningful way. Text-based interactions, such as many forms of social media, are often experienced as frustrating or distressing. Watching TV may be experienced as dizzying or disorientating. Autistic people who experience text or visual-processing challenges may find it more accessible to engage with spoken content such as podcasts or music rather than blogs or videos. They might listen to audiobooks instead of reading books, or find it easier to interact through voice messages instead of text messages. They may find emails confusing to understand and prefer planned phone calls or voice messages. They may find it disorientating moving in busy environments and talking at the same time. For example, in The Adult Autism Practice, some clients find the online intake forms that require text-based responses to be daunting. Using voice-to-text or scheduling a phone or video call so they can tell the other person the answer and they can fill it in for them can help a lot.

In contrast, some Autistic people may sometimes experience audio-processing issues and might experience audio communication such as phone calls, voice messages or talking as draining, distressing and/or difficult. Sounds and tone might be distorted, voices may feel merged together, and words might become unrecognizable so they may prefer email or the written word. They may find it hard to talk to people offline and find it much easier to connect though text-based social media platforms. Some may find it easier to explain themselves by writing it down, and find online booking systems much more accessible than booking by phone. In The Adult Autism Practice, we have found a significant number of clients prefer to use text communication to engage with the assessment. Some have benefited from conducting the entire assessment this way, for example primarily through email.

Reflection Point

Much of the terminology used to talk about Autistic sensory processing comes from the stance of an ableist and biased perspective of neurotypical sensory processing being the 'gold standard', and anything diverging from this as being disordered. Terms such as 'over' or 'under'-responsive are not Neuro-Affirmative and are not based on some objective measure of reality and correct response but again, are judged against what is typical for neurotypicals. It makes little sense to say Autistic people are 'over'-responsive to auditory information when they can hear sounds that do exist but that neurotypicals cannot hear. This type of judgement lacks reason but regardless, it is a judgement that is often made when talking about sensory processing.

In reality, Autistic sensory systems are different. It is not that that Autistic people have too much or too little of a reaction, but that their responsivity to the sensory stimuli is different to neurotypicals because they have different brains and different perceptual mechanisms. It is not a sensory problem out of context. Yes, it can be a sensory problem because of how society and the environment is designed, but internal to the Autistic person it is not that they have a deficit or malfunctioning sensory system; they just have a different sensory system.

The Process of All-Human Perception

Humans create perception through predictive coding. This means that our perception of the world is based both on external information we perceive through our senses as well as predictions we make based on our individual experiences. Our brains combine these two sources of information to create perception (Friston 2018; Friston et al. 2017; Friston and Kiebel 2009; Schneebeli et al. 2022).

For example, when we hear a sound, there are two different inputs interacting to create our perception: (1) the sound we hear through our ears and (2) our individual predictions of what the noise will sound like based on our past experiences.

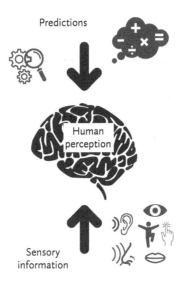

Another key part of human perception is prediction error. In every experience there is always some prediction error because no two situations are ever precisely the same (Friston and Kiebel 2009).

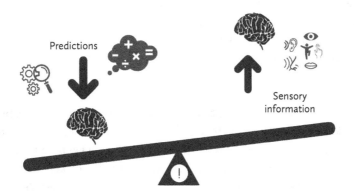

Prediction error is essential to our growth and development as it enables us to understand and learn. However, human brains do not cope well with surprise as too many prediction errors disrupt our equilibrium (Friston 2010).

Uncertainty and surprise are not inherently bad, and with support they can lead to human development, but prolonged exposure to uncertainty with no support can be damaging. The ability to self-regulate to reduce prediction error and to maintain balance is vital.

How predictive coding processes differ in Autistic neurology

One popular theory, within the Autistic community, suggests that the Autistic brain has a specific perpetual mechanism which is distinctively different to that of the neurotypical brain (van de Cruys et al. 2014).

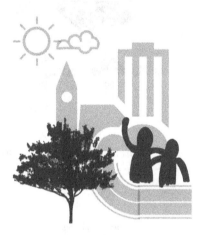

This can be easier to understand if we use an example of perceiving something in the environment, such as a tree. Both Autistic and neurotypical brains are likely to have a similar experience of the first perception of this tree. Both are likely to perceive the tree in a lot of detail. Subsequently, however, the experience for Autistic and neurotypical individuals differs significantly.

After the first viewing, a neurotypical person recognizes the tree, but are less likely to notice all of its details. Any surprises (prediction errors) that the neurotypical brain registers about the tree are likely to be judged as unimportant. Therefore, neurotypical people are more likely to have a generalized understanding of the world that incorporates less detail. Neurotypical people are much less likely to experience perceptual overload because their brain naturally ignores much of the uncertainty that exists in the world (van de Cruys et al. 2014).

Each time an Autistic person perceives a tree, they are likely to perceive it in all its detail. Even the smallest surprise (prediction error) is likely to be noticed and judged as important and relevant for learning. Each surprise is categorized as its own individual scene or whole new 'picture', which is perceived separately and as new in all its details. Therefore, Autistic people are more likely to have a more complex and rich understanding of the world that incorporates much more detail (van de Cruys et al. 2014).

Neurotypical people might feel like they process information faster and in a more automatic and effortless way, but consider that they are not perceiving as much information, that their brain is automatically ignoring a lot of information, while Autistic people perceive much more of the richness and details of the world. So it's not that Autistic people have slower processing, but rather that they process more, and that naturally takes longer.

Stimming and the role of the environment

One function of self-regulating actions such as stimming is that it provides controlled predictable feedback (van de Cruys et al. 2014). Stimming functions as an adaptive strategy to reduce prediction error in the same way that ignoring prediction error works for neurotypicals. Autistic individuals often seek out predictable environments with less likelihood of a bombardment of prediction error. However, in volatile environments, continuous exposure can lead to damaging sensory overload (van de Cruys et al. 2014).

Shutdowns

Prolonged exposure to volatile environments means Autistic people are vulnerable to experience shutdown (Bogdashina 2016). This is where somebody loses their ability to function. Shutdown is both physically and emotionally exhausting. It can happen in all the senses at once, or just some of them. For example, if an Autistic person experiences too much noise, then a coping mechanism in their brain might switch off the auditory sense. Or perhaps every other sensory channel will shut down to limit resources spent elsewhere. This is something an Autistic person can develop as a child – it can be seen as withdrawing into their own world to regain some sense of control. This may mean retreating away from sources of unpredictable stimuli (such as other people) for hours or even weeks to recharge after pushing Autistic sensory perception to its limits.

A downloadable deep dive into Autistic perception is available at https://uk.jkp.com/catalogue/book/9781839971662 – here you will find a more in-depth exploration of the predictive coding process of human perception, the critical role of stimming in maintaining homeostasis, the consequences of perception overload and the role of the default Autistic cognitive style.

Research

Research into Autistic sensory perception has found that throughout lifelong Autistic development there can be a variety of influences across different adult milestones and life events that present with unique sensory experiences. For example, thematic analysis found that barriers in relationships include different experiences of sexual activity due to sensory perception (Barnett and Maticka-Tyndale 2015).

A Swedish study exploring Autistic sexual expression and relationships found that there was a qualitative difference in sensory perception in relation to Autistic compared to neurotypical sexual difference. It found that Autistic people often experience physical pleasure differently, and also that tactile sensitivity could be an issue in experiencing physical pleasure. It was noted that with awareness and the right strategies, many of these things can be adapted for (Bertilsdotter Rosqvist 2014).

Other research exploring Autistic perspectives about the impact of sensory perception and sexuality and relationships found that a combination of sensory sensitivity (heightened awareness and experience of sensory stimuli) and sensory seeking (actively seeking out stimulating and pleasurable sensory stimuli) across the senses had an impact on such experiences, and a lack of awareness or a mismatch between sensory needs and preferences could prove challenging (Gray, Kirby and Graham Holmes 2021).

Gender, Sexual and Relationship Diversities (GSRD)

Research in the area of sexual expression is sparse, and our experience in practice at Thriving Autistic has aligned with some of the findings of the literature, in that Autistic people can experience sexual arousal and enjoyment in a qualitatively different manner from non-autistic people. Scantling and Browder (1993) wrote *Ordinary Women, Extraordinary Sex,* which introduced the concept of peak experiences in sexual activity. These were moments when the woman entered a 'flow state' and became completely absorbed in the sensations and experienced a profound sense of joy and fulfilment. Given that Autistic people appear to more easily enter flow states, we can perhaps appreciate the possibility that the right combination of sensory stimuli for the individuals engaged in sexual activity may contribute to heightened positive sexual experiences for some.

Another significant developmental event where sensory perception and sensory sensitivities can have a specific influence is during pregnancy, although there is limited research into Autistic experience of pregnancy and parenthood. One reason is that many Autistic parents are identified as being Autistic only after their children are diagnosed and they recognize similarities in themselves, meaning that many remain undiagnosed throughout pregnancy and early parenthood. A small thematic analysis by Talcer, Duffy and Pedlow (2021) into the experiences of Autistic mothers found that in the antenatal stage of pregnancy, all participants reported an increase in their sensory sensitivity, and in some cases, some of the Autistic mothers felt that after the birth of their child this did not go back to their prior baseline level of sensory perception. One mother described the feeling of her child moving inside her as feeling sensorily unbearable. Autistic mothers also reported experiencing what they described as a different level of sickness throughout their pregnancy compared to neurotypical mothers they knew, and felt that it was hard for other people to understand as the neurotypical mothers weren't able to detect the same level of sensory stimuli as the Autistic mothers. In terms of giving birth, some felt they were able to prepare and ask for sensory adjustments to be made while others felt that the doctors didn't take them seriously or that they couldn't understand their perception. They felt that their requests for physical sensory environment changes impacted their experience and they had insufficient pain management. Others also reported that they found planned caesarean sections and having consistent staff to be particularly helpful, as this provided predictability (Talcer et al. 2021).

It is important to note that as there appears to be a significant overlap between gender variance and neurodivergence, pregnant Autistic people may have additional barriers accessing appropriate and respectful healthcare during the perinatal period. At Thriving Autistic, our experience shows that consistency and predictability is key, alongside a psychologically safe, sensory-adapted environment. Individual preferences must be explored and respected. For some pregnant people, the predictability of a scheduled caesarean section will have beneficial consequences; for others, home birth with a midwife who has developed a relationship with the pregnant person and is able to offer consistent care in their own environment will be the most appropriate avenue. A sensory-adapted environment for perinatal medical appointments can offer pregnant people the equitable access to healthcare they need, and potentially transform their entire experience entering parenthood.

Birth Trauma

Autistic mothers and pregnant people may go through pregnancy and labour not yet having discovered that they are Autistic. Without this self-knowledge, it is challenging to identify, communicate and receive the support needed during this time. Coupled with the stressors of the sensory environment, this can make it extremely challenging to advocate for one's needs at such a vulnerable time, leaving Autistic birthing people unheard and not taken seriously when expressing concerns or describing their birth experience. Even with knowledge that someone is Autistic, delivery can be a traumatic experience. Coupled with the increased likelihood of hypermobility and different responses to anaesthetic, there exists the melting pot of potential for a traumatic birth or postpartum experience. Clinicians need to be mindful of this and pay this due regard. One option for low-risk birthing people is home birth with a qualified midwife. Home birth offers the opportunity for the person to be in their own surroundings, in an environment that is suited to their sensory needs, and the intimate, 1-1 care provided by a midwife over the entire course of the pregnancy and postpartum period can be liberating for an Autistic person. They can specify clearly in advance what their needs and wishes are, they can develop a plan with their midwife for what will happen in the various scenarios, and be prepared for hospital transfer if necessary. If a hospital transfer is required, they can have prepared a sensory toolkit to bring with them and have an advocate to communicate on their behalf if necessary. Providing the Autistic birthing person with as much control and power in decision-making as possible is paramount.

In terms of the experiences of being a mother, one study found that a significant number of their participants showed an increase in auditory and tactile hypersensitivity, which had a negative impact on stress – for example babies crying and children making a noise was felt by some as excruciating. Some of the mothers explained issues with touch and tactile hypersensitivity; they explained how being a mother involved a lot of tactile input and how this could be incredibly overloading. One mother described it as if she was torn because she loved her child, but all of the affection just felt too much like a painful fullness, like her skin was going to burst. Breastfeeding was also noted for those who had tactile hypersensitivity as being painful and overloading (Talcer et al. 2021). Participants in Talcer et al.'s (2021) study reported strategies they used to attend to the competing needs of their sensory systems. One Autistic mother reported that she used the same strategies that calmed her children down to also calm herself down; others reduced lighting by adding lamps and keeping bright overhead lights off; while others engaged in exercise and stretches to increase relaxation. Participants reported that time in solitude recharged and recouped their sensory systems. Barriers to achieving this restorative time alone were also expressed (demands of parenting, lack of understanding from others, etc.).

Participants in Talcer et al.'s (2021) study reported that peer support from other Autistic mothers was the most helpful, as they did not feel judged and had a shared experience. Many reported barriers to seeking help included concerns about judgement on their parenting abilities and about receiving a misdiagnosis. Most of the participants wanted something like a face-to-face Autistic mothers' group, but found it very difficult to access anything like this. All of the participants in Talcer et al.'s (2021) study were undiagnosed at the time of giving birth, and while many of the Autistic mothers found that being diagnosed later in life felt odd, they all felt that it was also a really significant and crucial part in understanding their authentic self and how they experienced the world. They reported that having a diagnosis meant that they could stop trying to fit into the neurotypical way of being, and were instead able to embrace their sensory differences and felt more open to talk about them. Similarly, participants explained how getting a diagnosis and building that understanding of their sensory perception and sensory needs allowed them to begin to stop masking and to figure out who their authentic self was (Talcer et al. 2021).

It's important to note that only the negative sensory experiences of parenthood have been investigated thus far, and in our experience with clients at Thriving Autistic, as well as the experiences of the Autistic authors of this book who are parents, the research outlined here portrays only a very limited glimpse into the nuanced sensory experience of pregnancy, birth and parenthood. The sheer sensory joy of the smell of our babies' heads as we snuggle them down for a feed, the overwhelming rush of love that flows from the sense of connection during skin-to-skin contact and the weight of their bodies as we carry them close to us are hugely regulating, joyful and positive experiences. While there are, of course, times that the sensory experience of parenting, particularly in the early years, provides many challenges to navigate, there are also many opportunities to experience sensory joy and deep connection.

While research overall into Autistic later years life is limited, there have been some studies that identified factors in later years Autistic life relating to sensory perception. Studies exploring the use of assistive technology (AT) in later life have found that technology that allows someone to manage the sensory environment is particularly important to older Autistic adults. Sensory-specific AT includes noise-reduction earphones, smart lighting, control over audio environments and hearing aids (Zheng et al. 2021). In a report by Crompton et al. (2020c), 10 topics were identified as being important for residential care for older Autistic adults. One was sensory sensitivities and considerations relating to the sensory environment. Crompton et al. (2020c) noted that visual and auditory age-related changes, and also postmenopausal changes, are likely to affect Autistic sensory systems, and that a residential care setting needs to be designed to be controllable and adaptable for each Autistic individual. They suggest including a reduction in smells, lights and visual information as well as auditory information from other people, but also from equipment and the proprioceptive barriers of furniture. They note the importance of increasing sensory stimuli that is soothing and regulating, such as soft lighting, deep pressure aids and weighted blankets, and also the importance for increased awareness of the effect of the design of the environment on Autistic older people, and for suitable accommodations and accessibility to be made (Crompton et al. 2020c).

Sensory Integration

'Sensory integration' is used to refer to the processing, integration and organization of sensory information for the body and the environment. 'Sensory integration' and 'sensory processing' both refer to brain processes that take the information provided by our different senses, and play a role in making sense of that information and in influencing our responses. Dr Jean Ayres first described the concept of sensory integration in the 1970s, defining it as the 'neurological process that organizes sensation from one's own body and from the environment and makes it possible to use the body effectively within the environment' (Ayres 1972, p.11).

Sensory integration therapy is a specific approach to supporting people with sensory processing differences and it can be used in conjunction with the sensory profile tool to help individuals understand their own sensory system and make adaptions to their environment and routine to help them get the best from their sensory environment. The sensory profile highlights each individual's pattern of sensory processing, and ways in which they respond and notice sensory information (actively avoiding, passively sensing, actively seeking or passively low registration) (Dunn 2001).

Sensory integration therapy can involve activities such as developing a 'sensory diet', learning new ways to self-regulate, movement and balance activities, and exploring adaptions that can be made to an individual's sensory environment and daily routine.[1]

Sensory integration therapy has been criticized for its deficit-based language and its promotion of 'adaptive responses' to sensory information. However, Spielmann (2021) outlined how it can be delivered through a Neuro-Affirmative lens, ensuring that practitioners dismantle ableist assumptions and listen to the voice of the person with whom they are working. Spielmann (2021) explains that sensory integration therapy **should** be delivered through the therapeutic relationship, forming a respectful relationship with the person in a way that allows them to self-actualize and honour their spirit.

Our recommendation is that anyone considering sensory integration therapy (or indeed, any therapy) should first ask a series of questions of their provider to assure themselves that the provider is fully trained and that their ethos is aligned with the Neuro-Affirmative approach, as outlined in this book.

Practice-Based Recommendations

- Explore and consider each client's unique sensory perception and adapt the environments of the assessment (including the information given before, waiting room options and information provided after assessment) to be as accessible as possible to each client's sensory perception of the world.

- Conduct a sensory audit of the assessment space (including if this is an online space) to identify environmental sensory barriers in your environment as well as elements that need new design and elements that can be adapted to be accessible.

- Having elements in the environment that can be controlled and adapted, such as smart lighting, curtains, temperature control, space to move around, the option of sitting in a rocking chair or on bean bags, or even the option to do the assessment while going for a walk instead of having to sit down, can be useful in creating a space that can be altered for a diversity of sensory perceptions.

---

1   www.sensoryintegrationeducation.com

- It is important that you consider the client's sensory perception throughout the assessment journey, including getting to the assessment and in the waiting room for in-person assessments. Have an accessible waiting area with low lightening, reduced sensory input such as switching off televisions, comfortable sensory seating options, such as rocking chairs and swivel chairs, as well as sturdy, solid chairs, making sure your waiting space is an inclusive space where clients feel comfortable to get up and move around, where they can feel comfortable to wear hats or sunglasses inside or use ear defenders or headphones.

- Providing clients with information prior to arriving can also help. This can include pictures of the waiting area and assessment space, and letting the client know who they will need to interact with before the assessment (such as how the admin will work, the receptionist, etc.).

- Having appointments on time is important, but in unavoidable situations, if services tend to run late, it is good to let the client know this so that they can be prepared.

- Conduct a sensory audit of your assessment space. You can use a free tool such as the BBC environmental checklist.[2] It helps to get the input of an Autistic professional to oversee the audit as they are likely to notice stimuli that a neurotypical professional may not.

- In an online space, reduce the clutter on your screen background, make sure you test your microphone and the acoustics of your environment before a meeting (e.g., turn on the background noise reduction in your settings), and regularly change light bulbs and check to make sure there is no flickering in the background.

- Creating accessible online spaces where a client's communication needs are respected and they feel comfortable and know they have the option to turn off their camera or use the text box, to close their eyes when talking or to move around, or not feel they must look at the screen, can be beneficial in making the online sensory environment accessible.

- It is important to note that creating an accessible sensory environment is not all about reducing sensory stimuli, but is much more about balance, and having available pleasant and useful stimuli that is tailored to each individual, such as natural lights, plants, pops of pastel colour, textures that are

---

2   https://bbc.github.io/uxd-cognitive

available to touch but that can also be avoided, space to stim, colour lights or visuals that can be turned off.

- The element of control is important here. An environment entirely void of any sensory stimuli can be just as overloading and uncertain as one that is bombarded with sensory stimuli.

- Change and adapt the environment, not the Autistic person.

- It's not all about reducing – too little sensory stimuli can be just as overloading as too much sensory stimuli. It's about balance. And each individual has their own balance and their own sensory profile. In sensory design it is important to have a balance that includes a reduction of distressing stimuli and an increase of pleasurable and soothing stimuli, which can be adaptable for individual clients' needs.

To be truly Neuro-Affirmative we need to actively work to make this world accessible; we need to step toward each other and work collaboratively to make a world that is inclusive for all, for all life's neurodiversity. From challenge with support comes growth, but threat divides and adds barriers. Today, there is still too much threat for Autistic people to continue down this route where the neurotypical society and the neurotypical professional community continue to ignore the noise that difference makes by explaining it away with the belief that there is one normal and one 'gold standard' neurotypical way to experience the world. Continuing to do this leads to too much suffering and distress. With collaboration we can support each other's communities to truly embrace human diversity and celebrate difference, and act to acknowledge, embrace, accept, design and adapt for neurodiversity without being swayed by a want to reduce uncertainty by ignoring it.

7

What Does It Mean to Be Neuro-Affirmative?

Introduction

First off, it's important to be aware that there is a distinction between neurodiversity as a neutral descriptor, the neurodiversity movement and the neurodiversity paradigm.

The word **neurodiversity** by itself is a neutral term, coined by Judy Singer, that refers to the vast variety of human brain types, how brains are structured, how they perceive a reality, process information and interact in the world. This is the same as how biodiversity refers to the biological variety and variability of every living thing on earth. **All** brains, including neurotypical brains, are considered to be part of neurodiversity.

People whose brains are considered **different to the majority** are considered 'neurodivergent' (a term coined by Autistic activist Kassiane Asasumasu). Included in this neurodivergent umbrella are, for example, autism, Dyspraxia, Dyslexia and ADHD. The broadest conceptualization of neurodivergence includes **all** brains different from neurotypical brains, including people with cluster headaches, acquired brain injury, post-traumatic stress, depression, Tourette's and OCD.

Neurodivergent people have always been part of the fabric of our society, and are now mobilizing as communities to raise awareness of Autistic people as a **minority group** and claim the equal rights owed to them. This is termed the **neurodiversity movement**, which is a growing human rights, disability and social movement aligned with and part of the broader disability rights movement. It was started by Autistic advocates (many of whom have additional, quite significant, support needs).

Key goals of the neurodiversity movement specific to Autistic advocacy (adapted from Bettin 2022) include:

- Appreciation of Autistic ways of being as equally valid to non-autistic ways of being.

- For the Autistic neurology to no longer be described and constructed as a pathology.

- For non-autistic people to receive education about Autistic people, including how they can communicate with their Autistic peers.

- For the Autistic community to be recognized as a minority group.

- The creation of Autistic-led organizations, events, conferences, social networks, etc., which allow Autistic people to collaborate and socialize on their own terms.

The **neurodiversity paradigm** is the philosophy behind the neurodiversity movement. One of the most important messages arising from this paradigm is that all neurotypes are equally valid, that no Autistic or otherwise neurodivergent person needs to spend their lives attempting to conform to a neurotypical standard based on the faulty premise of a normative agenda. There is no **one way** of being in this world.

Here are some key takeaway points of the neurodiversity paradigm, **as it relates specifically to Autistic experience**:

- Humans are a neurodiverse population. Neurodiversity, like biodiversity, is a wonderful and integral aspect of life. There is immense benefit and beauty in diversity itself.

- Autistic people are not broken versions of neurotypical people. The Autistic neurotype is as equally valid as any other neurotype, including a neurotypical one.

- Subcategorization of the Autistic community (e.g., through 'levels' or subcategories of Autistic people) is detrimental, simplistic and unhelpful in relation to understanding the Autistic experience. It also divides the community unnecessarily, and erases the difficulties that some Autistic people experience and the strengths that other Autistic people may experience.

- Autistic people **are** disabled not by being Autistic, but by living in a world that is designed primarily for neurotypical people.

- Neurotypical people have historically not understood Autistic developmental trajectories, needs, communication styles, perceptions and experiences, or taken action to meet them. This has been, and continues to be, disabling.

- All humans, regardless of their neurotype, support needs, communication style or independence levels have the right to autonomy and the same human rights as everyone else.

- Autistic people (like all minority groups) have the right to make decisions for themselves and their community in relation to how they are spoken about, treated and supported.

- The neurodiversity movement is deeply concerned that a focus on a cause, cure or prevention for Autistic people, or certain Autistic features, will lead to eugenics. These concerns are real – for example, prenatal testing has halved the number of babies born with Down syndrome in Europe (de Graaf et al. 2020). Research priorities need to be defined by the Autistic community, and the community majority wants a focus on research to help Autistic people thrive as they are. This means that the focus of funding for therapy, support or research in relation to the Autistic community (for children and adults) should focus on Autistic people exploring, developing and thriving through their authentic Autistic selves while also accessing support to navigate environmental barriers and co-occurring challenges that they want support with (e.g., misophonia and Ehlers-Danlos syndrome).

Ways to Be Neuro-Affirmative

1. Reframe autism from a disorder to a neurotype

A vital and essential part of being truly Neuro-Affirmative is to reframe the Autistic experience as a disorder (which is how many of us have traditionally been taught to understand and categorize it) to a different, valid **neurotype** with a distinct Autistic developmental trajectory.

As a neurotype within the greater tapestry of neurodiversity, it is a naturally occurring brain difference that leads to a different way of experiencing the world. Being Autistic is also a culture, an identity, and as a group, Autistic people are a minority.

2. Don't pathologize Autistic ways of being

Current autism assessment procedures and tests are at their core ableist and based on the pathologization of Autistic ways of being. Their goal is to measure how the person is failing as a neurotypical person, and just how significant these perceived deficits are.

So, for example, the ability and desire to engage in back-and-forth, spoken word, social chit-chat is held up as a 'gold standard' and 'normal' way to interact, while a dislike of social chit-chat and a preference to speak about one topic for an extended period of time about matters of great importance to the person is considered a problem, deficit or symptom. Within the Autistic community (and for many non-autistic people) communicating at length on one topic is a perfectly valid and valued method of communication, and has made for many an Autistic podcaster, professor, lecturer, teacher or friend. For the dominant group (i.e., neurotypical people) to judge that this way of expressing yourself is unacceptable and 'disordered' is itself unacceptable, prejudiced and judgemental.

3. Use supports and follow recommendations that target Autistic people's needs and challenges and not their Autistic ways of being

Being truly Neuro-Affirmative means not pathologizing Autistic ways of being (e.g., stimming, Autistic developmental trajectory, ways of learning about the world) or communicating (e.g., differences in eye contact or monologuing). Leading on from this, follow-up supports for Autistic people (including therapy and report recommendations) should never focus on changing or 'treating' the person's neurotype, but should instead focus on what that particular person actually wants support with, such as their mental health, validating their authentic ways of communicating, help with building sensory self-awareness and adapting the environment to suit their sensory perception, or help educating their workplace or family about more modern ways of understanding the Autistic experience.

4. The Autistic voice should be at the centre of everything you do

The Autistic voice being at the centre of everything you do is a non-negotiable aspect of being truly Neuro-Affirmative. This does not mean a tokenistic 'listening to', because being 'listened to' implies a power dynamic of the dominant group making the magnanimous choice to listen to the group with no power and then carrying on as before. It means the Autistic community having the agency and power to choose for themselves how their Autistic experience is explored, understood, assessed for and supported.

One example of putting the Autistic voice at the centre of everything you do is to use (and encourage others to use) the language of choice of the community when talking about autism. If you are a professional currently undertaking autism assessments (for adults or children) and you are not aware of the Autistic community's voice, culture, recent Autistic-led research and publications and the community priorities for future research and support, then you are not serving the population you are being paid to serve. In addition, as you will see throughout this book, it is not possible to undertake a truly Neuro-Affirmative, best practice autism assessment without understanding the Autistic experience and Autistic identity as told by Autistic people.

5. Respect Autistic culture and identity

This involves professionals putting effort into being aware of, researching and making their best efforts to understand a constantly growing and shifting Autistic culture and identity. The idea that there even exists an Autistic culture, communication and identity is very new to the vast majority of professionals working with Autistic people.

Some examples of this culture include the symbols that the Autistic community choose to identify with (e.g., many like a gold infinity symbol) and the ones they firmly reject and consider insulting in their use (the puzzle piece and the colour blue to represent them). Other examples of respect include using the language preferences of choice of the community and embracing Autistic ways of communicating (e.g., a preference for honesty and a dislike of superficial chit-chat) and Autistic play (e.g., lining up and categorizing, although Autistic play can also, of course, be highly imaginative). It involves recognizing that Autistic people have distinct ways of exploring and learning about the world. It also involves Autistic memes, humour and jokes. The only way to become and keep up to date with any of these is by listening to Autistic people.

6. If you have the power, employ Autistic and otherwise neurodivergent team members; if you don't have the power, advocate others to do so

■ **Important note:** It is vital to highlight here that Autistic people are employers and leaders too, and so this call to action is for all people regardless of their neurotype. For example, Thriving Autistic is led by Autistic people, as well as employing many other Autistic people.

Being Neuro-Affirmative does not just mean changing your language to be more respectful of the neurodiversity paradigm while keeping all else the same; it means making systemic changes across workplaces, healthcare systems, communities, and society, so that Autistic and otherwise neurodivergent people have the equal rights they deserve. For this to come about, there need to be community allies as well as advocates. Outside of being a basic human right to have a voice and a place at the table regarding what is about them, diversifying teams in this way leads to better care and support to the Autistic clients you are aiming to support. The Adult Autism Practice would not be the team it is today without our Autistic team members patiently helping the neurotypical team members to grow and learn, and they have revolutionized how the team understand the Autistic experience and how we conduct our assessments, leading to the overwhelmingly positive experience our clients report. Learning and growing from collaborative teams benefits **all** members of the team.

7. Recognize that there is immense value in diversity

This means recognizing the inherent value in diversity in and of itself. For example, we have seen the significant negative impact that a reduction of biodiversity can cause to our planet and ecosystems. As with biodiversity, all humans are part of a tapestry of neurodiversity, and we are all connected to each other. We need all kinds of people and minds in order to flourish as worldwide societies. Being Neuro-Affirmative is to see and celebrate the value of this diversity.

8. Recognize that there is value in living a disabled life

To see the value in disability and living a disabled life necessitates becoming aware of just how tied our views on disability are to capitalist ideals of being 'productive' (i.e., making money for yourself so that you don't cost the system money) and independent (i.e., needing no outside help or support so that you don't cost the system money). It also necessitates examining the feelings of shame associated with being disabled, and unpacking what external factors are causing these feelings.

All humans have intrinsic value regardless of how much it costs to care for them or how much money they can make through their productivity. Many disabled (including Autistic) people **will** need ongoing support from others throughout their life and may never have a paid job, but this does not mean that they cannot or should not live a meaningful life that has value. There are, for example, democratic socialist countries in which the care economy is healthy and well-funded, and disabled people are supported to be integral members of their communities without being seen as a burden.

Seeing the value in disability and a disabled life requires ongoing reflection and unpacking of ableism for those who are not disabled and internalized ableism for Autistic or otherwise neurodivergent or disabled professionals. It means all of us challenging the many views and assumptions that we collectively hold and that we have learned over a lifetime of both implicit and explicit messaging that exist from the people and societal structures around us. In order to change these external messages and forces, we need first to reflect and change ourselves.

It also includes changing our definition of what 'being productive' means and broadening this from only producing something of monetary or other value to society to include production of something of value to that individual person, or the production of calm, joy or connection with life.

Disability is not a 'dirty' word (and if you feel it is, then this is an indicator that you have some internal unpacking to do in these areas). People should be free to choose to declare themselves disabled, receive the supports they need, and not be shamed or be reacted to negatively for doing so, either from individuals or societal structures.

9. All neurodivergent people (including those with significant intellectual disability and high support needs) have power, a place at the table, and are supported and advocated for

Being Neuro-Affirmative means that **all** neurodivergent people, no matter how high their support needs are, or how they communicate, have an equal voice and agency in relation to their own lives and communities. The neurodiversity movement was born out of the wider disability movement and has always (and continues to) encompassed, embraced and advocated for the voices of **all** disabled people.

Traditionally, little effort has been made by researchers or clinicians within healthcare systems to access the voice of Non-Speaking or sometimes Non-Speaking Autistic people, with or without an intellectual disability. But it **is** possible to capture these voices. There is a large online community of Non-Speaking or minimally speaking Autistic adults (with and without an intellectual disability) who interact online on Twitter, other social media platforms and safe online spaces. They often speak out there about what is important to them, how they want to be spoken about, their priorities for research, and how they want their care to be managed. These voices need to be listened to and taken seriously in terms of service planning and supports.

10. Reject behaviour-based compliance approaches (e.g., Applied Behaviour Analysis)

Behaviour-based compliance approaches are fully rejected by the Autistic community and the neurodiversity paradigm, with comparisons being drawn between them and gay conversion therapy. This is because (despite some recent reported industry changes and a great many kind and well-intentioned practitioners) ultimately the end goal of true ABA is an Autistic child and adult who is indistinguishable from their neurotypical peers, who looks and sounds like a neurotypical child. And the methods to get to this point are based on compliance. Behaviour-based compliance approaches have significant, negative, long-term effects on people's mental health. They are counter-intuitive to a human rights model emphasizing the vital importance of self-advocacy and self-determination. Besides this, the fact alone that the Autistic community rejects them should be enough (see point 1). There are newer versions of ABA, for example, which claim to be different, but if a method is based on compliance through behavioural means, it is not Neuro-Affirmative.

11. Reject neurotypical social skills training

Neurotypical social skills training is also fully rejected by the Autistic community and neurodiversity paradigm, where again, legitimate comparisons to the practice to gay conversion therapy are made. Like ABA, neurotypical social skills training encourages neurodivergent people to hide their true selves (which decades of psychological research has shown us is a core element of positive mental health), and instead promotes masking and the presentation of an inauthentic self. It leads to internalized feelings of shame and ableism, and the person's core ways of being and interacting are presented as something to hide and change.

Besides being disrespectful and pathologizing of Autistic ways of being, and the large body of research indicating that neurotypical social skills training is ineffective anyway, there is a growing body of research showing links between masking or camouflaging (which is what neurotypical social skills training promotes) and poor mental health, self-harm and suicide. Neurotypical social skills training is a barrier to connection, and increases loneliness and isolation. It prevents full exploration and development in the world as the person's authentic self is not able to explore, discover or grow, but is instead kept hidden away. It leads to feelings of rejection, hurt and devaluation. A similar body of research can be found for the LGBTQIA+ community related to levels of masking of authentic sexuality and gender.

This is not to say that neurotypical social skills training never achieves its goals. In the past left-handedness was looked on as inherently 'wrong' and outside the norm, and left-handed children were forced (with much discomfort and shame) to write with their right hand. But while these people may have learned to write with their right hand, they were still inherently left-handed people, and at what cost did they learn to write this way?

Neurotypical social skills training does not take into account up-to-date ways of understanding Autistic communication, such as the double empathy problem. Communication and social interactions are complex and involve more than one person. While Autistic people communicate and interact in different ways to neurotypical people, research indicates that Autistic people understand, communicate and socialize just fine with other Autistic people. So we need to ask ourselves, where does the problem lie? The answer is in the interaction between the two groups. As communication has been shown to be bi-directional, responsibility lies with both parties in a communication interchange. The emphasis should be on **both** Autistic and neurotypical people developing an understanding as to how the other experiences the world and interacts, and both groups working to find ways to best interact with **each other**.

Therefore, the onus should not be just on the Autistic person to change their interaction and communication style, but instead there needs to be a joint effort. Neurotypical people need to learn about Autistic ways of communicating, and Autistic people need to learn about neurotypical ways of communicating. A new middle ground needs to be created where a new way of communicating is developed that incorporates and allows room for all styles of communication, with neither fundamentally changing for the other. There needs to be a mutual respect for the diversity of communication between humans.

12. Advocate for systems and environmental changes

Some of the biggest barriers right now for the Autistic community in relation to a good quality of life and mental health are the systematic, cultural and environmental factors that have led to Autistic people being misunderstood, misdiagnosed, mischaracterized, rejected and not listened to as a group.

Professionals wanting to make positive changes for their Autistic clients will need to move beyond just assessment, diagnosis and individual therapy, and also engage in the more wide-reaching work of combating systemic ableism by advocating for change within the systems around their clients. This means (if you are not Autistic yourself) learning to be a true ally, and using your privileged position to stand with Autistic people in helping to change these systems.

As professionals (whether we are Autistic, otherwise neurodivergent or neurotypical), we all need to make sure we are upholding the disability rallying cry of 'Nothing About Us Without Us'. Here are a few practical ways you can do this:

- If you see a conference that involves autism in any way, make sure that there is a significant percentage of Autistic people presenting and involved in its aims and goals. If this is not clear, contact the organizers to ask.

- If you are neurotypical and asked to present about Autistic people at an event, ensure that you have Autistic colleagues also presenting with you. Or even better, do you have an Autistic colleague who may know the topic better and do a better job?

- If you are supporting or recommending an organization or charity claiming to support Autistic people, first check: how many board members are Autistic? No Autistic board members is a huge red flag for any non-profit organization claiming to support Autistic people. Investigate their goals and aims, and whether they align with the Autistic community. What does the Autistic community feel about this organization, and do they believe they align with them? If you believe the organization is not truly Neuro-Affirmative, send your support elsewhere and encourage others to do so also.

- When evaluating research or academic articles, check to make sure that Autistic people are involved, and their voices heard, from the outset. Are the research goals aligned with community priorities? If it is a piece of research, were there Autistic people on the steering committee (for example), or did the research use scales and materials designed with Autistic people and validated with Autistic populations? If it is an article about the Autistic experience, were Autistic people interviewed and given prominence in the article? If these factors are not present, this is not a high-quality piece of research in relation to the Autistic experience.

- If you are reading a policy related to Autistic people, check if Autistic people were involved in developing it. If it is not clear, contact the developers of the policy to ask. Without Autistic involvement, the decision-making of policy documents related to Autistic people is inherently prejudiced.

The more that professionals advocate and look for these factors, the greater and quicker the organizational and societal changes will be for Autistic people.

13. Fostering a positive Autistic identity is a priority goal

Fostering a positive Autistic identity in your clients should be the number one goal for all professionals working in this area. Support clients to have pride in their culture, value their own personal communication style and recognize and increase their own personal strengths. Help clients to promote their own self-autonomy and self-advocacy. Perhaps most important of all, link them in with Autistic peers and community. Help them to understand what it means to be Neuro-Affirmative alongside an in-depth understanding of the social model of disability, identifying **for them** what the components of a good and valuable life are, and how they can advocate for these things. Support them in understanding the importance of environmental fit to their overall wellbeing.

8

Current Adult Autism Assessment Guidelines

Introduction

Within any healthcare setting, best practice guidelines are extremely important in terms of maintaining a safe and helpful experience for all. They help to ensure consistency in approach, an efficient use of resources, and that the best possible outcome is achieved for people who are accessing the service. They outline information about a standard of care that needs to be provided, and they support clinicians and services in making decisions about and being confident in the service they deliver, while helping to identify service gaps. For people accessing a service, best practice guidelines offer information about what a person should be receiving from a service and empower people in making informed decisions.

However, while best practice guidelines are important and helpful, there are also potential limitations that need to be considered. Of primary concern, guidelines can rapidly become out of date as new information and research comes to light. They require regular review and updating in order to be effective. Guidelines that are out of date can inadvertently promote at best ineffective services and at worst harmful practice. Furthermore, guidelines that are particularly restrictive can make it very difficult for services to tailor an approach to match the specific needs of a person accessing the service.

Best practice guidelines for autism assessments with adults vary across countries and jurisdictions, and many countries do not presently have any best practice guidelines for assessments with adults. In some countries there are only guidelines for assessment with children, with no consideration given to the assessment process for adults. As a professional, it is important to be aware of the guidelines that are referred to in your locality, and to consider whether they are up to date and in line with current research and knowledge in relation to Autistic adult experiences.

American and Canadian Guidelines

At present, it appears that there are no specific guidelines for autism assessments with adults in either the USA or Canada. The American Academy of Paediatrics published guidelines for the assessment process with children, but there are no equivalent guidelines for adult assessments, either from the American Psychological Association or any other regulatory authority. There is a similar scenario in Canada, with guidelines available in some states for child assessments, but no such provision for adult assessments. Anecdotally, there appears to be much variability among professionals within these jurisdictions in relation to how adult assessments are conducted.

UK NICE Guidelines

The National Institute for Health and Care Excellence (NICE) produces evidence-based guidance and advice for health, public health and social care practitioners in the UK. The NICE guidelines for Autistic assessment with adults were, at the time of writing, last updated in June 2021. While there are many positive aspects to this, there remain areas in need of review and updating to be in line with a Neuro-Affirmative framework.

From a Neuro-Affirmative perspective, the guidelines primarily use identity-first language. They outline how the process should be carried out 'in **partnership** with Autistic adults and, **where appropriate**, with their families, partners and carers'. This means that the assessment process should be collaborative and the inclusion of others within the process only occurs 'where appropriate', with what they mean by 'appropriate' being left open to interpretation. This can and should be interpreted as the need for there to be choice for the person in relation to whether a family member is involved in the process or not. The guidelines talk about respect, trust and non-judgement as being core aspects of the process, and they advocate for accommodations to be made within the environment where the assessment will occur. When referencing the actual assessment process, the NICE guidelines hold that a number of different assessment tools can be 'considered', but none are prescribed. There is comprehensive provision for consideration of a person's mental health needs and the need for accommodations when accessing healthcare. The guidelines do not state that a cognitive assessment needs to be carried out as part of the assessment.

One of the most significant issues with the NICE guidelines in their current format is the deficit-based language throughout. There is mention of 'persistent difficulties with', 'rigid and repetitive behaviours', 'resistance to change', 'restricted interests', 'behavioural problems' and 'behaviours that challenge'. This language and framing of Autistic experiences within the NICE guidelines is within a medical model paradigm that is grossly outdated and out of step with current understanding. The guidelines also advise to 'carry out direct observation of core autism features especially in social situations', which is problematic as due to masking the need for such 'direct observation' results in missed identification of Autistic identity.

Australian Guidelines

Australia's guidelines are termed the 'National Guideline for the Assessment and Diagnosis of Autism Spectrum Disorder'. These were the first attempt at developing guidelines, and were launched in 2018. The most recent update at the time of writing was in December 2020. They state that they do not redefine or change Autistic criteria, but outline a clear, step-by-step process for assessment. The guidelines pertain to the assessment process with children, adolescents and adults.

From a Neuro-Affirmative perspective, the Australian guidelines are strengths-based in their approach. They provide a comprehensive outline of Autistic specific strengths and general strengths to consider as part of an assessment process. Collaboration with an individual is also advised, and the guidelines state that assessment tools are not to be used as the primary or sole source of information in an assessment process. Equity of access to assessment is promoted across age, gender, cultural background, etc., and consideration of needs across a person's lifespan is advised. Within an adult assessment process, the guidelines also state that it is important to 'ask the individual' if they would like family member involvement. The Australian guidelines make clear reference to the importance of clinicians and services having an understanding of gender identity, racial and ethnic backgrounds, cultural factors and trauma history.

The Australian guidelines are problematic in relation to the widespread use of person-first language and language that is couched in the medical model. They contain language such as 'symptoms', 'disorders' and 'concerns', 'reduced ability to...', and widespread use of 'ASD' throughout, which again is hugely problematic in relation to the clear preference of the Autistic community as regards how they request to be spoken about. The guidelines also stipulate that the assessment must include a minimum of one face-to-face session and cannot be carried out exclusively via telehealth. In our experience, this is a redundant requirement and is not in keeping with a Neuro-Affirmative approach where there is no need to 'observe' Autistic traits, but to understand the inner experiences of a person, which can very effectively be carried out via telehealth. Telehealth options, if a person chooses to avail of them, also mean that a person can control their environment while undertaking the assessment, resulting in a much more comfortable and less stressful process for many.

There is an emphasis within the guidelines on the observation of Autistic characteristics, which again will result in missed identification due to masking. Such rigid limitations place the person in the position of 'proving' through demonstration that their identity is neurodivergent. From an identity perspective, this would be akin to asking someone to prove they were gay – how would such observations be conducted then? Such insistence on direct observation of Autistic traits can only further lead to stereotyping and indeed limited diagnoses due to not fitting the stereotypes of being Autistic that are perpetuated, however inadvertently, by such guidelines.

Scottish SIGN Guidelines

The Scottish Intercollegiate Guidelines Network (SIGN) first issued guidelines for Autistic assessments in 2007. At the time of writing, the most recent update occurred in June 2016. SIGN refers to assessment processes with children, young people and adults.

SIGN recognizes that there are gender differences in Autistic experiences, and states that professionals need to be aware of these differences. Although the guidelines don't clearly state that the involvement of family members is optional, they do make reference to how information 'could be sought' from a family member, and that an assessment should proceed in the absence of information about a person's early developmental history. While there is reference within the guidelines to 'adapting' the environment for Autistic children and people, guidance in relation to this is weak as it states it 'may be of benefit' rather than reflecting the basic human right of having access to an environment that is adapted according to a person's needs.

As is the case with all other best practice guidelines, SIGN contains problematic language throughout. The language is reflective of the medical model paradigm, with mention of 'ASD', 'patient', 'regression', 'delay', 'symptom', 'affected by ASD', etc., and it also contains person-first language, that is, 'person with ASD'. Again, this language is not in line with the clear preferences of the Autistic community, and is outdated in terms of current understanding of Autistic experiences. SIGN recommends 'direct observation' of a person's social and communication skills and their behaviour, and advises intellectual, neuropsychological and adaptive behaviour assessments. Finally, of huge concern within SIGN is a strong recommendation that access to support from staff trained in ABA interventions **should** be considered, with reference to the goal being to build independence in adaptive, communication and social skills, rather than the being about supporting people and adapting to their needs in relation to these areas. Given the significant harm and trauma that the Autistic community have experienced as a result of ABA approaches and practices, having a recommendation within best practice guidelines such as this is both hugely problematic and harmful.

9

Medical Model Assessments

In this book 'medical model assessments' is used to refer to how the vast majority of autism assessments undertaken with children and adults have been conducted until very recently, when pockets of professionals began to undertake Neuro-Affirmative assessments instead.

In this chapter, we will briefly outline how these medical model assessments have generally been conducted **purely for educational purposes**, in order to provide information and contrast with how we recommend they be done. Please take note – we are **in no way** endorsing that this is how assessments should be completed. Please see Chapter 12 on conducting a respectful, Neuro-Affirmative assessment for how an assessment **should** be undertaken.

Introduction

In a medical model assessment, professionals come to a diagnosis by collecting information about the 'deficits' and 'symptoms' outlined in the current 'best practice' guidelines and classification systems, the DSM-5-TR and ICD-11, in addition to non-Neuro-Affirmative training, diagnostic manuals and autism tests. And while the subsequent reports and recommendations following this assessment **may** list strengths as well as deficits (and professionals may believe they are undertaking 'strengths-based assessments'), the focus of the assessment is still on 'deficits' in relation to formulating the diagnosis, and subsequent recommendations focus on how best to 'remediate the deficits'.

As this is how our diagnostic manuals are framed, medical model assessments are also based on the **observable behaviours** the diagnosing professional can actually **see**, and what caregivers have **seen** in the past. By conducting assessments in this way, an actual person's story, history, experiences, feelings and their own thoughts on how their experience may align with the Autistic experience are ignored instead of being the **most important** aspect of any assessment. As clinicians we need to constantly reflect on who it is we are supposed to be supporting, and what the **purpose** of any assessment we undertake is.

It is understandable up until this point that professionals have traditionally taken these medical model methods of assessment and report writing, as this is the way we have been trained in the past. But it is part of our role as healthcare professionals to continually question if what we are doing is ethical and **truly** best practice, and to advocate for change if we believe it is not. We were doing our best with the information we had at the time, but now that we know better, we need to do better.

Reflection Point

As you read the following about **why** and **how** medical model assessments no longer merit our attention, we urge you to be gentle with yourself if you see your previous practice being described. We present the information below to **support** learning, not to criticize past practice. Knowledge and practice shift over time, and it is only by revisiting our practice that we develop as clinicians. We do what we do, and how we do it, for good reasons. We are constantly learning and reflecting, and this is what makes us better clinicians. You are here, learning, moving forwards.

The traumatic nature of medical model, deficit-based, adult (and older child) autism assessments is something that is frequently spoken about online between community members, as well as by Autistic clients, friends and colleagues. In Thriving Autistic, we hear on a daily basis from people who are self-referring to us for support following a traumatic diagnostic experience. This trauma and the inappropriate nature of medical model assessments is something that needs both research into and immediately addressing. Common experiences reported include that the assessment was adversarial, demeaning, infantilizing, insulting and invalidating, and it is **very** common to hear that the person being assessed did not feel that they were being listened to by the diagnosing clinician/s. In fact, many of the people who come to us for assessments have told us that this is the first time they have felt that they were being listened to by a professional, and they have generally seen many professionals before coming to us. It is no wonder that so many Autistic people choose to self-identify rather than put themselves through a potentially traumatizing assessment. However, as well as being unacceptable, it is **completely unnecessary** for autism assessments to be traumatizing in this way, and we plan to conduct research in this area in the future to support this.

While there are, of course, pockets of excellent practice, and we have noted a huge interest and enthusiasm for non-autistic professionals to learn about the **real** experiences of Autistic people **in Autistic people's own words**, there continues to be a large percentage of non-autistic diagnosing or screening professionals who have not received updated training in relation to Autistic people. This lack of up-to-date training leads to poor practice in relation to assessment, and diagnosis being gatekept erroneously, based on outdated information.

In The Adult Autism Practice we have seen many clients who, prior coming to us, had a potential diagnosis dismissed by their doctor or did not receive a diagnosis from a further professional, because (for example) they showed good eye contact, had a family and/or a job, a good sense of humour or did not show distress during their appointment. Yet, following in-depth assessment with the person, it is **very clear** that they are Autistic and that they meet the criteria for autism across both the DSM-5-TR and the ICD-11.

In order to stay within best practice, most professionals in the UK and Ireland (for example) reference the NICE guidelines when planning their assessments. As outlined in Chapter 8, while there are some helpful and respectful aspects to these, they are still firmly within the medical model of disability, largely ableist, not up to date in relation to current thinking in relation to the Neuro-Affirmative paradigm or double empathy problem, and there are many other highly problematic areas from a Neuro-Affirmative standpoint. In Canada and the USA there are no overarching best practice guidelines to support professionals.

Adult autism assessment is such a new area that there is no best practice, generally agreed upon **standard operating procedure** around conducing them. In the absence of this, most services and professionals have (understandably, but inappropriately) taken the approach to adhere to the methods designed for child assessments and to extend them to adults. Exactly which tests or procedures are used for which people can then vary between services and diagnosing professionals, but there are commonalities in approaches.

Currently, most professionals undertaking adult autism assessments across Ireland, the UK, Canada and the USA appear to be taking the approach of screening with, for example, the self-report Autism Quotient 10 (AQ10) and/or the Social Responsiveness Scale (SRS), and the subsequent use of a mixture of the Autism Diagnostic Observation Scale (ADOS-G) (still considered a 'gold standard test', despite its widely reported and significant limitations with an adult population), Autism Diagnostic Interview – Revised (ADI-R) or Ritvo Autism Asperger Diagnostic Scale (RAADS) (along with developmental history). 'Corroborating evidence' from caregivers is typically a requisite, with caregivers being expected to attend the assessment. Cognitive assessments can also often be conducted alongside these, as well as mental health screening.

It is therefore somewhat of a challenge currently for professionals wishing to work within a Neuro-Affirmative framework to find up-to-date, best practice information and assessment guidelines in this area (hence the great need for this book). However, as you will see in Chapter 12 in relation to how to conduct assessments in this way, it **is** possible to both stay within the parameters of best practice and up-to-date learning while also providing respectful, Neuro-Affirmative comprehensive assessments.

Here is some further information on some of factors related to medical model autism assessments.

Screeners

Many services use screeners in order to manage wait lists. However, using screeners to determine the need for an assessment will result in many Autistic adults not being brought forward for assessment or even being met by a professional, due to low scores on such screeners. While they may be useful as part of a full comprehensive assessment, we strongly advise against them as used for the purpose of inclusionary or exclusionary criteria to be assessed.

In addition, most screeners do not reflect Autistic experience and are often used in routine clinical practice without the background knowledge of Autistic experience to guide critical thinking. This means that the score is often taken as representing a fundamental truth about the person, whereas actually all it represents is a score on a measure. **As can be said for all screeners and tests, just because something is reported to be 'reliable' does not mean that it is valid.**

Tests

While we have valid concerns about the deficit-based nature of current 'gold standard' assessments for Autistic **children** (and indeed even the terminology of 'gold standard' in relation to these tests), they are generally thought of currently as being a reliable part of a comprehensive assessment in identifying Autistic children. **However, there are currently no standardized tests to assess if an adult is Autistic that are fit for purpose or reliable**, that is, there **are currently no** 'gold standard' tests to identify Autistic adults.

Ignoring for a moment the fact that the currently available tests are deficit-based and rely on an outdated understanding of what it means to be Autistic, these tests are unreliable for many important reasons, including a reliance on early developmental history (which may not be available) and caregiver recall, limitations in accurate diagnosis when co-occurring adult mental health conditions are present (as they very frequently are), and their inability to assess adults who have learned to mask over the years. The fact is that currently available instruments based on how Autistic children present are not going to be accurate for older adults who have learned to mask over the years, or who have developed mental health issues (as many have) from living in environments designed for neurotypical people. In the NICE guidelines the language around any currently available test is that these are tests professionals can 'consider using', that is, there is no onus regarding best practice to use any of them.

In addition, it is always necessary to critically evaluate the validity of any assessment. While it may be posited as reliable and valid, if neurotypical people design a test without meaningful engagement from Autistic people, and it is at its core ableist, then arguably, could it be said to be a measure of true Autistic experience?

One vitally important issue with assessments that put tests as the primary focus is the subsequent adherence to the scoring results. We have seen many adult assessments where, although there was a clear indication that the person was Autistic throughout the assessment, because the person's scores on the ADOS or ADI-R (for example) fell one point short of the cut-off they did not receive an autism diagnosis. In addition, we have seen many clients who have scored very low on either or both the ADOS and ADI-R and were in fact Autistic (the same is seen within a child population). Tests should always only be used to **support** an overall formulation, and **clinical judgement is key**. Test scores should never be **the** deciding factor in a comprehensive assessment, and should never take the place of clinical judgement and the client's own self-understanding and experiences.

Autistic experience cannot, and should not, be reduced to 'scores'. Tests can help guide our clinical thinking but are no substitute for thoughtful exploration with the Autistic person.

The Autism Diagnostic Observation Schedule – Generic (ADOS-G)

The ADOS-G is considered one of the 'gold standard' tests to assess for autism in **children**, and it is the test most reportedly used in adult autism assessments currently. However, in our experience, the older and more able a child or adult is to communicate about their experiences themselves, the less useful this test is, and it is recognized that it is **not a reliable test to use**

with an adult population. Many adults have told us they have found the experience of undertaking the ADOS-G humiliating and traumatizing. They report feeling unnerved by being clearly observed doing tasks that appear arbitrary, and have been provided no clear rational for undertaking them.

Reports

In reports following these medical model assessments, the language of disorder and disease is generally used, and explanations of tests are given with dehumanizing scores for each section and how and why the person met the criteria on those tests. Unhelpful 'levels of Autism' (as seen in the DSM-5-TR) are also often reported. These reports mirror those provided for children and are written **with other professionals** in mind, instead of what would be helpful for the person who has just been assessed. This negative, damaging language included in reports is often traumatizing for the person. A common narrative is that people do not look at their report again after the first read as they found it so upsetting. Many parents have said the same in relation to their children's reports.

Power Dynamics

One aspect seen in the majority of medical model assessments is the unhelpful power dynamics that are often present. Traditionally, assessments were undertaken with the person coming to a non-autistic 'expert', going through an assessment where they are observed, rated and coded using questionnaires they don't identify with or understand, and then being 'told' whether they are Autistic or not. There is often little sense of collaboration or of the person and the professional coming to a **mutual**, **shared** understanding of what might be going on for them. Unfortunately, in our experience many professionals can mistrust Autistic people who come to the assessment with strong (or otherwise) beliefs that they are Autistic (this may be particularly true for clients with a long history of service involvement and previous diagnoses such as 'personality disorder'). Many people have felt a sense of the professional trying to 'disprove' their belief that they are Autistic rather than showing a warm curiosity for where they are coming from, and working towards a mutual understanding.

Involving Caregivers and Early History

In the UK, the NICE guidelines say to involve a family member, partner, carer or other informant 'where possible', or to use documentary evidence such as old school reports of current and past behaviour and early development. However, having a family member attend the assessment has, unfortunately, been taken on by many professionals providing them as an absolute requisite, with many private practitioners excluding clients from accessing assessment otherwise.

Typically, the reasoning given for this is the 'requirement' for evidence of developmental differences in the early developmental period, although there is much emerging research to indicate that clear 'signs' of being Autistic are not present in many children at that age. In addition, it was added to the DSM-5, for example, that signs may not fully manifest until later in life because of increased (neurotypical) social demands or due to masking. Caregivers may either (a) not have noticed developmental differences as they, too, may have been Autistic and experienced the same developmental trajectory or (b) may have cultivated a rigid structure within the home environment where the child had been taught to mask from such an early age that there were no evident differences.

For people who have fractured relationships with their parents, having to include (and therefore be in contact with) these family members can itself be traumatizing. It is also common for these parents to hold the old school reports or other 'acceptable' documentation from early childhood, and so for those who are estranged from their parents it is not possible to access them (never mind that for most these documents have been lost). It is also a common (and unacceptable) experience for people to feel that their own experiences and beliefs about themselves were discounted and not believed, and parents' views were given priority in the assessment.

The practice of insisting on caregivers being present for assessments is infantilizing and disrespectful, as well as unnecessary. Denying someone self-understanding via formal identification of their Autistic self because the involvement of family members is not possible is also potentially unethical. People also often take a huge emotional risk coming for their assessments, and sometimes sharing this information with family members is either not safe or just too overwhelming to contemplate. In addition, many adults' parents are deceased, and this should not be seen as an exclusionary factor in assessment.

Learning Through Practice

In The Adult Autism Practice there is no requirement that people bring along a family member or for information to be 'corroborated', and it has in no way affected the quality or comprehensiveness of our assessments, although we give clients the option if they wish for someone to attend with them, and many choose to do so. Clients have reported feeling relieved and respected, which has greatly helped the therapeutic relationship during the assessment. As discussed later, many of our clients choose to independently have informative conversations with family members about their early lives (choosing themselves to disclose the purpose of these conversations or not), and bring to their assessments a wealth of information. For some people who have no recollections or information from early life, we have on a case-by-case basis looked at all of the evidence and the diagnostic criteria and mutually come to a shared understanding of the likelihood that the person is Autistic (see Chapter 12 on how to conduct Neuro-Affirmative assessments).

Cognitive Assessments

We have noted that many services insist on cognitive assessments being undertaken with adult clients, although it is not indicated in the NICE guidelines. Cognitive assessments are often part of a comprehensive child autism assessment, although at times, where it is clinically not indicated (e.g., if the child is doing well academically in school), it is often not conducted.

However, there are many professionals and practices still unnecessarily insisting that adults undertake cognitive assessments (most likely because of their use in child assessments). One proposed rationale for doing them is to differentiate between 'giftedness' and being Autistic. While there are strong links between giftedness and neurodivergence, there are clear diagnostic criteria (e.g., sensory differences) present for Autistic people that are not related to being gifted, and cognitive assessments in this case are not a diagnostic necessity. In addition, the additional stress of undertaking a cognitive assessment may serve to further demoralize the client, which is entirely unnecessary, unhelpful and ultimately void when an adult is working or otherwise engaging in activities of daily living or independence that rule them out as presenting with likely intellectual difficulties, which would be the only rational reason to conduct a cognitive assessment to begin with.

Neurodiversity-Lite Assessments

What some services currently do is undertake a medical model assessment using deficit-based tests, but then when the diagnosis is made, describe the diagnosis to the client in strengths-based, positive terms. However, this is not good practice, and could be described as a 'neurodiversity-lite' assessment (i.e., there is a pretence of being Neuro-Affirmative, but ultimately the change is only in the words used and no real changes have been made to practices). Assessments should be therapeutic and support a person to reframe and understand their life and neurology better. We need to 'hold' our clients gently throughout the whole assessment and identification process. Framing our assessment questions as deficits is not gentle. We have had many conversations with parents coming to assessments with us who are very aware that they do not want to experience an assessment process that they leave feeling 'less than' or flawed, having gone through that exact process with their Autistic child's previous diagnostic assessment.

Every question or activity posed by an assessor is giving that person a value judgement about what is being assessed. This means that if every question posed to a person is something like 'Do you have a problem with X?' it is facetious at the end to talk about how positive being Autistic is. Every question you ask, every screener and test you use, is proving to the person how you frame what they are being assessed for, and tests need to be Neuro-Affirmative from the very start (if they are to be used at all). Otherwise, people are just left with the message 'And now isn't it amazing that you are Autistic after I have left you painfully aware of all you can't do?'

Reflection Point

We urge non-autistic clinicians to imagine themselves attending a potentially life-changing health-related appointment. You have lived with this experience (and for this hypothetical scenario we suggest thinking it relates to a chronic pain issue) for a very long time, you have waited to see the professional for some considerable time, and have had to advocate vigorously for your right to do so.

You have invested a great amount of time and energy in researching what you think is causing your pain. Finally, the appointment comes. You attend with trepidation, but with great anticipation that finally someone knowledgeable is going to help. You have thought very carefully about how to explain your experiences, what you think is a possible explanation, and have a good sense of how you would like the appointment to proceed. You decide to take a close friend or partner with you for moral support and to share a coffee and debrief with afterwards.

The appointment does not proceed as you expected. Instead of asking you to describe what has been going on for you, the professional talks predominantly to your friend or partner, asking them what they have noticed about your pain and how it impacts you. This makes little sense. How can they possibly describe what if feels like? How can they know what it feels like? Pain is an embodied experience – no one can describe for us if it is an aching pain or a stabbing pain, and even if they know it is a stabbing pain, they have no felt sense of its nature or degree. Is it is stabbing like a small needle, or more akin to a knitting needle or even a sword? How can anyone but us describe the intensity, or how the pain radiates throughout our body?

Even though you filled in a pain rating scale yourself, the rating scale that your friend or partner filled in was given equal or even more weight.

Next, the clinician decides to ask you about pain. Except, they ask you to do some simple tasks and then rate your pain for you. They do not ask how it feels as you do the task, what happens in your body, or whether the task even makes sense for you in the context of your lived pain experience. The clinician focuses far more on your outward expression of pain (i.e., how your face and body looks) rather than what you try and tell them is going on or the form that you fill in. The appointment concludes. The professional tells you that based on what they observed and what your friend or partner told them, it does indeed appear that you are in pain and your suggested explanation might be correct.

Would this have felt a successful appointment? After all, the professional agreed you are experiencing pain and that all your careful research about possible causes or explanations is probably right. And yet, you leave distraught. Why might this be?

After the appointment you receive a clinic letter. It describes everything that your friend or partner said in detail, but less of your own information. You are described only in negative terms. How can you use your reflections to guide clinical work and the stance that you take?

10

Important Considerations

This chapter summarizes the multiple considerations that must be held in mind while working with Autistic people, and especially when undertaking adult autism assessments. While we present each consideration separately for clarity and ease of reference, clinicians need to centre all of these during the assessment process, paying due regard to every aspect of clients' experiences and needs, the stories that they have been previously told to explain their needs, and how all these areas combine and interact to create a unique Autistic way of being in the world for each person.

We can see there are multiple threads that we must consider when exploring Autistic experience and identity. Often clinicians and mental health services focus on seeing only the 'complexity', and we hear time and time again about people being told that they are too 'complex' for a service and becoming 'bounced' between different services in a ceaseless game of 'pass the parcel' while the person goes unsupported and their needs unidentified. Or the 'complexity' is seen as indicative of a 'personality disorder'.

We need to understand all the threads contributing to what is labelled 'complex'. If we see 'complexity' as being a tightly tied knot (and only look at the knot itself), we miss the beauty and colour of the intertwining contributing threads, all the ways they entangle each other, and that the unique nature of each knot is itself beautiful. We urge clinicians to thoughtfully untangle the knotted threads, wonder at the beauty and richness of each strand, and celebrate how each has contributed to the person's story. The identification of Autistic identity gives an opportunity for the person to untangle the threads of their stories and understand their experiences and needs in a new light. The clinician's role is to support this process by thoughtfully paying heed to all the issues outlined here.

Intersectionality

Too often the research and clinical literature approach autism as if all Autistic people are from similar social groups, cultures, ethnicities, gender orientations and sexual orientation, with standard assessment approaches and measures typically ignoring the multiple identities and experiences that someone brings with them. Intersectionality takes into account the complex and multiple identities that a person may have, the combination of which will shape their individual experiences. Being a white, straight, Autistic cis man will be a different experience to that of a Black, gay, Autistic woman. Yet standardized assessment protocols and diagnostic criteria do not take into account all those factors that impact on both the individual's lived experience, route to assessment and understanding of the their autism in the context of their intersectionality.

People with multiple identities and subsequent multiple marginalization can be at greater risk of mental health problems (Snapp et al. 2015). This can be understood through minority stress theory, which sets out how minority groups can be at risk for negative physical and mental health outcomes from cumulative experiences of stigma and discrimination (Chiang et al. 2017; McConnell et al. 2018).

Mallipeddi and VanDaalen (2021) highlight intersectionality as a critical concept in considering the experiences of marginalized groups within the Autistic community, for example, people of colour, women and LGBTQIA+ people. They point out the greater intersectional analysis of autism in the context of gender (although this often focuses on white women rather than women from marginalized groups) and sexual orientation compared to race and ethnicity. They found only 1 of 11 articles they reviewed explicitly assessed the experiences of people who identify as Black and Autistic.

Clinicians need to centre intersectionality in their assessments, heeding Gillespie-Lynch and Botha (2021), who stress that we must understand differences **within** the Autistic community to support all Autistic people to have the dignity that they deserve. Taking an intersectional approach means recognizing that we do not have a single identity or community; rather, we may have multiple ones, perhaps simultaneously. Clinicians need to heed the existence of multiple identities in the people they are working with, and in the assumptions and experiences that they themselves bring to their clinical work.

This involves a process of acknowledging, sitting with and actively confronting our previous practice where we have not actively attended to intersectionality. Our work is to reflect on the shift and evolution of our learning and to hold the space for our discomfort. Within this section, we acknowledge the diversity within the communities that we serve, and do not seek to claim any privilege when discussing the issues below.

◾ **Important note:** Discomfort means we are heading in the right direction. But we must also remember we will never arrive. If we think we have, our learning has stopped.

Cultural Competence

Definition

Cultural competence is multidimensional and refers to a person's cultural sensitivity and attitudes, cultural awareness, and cultural knowledge and skills (Kaihlanen, Hietapakka and Heponiemi 2019). We need to attend to how our cultural beliefs and awareness shape our clinical assessments and decisions. Being culturally competent goes beyond simply respecting the different cultures of the individuals with whom we work; it's also about having an understanding of how we work, and responding to the needs of our diverse clients.

Research

Reading the research and clinical literature you might sometimes assume that all Autistic people are homogeneous. The reality is, of course, far from that. In a powerful and passionate article, Giwa Onaiwu (2020, p.270) writes that:

> When it comes to autism, either they – or should I say you all – do not know, do not show, or do not care about Black, Indigenous, People of Color (BIPOC) very much. The typical 'face' of autism tends to be that of a little white boy, regardless of autism's actual prevalence in all racial, age, and gender groups. These are the individuals and institutions within the autism community who 'don't show'. They do not adequately show what is going on with regard to the diagnostic, access, outcome, educational, psychosocial, economic, and other gaps between races.

Stoll, Bergamo and Rossetti (2021) recently explored autism assessments from a multicultural perspective, reviewing both the literature and commonly used assessment measures. They point out that there is little information around approaching assessments from a culturally sensitive perspective, further noting that the focus of extant research is on discrepancies and disparities in diagnosis rather than exploring the causes and maintenance of these. They further stress the need to evaluate the 'gold standard' assessment tools considering cultural (in)sensitivity.

What we know from existing research is that identification of autism in certain ethnic groups can be missed or delayed (Tromans et al. 2021), meaning that already marginalized people are perhaps further marginalized through lack of access to appropriate sources of support. Tromans et al. (2021) suggest multiple explanations for the variation in autism identification across different cultural groups, including health-care related factors, environmental factors and the belief systems operating within specific ethnic groups and how this may impact on autism identification.

Autism is under-diagnosed in Black and Hispanic children (Jones et al. 2020), for example. Kandeh et al. (2020) explain that anti-Black racism is a pervasive issue, impacting the whole pathway from identification of concerns to navigation of services. Black Autistic children are 2.6 times more likely to be misdiagnosed than white Autistic children, and are more likely to be given a misdiagnosis of adjustment disorder or conduct disorder (Mandell et al. 2007; Straiton and Sridhar 2021), with longer wait times and later age of diagnosis. Straiton and Sidhar (2021) further explain that Black families not only encounter a racist system that perpetuates disparities, but also typically experience a poorer quality of care accessing services.

Little attention has been paid to the intersectional experiences of Black Autistic women and girls in autism-related research, policy and practice (Mandell et al. 2007; Straiton and Sridhar 2021). Furthermore, while culture plays an important role in expectations about and demonstration of social communication, little attention is paid to this in the autism research literature (Golson et al. 2022).

In 2018, Autism Voice UK, the Participatory Autism Research Collective (PARC) and the Critical Autism and Disability Studies (CADS) Research Group held a symposium at London South Bank University. The symposium highlighted the limited understanding of the cultural context of language and autism between professionals and families, stressing that many languages of the BAME (Black, Asian and minority ethnic) community[1] have no word for 'autism'. The symposium also focused on how professionals often ignore cultural, ethnic and religious sensitivities that may impact on all facets and stages of an individual's and family's journey (Kandeh et al. 2020).

Irish Traveller Community

Irish Travellers are a minority ethnic and socially excluded group, facing considerable barriers and stigma, discrimination and reduced educational

[1]   Please note that this is now seen as an outdated acronym and is generally no longer in use.

opportunities. They have a high prevalence of mental health problems, and suicide rates are six times higher compared to the general Irish population (Villani and Barry 2021). Quirke et al. (2020) explain that Travellers experience high levels of discrimination with a negative impact on engagement with health services, stressing the need to develop culturally competent services. The Traveller community has a low uptake of mainstream services, which is unsurprising when lack of cultural awareness can give Travellers the same experience of being misunderstood as in their daily lives. Non-Travellers need to consciously attend to the barriers their services present, and take action to make changes at both systemic and personal levels.

Rose Marie Maughan is a mother of two and autism activist who is a member of the Traveller community in Ireland. She created the Celebrate Autistic Travellers campaign after finding autism was not widely spoken about within her community yet was hearing about more Traveller children being recognized as Autistic. A recent study highlighted that the lowest autism prevalence was in Roma and Irish Travellers (0.85 per cent), which the authors attribute to diagnostic bias (Roman-Urrestarazu et al. 2021). While the study conflated Roma and Irish Travellers, it highlights the need to actively make changes to better serve the Traveller community to avoid contributing to the further marginalization of Autistic Travellers. While it is encouraging that the authors report prevalence rates for Roma and Irish Travellers, we should be mindful that Roma and Irish Travellers are two different communities, and will have different needs.

Frameworks to support understanding

Writing about neuropsychology, Cory (2021) pointed out that extant validated instruments and norms remain ill equipped for increasingly culturally or linguistically diverse populations. He draws on McIntosh's paradigm 'of unpacking the invisible knapsack of white privilege', suggesting that white privilege within neuropsychology may perpetuate healthcare disparities. Commenting on Cory's article, Postal (2021, p.224) argued that the field of neuropsychology requires 'immediate, disruptive, organization-level actions to place assessment methods and research paradigms that reflect the racial, cultural, and linguistic diversity of our society at the heart of our education, training and practice models'.

Reflection Point

It is important to remember that validated instruments typically do not represent cultural diversity among Autistic people. While there is a need for a systemic shift in ensuring that standard assessment measures adequately address cultural diversity, individual clinicians must ensure that they utilize existing measures through a critical cultural lens, unpacking their own cultural assumptions and experiences and how these impact on how they both approach assessments and understand an individual's needs in view of their cultural background and experiences.

Milton (2012) has written extensively about the 'double empathy problem'. As we saw in Chapter 4, the essence of this is that any difficulty in social communication arises from the interaction between Autistic and non-autistic people. The challenges are dynamic and not located in either individual, but rather are dependent on both partners in any interaction. Here we propose that we should conceptualize this as 'multiple empathy' when considering intersectionality. Rather than focus only on differences between neurotypes, we need to pay effortful attention to using multiple lenses to examine our clients' complex and multiple identities and marginalizations, reflecting on all identifies across the communication partners.

Bordes Edgar et al. (2021) suggest using Fujii's (2018) ECLECTIC model during assessments to enhance clinician awareness of potential biases during their clinical decision-making and in making culturally relevant recommendations. Their report focuses specifically on paediatric assessments, but is pertinent for all age groups. Fujii's (2018) framework considers a range of individual components: **E** (Education and literacy), **C** (Culture and acculturation), **L** (Language), **E** (Economic), **C** (Communication), **T** (Testing situation), **I** (Intelligence conceptualization) and **C** (Context of immigration). This framework can serve as a helpful guide to understand an individual in the context of their intersectionality.

Straiton and Sridhar (2021) suggest drawing on the critical consciousness of an anti-Black racism model (Mosley et al. 2021) to inform clinical practices with Black Autistic individuals. This highlights the importance of approaching clinical work with cultural humility, which they explain as a process of self-reflection, including examination of one's own beliefs and cultural identities, and having genuine regard and curiosity for other cultures, in addition to paying attention to intersectionality.

What we recommend

- Actively acknowledge, and seek to challenge, how your profession perpetuates racism or cultural insensitivity, and embrace a position of cultural humility (Straiton and Sridhar 2021).

- Actively reflect on intersectionality, and be mindful that it includes a broad range of marginalization (e.g., in Ireland, paying respectful attention to the needs and challenges faced by Autistic members of the Traveller community).

- Be mindful of all the complex pathways that individuals and families navigate when accessing services, explicitly naming and holding a space for these to be heard.

We end this section as we started, with the powerful words of Giwa Onaiwu (2020, p.270):

> It is a lot safer to maintain the status quo, to 'go with the flow' and to pretend not to notice. It takes courage and integrity to have to initiate difficult conversations. It takes time, and energy, and resources to make the efforts required to transform our spaces, our policies and our practices to make them more inclusive. It takes self-awareness and strength to yield one's privilege: to ask hard questions, to make space for others, to work towards restoration, and to unlearn and re-educate ourselves.

Addiction

The DSM-5 outlines 11 criteria for substance use disorders, focusing on **impaired control** (using more of a substance than intended, or more often than intended; wanting to cut down but not being able to); **social problems** (neglecting responsibilities or relationships; giving up previously cared about activities because of substance use; inability to complete tasks at school, home or work); **risky use** (using in a risky situation; continued use despite known problems); and **physical dependence** (needing more of the substance to get the same effect, i.e., tolerance; having withdrawal symptoms if the substance is not used) (Addiction Policy Forum 2020).

The DSM-5-TR does not use the term **addiction**, although this is characterized by a person's inability to control the impulse to use drugs (either illegal drugs or using prescription drugs other than prescribed or otherwise obtained), even when there are negative consequences.

Until recently research suggested that substance use-related problems were relatively uncommon in Autistic people. However, Chaplin, Spain and McCarthy (2020) suggest that while substance misuse within specialist services is seen in Autistic people (Murphy et al. 2018), clinicians in non-specialist services may not recognize that clients are, in fact, Autistic, and this may be why there has, to date, been little evidence regarding prevalence, assessment and treatment of substance use issues in Autistic people.

Chaplin et al. (2020) also point out that it is difficult to conclude how representative extant research findings are of the Autistic community because existing studies are difficult to compare due to, for example, different methodologies or samples, varied definitions being used to identify Autistic participants or substance use problems, different designs and use of small samples.

Butwicka et al. (2017) found that a doubled risk of substance use disorders in their Autistic participants compared to the general population. Szalavitz (2017) suggested that Autistic people may use alcohol and drugs as a means of self-medication, to relieve anxiety, manage insomnia and their sensory needs, for example. Huang et al. (2021) found that there was an increased risk of substance use disorder in their Autistic participants compared to non-autistic participants. Palmqvist, Edman and Bölte (2014) suggest that high rates of substance use problems may be attributed to the co-occurrence with ADHD.

Weir, Allison and Baron-Cohen (2021a) reported that while Autistic people were overall less likely to use substances compared to non-autistic people in their study, those who did so were more likely to do so in order to self-medicate their mental health needs. Autistic participants also described using drugs to reduce sensory overload, help with their mental focus and provide routine.

Kervin et al. (2021) conducted a systemic literature review exploring the prevalence of behavioural addiction (e.g., internet, gaming and gambling). They identified 27 studies reporting a link within behavioural addictions in Autistic people, but noted that many studies did not provide the statistical analysis showing if the correlations were significant, and that in many of the studies, Autistic people had other co-occurring mental conditions, making interpretation difficult.

Brown (2020) points out that little is known about what is helpful for Autistic people with substance use disorders. She highlights that many interventions are group or community-based, which may be anxiety-provoking and present a significant barrier. She points out that this could trigger further feelings of failure and alienation and become a self-perpetuating cycle. Chaplin et al. (2020) suggest a further barrier to Autistic people with substance use issues receiving the help that they need is the continued unwarranted belief of many clinicians that substance use is not common in Autistic people, despite recent research clearly showing that this is not the case.

Women

Research

There is considerable debate about the gender prevalence in Autistic people. Back in Kanner and Asperger's time, when autism was first identified, it was estimated that there was a 4:1 ratio in favour of males. With more understanding of different gendered presentations of autism, and acknowledgement of the apparent bias in research about Autistic people, identification and diagnosis towards a limited, stereotypical male presentation, we are now beginning to fully understand the limitation of previous estimates of gender prevalence among Autistic people. Only recently has our understanding of the nuances of gender experience been recognized as not always subscribing to a binary split between girls and boys in the neurotypical population. While there is clear evidence of increased variation in gender experience in Autistic people, much autism research continues to rely on this strict binary gender divide.

It is still typical that from birth people are identified as a boy or a girl. This understanding of their gender may change as they develop throughout life, but from birth, someone else makes that decision. This will then often have an influence on how society sees a child, and how that child is socialized by society, from their home environment to wider social practices and values. Women and men continue to be socialized differently in Western society. While this distinct gendered socializing is reducing, it is still present in more subtle ways and strongly influences development (Solbes-Canales, Valverde-Montesino and Herranz-Hernández 2020).

The bioecological systems model shows clear evidence that several systems influence development, how a person is socialized and presents – from the microsystems, where the person spends most of their time, such as school, home or the work environment (Tudge et al. 2009), to the macrosystem, contexts regarding different human groups, such as a person's ethnicity and gender. The core feature is that they share the same beliefs, for example, gender beliefs about what genders exist and how they should present, that schools should teach boys differently from girls, which affects resources and pathways that society provides for different genders (Hwang and Francesco 2010).

This is also a factor in considering the different presentations of birth-identified Autistic men and Autistic women, which is further complicated by recognizing that experience of gender and gender variation is not as clear-cut in the Autistic population as it appears in the neurotypical population (Kourti and MacLeod 2019; Walsh et al. 2018). However, the effect of socialization on children continues to have influence (South, Costa and McMorris 2021). Boys are more likely to be socialized to express their behaviours openly. There is more social approval for boys to respond with externalizing behaviour than girls, which affects different behaviour presentations (Solbes-Canales et al. 2020).

These different ways in which boys and girls are socialized across different levels influences behaviour presentations, and thus influences how girls who are assigned female at birth present, and how often they are missed when practices rely on stereotypical male presentation to identify autism (Carpenter, Happé and Egerton 2019).

Rose (2020) points out the importance of remembering that 'Autistic women and girls don't experience different Autism, they experience different prejudice'. This means that while Autistic women and girls may have different social experiences and challenges, these are driven by gendered socialization rather than diagnosis or a different experience of being Autistic per se (Pearson and Rose 2021).

There is increasing awareness that there are different ways in which to be Autistic aside from the stereotypical 'male' presentation (Kourti and MacLeod 2019), which most theories, research, screening and diagnostic tools continue to be based on. One such difference is in females identified at birth. While often known as the 'female presentation', this is unhelpful given that there are many ways in which to be Autistic apart from the stereotyped 'male presentation', and it is not exclusive to women and girls. Rather than gendering the Autistic experience, it may be more helpful to consider internalized or externalized presentation.

In their recent publication, Wassell and Burke (2022) describe an external presentation as one that is more 'recognizable' to the majority of people, where the Autistic person behaves in a way (e.g., stimming, being Non-Speaking, showing distressed behaviour) that is considered different to their non-autistic peers, whereas an internal presentation is one in which their Autistic 'traits' are internalized and masked and so less visible. Autistic Girls Network stresses that both males and non-binary Autistic people may have an internalized presentation, noting that many Autistic people who express their Autistic self in an internal way may not be identified as Autistic until, and because, they have reached breaking point.

Community and practice-based learning

It is clear that every Autistic person has their own way of being Autistic, their own Autistic needs and experiences. There is no one way in which to be Autistic. It is important to recognize the complexity and richness of Autistic profiles that are not limited to the stereotypical white cis male that drives so much research and cultural narratives about Autistic experience. Many Autistic people mask, and this comes at a heavy cost to the person. There is prejudice against being an Autistic woman (or indeed an Autistic person, and particularly not being a cis white male) and about being Autistic with lower perceived support needs. Significant trauma is associated with being misdiagnosed by mental health professionals, and this has a lasting legacy (this is addressed further below, in relation to 'borderline personality disorder').

Our clinical experience is that many clients seeking identification with our practice are adult women, although clearly this is by all means not all clients. Many Autistic women describe 'people pleasing' and the emotional and energy-related costs of doing this. Other Autistic women describe experiencing emotional challenges around body changes related to ageing, both as younger and older adults. This may be linked to experience of eating disorders, and one of the factors for the development of eating disorders in some Autistic people may be due to a fear of physical changes associated with growing up and becoming an adult (Snouckaert and Spek 2020). Autistic women may describe struggling with the mismatch between their ageing external self and internal self. Ageing can represent a period of too much uncertainty and change.

Many clients internalize their Autistic characteristics and may express concerns that clinicians will find their Autistic self 'less visible'. Internalization can lead to misdiagnosis and inappropriate treatment for Autistic people attending their GP surgery and/or mental health services due to lack of knowledge from professionals. Many Autistic strengths are not described or captured by the DSM-5 or DSM-5-TR (e.g., commitment to issues related to social justice, richness of connections and relationships and hyper-empathy), and many Autistic people have experienced being dismissed by different professionals as their accounts of their strengths and difficulties are not taken into consideration. Autistic experience as described by the DSM or ICD does not reflect the richness of Autistic experience we both live and see in the people we work with. People who are not the stereotypical cis white male are often justifiability sceptical and distrustful that professionals will not recognize them as Autistic, and will, understandably, check for experience of identifying across a diverse range of experience.

Many Autistic women seek identification in later life. It may be that the menopause is a trigger as it serves as the 'straw that breaks the camel's back' and prompts seeking identification during a time in which the person feels burned out and no longer able to survive (Kelly et al. 2022). Too often, women will have their experiences dismissed as 'just' representing the menopause. Moseley, Druce and Turner-Cobb (2020) conducted an online focus group with seven Autistic women, who described increased challenges (sensory sensitivity, socializing with others and communication needs) during the menopause that led to 'extreme' meltdowns, anxiety and depression, and feeling suicidal. Groenman et al. (2021) suggest that Autistic women are more sensitive than non-autistic women to changes in their body during (peri) menopause due to overall increased sensory sensitivity, proposing that Autistic women may experience issues related to the menopause sooner, and for a longer period, than non-autistic women.

Important considerations for professionals are that women (and Autistic people who are not the stereotypical white cis male) often have the experience that they are not listened to, or even believed, by their mental health professionals. This has often resulted in misdiagnosis, typically 'borderline personality disorder', and an understandable and justifiable mistrust of professionals. As such, it is impossible not to consider autism assessment through the lens of gender and social norms culturally specific to a person's context, that is, Ireland, the UK, India, Africa, Asia, and so on. Women often report strained relationships with their own mothers, which is itself an area for exploration of potential intergenerational autism. Many Autistic women choose not to have children, which can be linked to a range of physical, sensory and social-emotional considerations that often leave Autistic women feeling like they 'cannot' or 'should not' have children, although for many Autistic women, this is simply their preference, as is true for their neurotypical counterparts.

Many Autistic women can over-empathize and may find themselves needing comfort when someone else becomes emotionally upset. Others may feel discomfort or not know what to do or how to respond to distress in others. This is compounded by non-autistic people often misinterpreting Autistic expressions of empathy and compassion. Indeed, bluntness itself is often seen socially as a negative trait in women of all neurotypes, and as such, Autistic women may be seen as harsh or cold or even hostile by others. Autistic women often report complete strangers on the street telling them to 'Smile, it might never happen' or 'Cheer up love' or 'You'll look prettier if you smile more'. Many report masking smiles in social settings, but when they are in 'resting face', that is, walking down the street, they often receive comments such as these. This is very much a female experience as it is quite rare for males to be directly spoken to in such personal ways by strangers in public settings. It is also worth considering media influences on female presentation, as many Autistic women report learning many social skills from films. An over-exaggeration of happiness and glee may be portrayed in public settings – the quintessential 'bubbly gentle female' is one such trope often employed by Autistic women to cope with the social demands inherent in being a woman.

The reading of sexual and romantic intention in others, that are so important for females in terms of sexual and personal safety, are often not as present for Autistic women. Many report having gone on dates without realizing that is what they were involved in. **We would like to emphasize the point that responsibility for these actions and events lies entirely with the perpetrator. It is a damaging narrative to frame Autistic women as being more 'vulnerable' in relationships. It is always the choice of the perpetrator.**

Being in Relationships

Autistic people may report struggling with expected relationship norms, not wanting to 'settle down', get married or form a civil partnership, or even share their space with another person in an intimate relationship. Many Autistic people describe difficulties in their relationships that often are underpinned by Autistic-related concerns (e.g., struggling to find common ground with their partner's relatives, attending partner-related events, parties and gatherings), and that these often give rise to relationship challenges. While some Autistic people find supportive and loving partners who cherish and support their Autistic ways of being, for others, relationships may be a challenge, particularly if their partner is non-autistic and does not respect and support their partner's Autistic needs. Autistic people may struggle to recognize, understand and express their own emotional upset, and may instead retreat to a quiet space. It can take hours, days or even months to figure out what has upset them. Equally, it may be **because** they understand their emotional upset and have identified that what they need in order to regulate is a quiet space. The challenge is not the need to retreat, but rather a lack of understanding of this between both partners.

Autistic Parenthood

Many Autistic parents come to identify that they are Autistic during the process of their child being identified as Autistic. Many describe learning about Autistic experiences and needs as they explore the possibility that their child is Autistic, and find themselves reflected in the description of Autistic experiences.

Autistic people who have children may describe feeling they are not fulfilling expected social roles (e.g., having difficulties talking to other parents in the school yard, avoiding children's birthday parties, struggling to allow their children to have friends visit the house, being excessively studious about parenting approaches). An interesting and enriching aspect of parenting is that for many Autistic people, they only come to know their Autistic selves following one or more of their own children being assessed for and identified as being Autistic. It is therefore important for all professionals assessing children to consider the possibility that one or more parents may also be Autistic.

Connecting with other Autistic parents can be challenging as they may not be 'out'. While there are many parent groups on social media, for example Facebook, these typically predominantly privilege the neurotypical parent voice. Many parent organizations endorse language and approaches that the Autistic community find problematic, and parent groups are often not a comfortable place for Autistic parents. Many continue to endorse compliance-based therapies despite the clear concerns raised by the Autistic community. Many such groups do not feel a safe space in which Autistic parents can celebrate their and their children's strengths and focus on supporting their children in a neurodiversity-affirming way. There is a real need to develop alternatives to non-autistic-led parent support networks and organizations. There are few in real life or virtual spaces that support Autistic parents in a way that are strengths-based and honour Autistic identity. Autistic parents offer a richness of experience to support Autistic children that typically goes unheard in a non-autistic space, yet we are the community to which our children belong. Autistic parents need a safe space to discuss supporting their children in a Neuro-Affirmative way. Our voices need to be heard. It is also an opportunity to challenge the narratives of deficit so often encountered when discussing the needs of Autistic children and families, and to work together to encourage services to support us while celebrating our strengths and richness of experience.

And there are, of course, many Autistic parents who have not yet identified their Autistic selves. They may be so deeply masked in living a normative life that they are fierce proponents of a normative agenda for their child to be indistinguishable from their neurotypical peers. They may cling passionately to narratives of deficit and not be ready to hear a Neuro-Affirmative message; indeed, they may fight it ever more fiercely. Thus, such spaces can feel unsafe for all parties: for the 'out' Autistic parents, for neurotypical parents who have their own experiences and priorities, and for those Autistic parents who have not yet started their own discovery of being Autistic, let alone seeing that there is a journey to take.

What we recommend

- Recognize and validate your client's struggles, especially if they have had invalidating experiences in relation to their Autistic needs and experiences.

- It is important to understand and tease out the nuance in people's stories and to see beyond the 'good, quiet girl' to support Autistic women to collaboratively make sense of their identity.

- Avoid getting pulled into false narratives about 'female Autistic presentation' and remember that Autistic experience is no more binary than gender itself. There are multiple genders and multiple ways of being Autistic.

- Be aware that the 'typical' description of Autistic experience relates to cis white boys. People are Autistic in a diverse and rich variety of ways, so do not constrain yourself to looking for just one externalized expression of Autistic experience.

- Listen to these stories and value the client's understanding and formulation to date of their experiences, knowing not to rule out autism because the client describes friendships and relationships. Develop clinical knowledge about these areas, for example, understanding that people often describe having friendships and relationships with other neurodivergent people, can often and do make eye contact, but do not enjoy it or feel comfortable doing so, and that they have empathy (often describing themselves as overly empathic and very sensitive to others).

- Many Autistic people describe not being heard, or those in helping professions having made their mind up about them based on outdated or stereotypical information about autism. It is important to listen to a person's internal experience of their Autistic identity.

- Be mindful of masking and how this may impact on the identification process if you are not knowledgeable about it.

Masking or Camouflaging

Definition

Masking, also called 'camouflaging' or 'passing', is the conscious or unconscious act of taking on a role and masking or hiding all or certain parts of oneself (Cage and Troxell-Whitman 2019). While masking **may** keep us safer, it can equally unwittingly lead us into unsafe situations (e.g., 'going along' with someone's risky suggestions or those that are not in our best interests because to do otherwise would be to drop the mask).

These terms are, however, not interchangeable. A recent Aucademy webinar (Mundy 2022) suggests that 'camouflaging' carries connotations of trying to blend in as neurotypical, whereas 'masking' is a survival strategy. We do not wish to be appear neurotypical or to blend in, but rather to feel **safe**.

Research

Research has found masking to be related to many adverse outcomes, including low self-esteem, isolation, loneliness, late diagnosis or misdiagnosis, decreases in psychological wellbeing, exhaustion, burnout and suicidality (Pearson and Rose 2021). It can create a barrier to authentic connection and authentic self-development, blocking natural responses and expressions (Lai et al. 2017).

Many neurotypical people consciously manage the way that they are viewed in social contexts. However, research has shown a considerable difference in the self-reported experience of Autistic masking compared to neurotypical masking. Masking for Autistic individuals is often exhausting and takes a lot of effort; it is often experienced as a full-body experience, where the mask entirely takes over, rather than a conscious, controlled strategy people choose and can easily take on and off (Bargiela, Steward and Mandy 2016). Research has found that the reasons why Autistic people mask range from the conventional to the relational – wanting to fit in and pass in a neurotypical world, a desire to connect with non-autistic people that requires masking to get past the first steps of forming relationships that involve surface-level social chit-chat, to avoid bullying and negative reactions from others, internalized ableism and stigma relating to shame about having an Autistic identity, and out of habit, without consciously wanting to (Cage and Troxell-Whitman 2019).

Research shows that society often encourages masking in both subtle and overt ways, from subtle societal pressures to direct social skills training. Hull et al. (2017) found that motivations for masking included societal expectations that Autistic individuals had to change to be accepted by others, and that the neurotypical population viewed 'sticking out' or being different as unacceptable, leading Autistic people to feel they had to change how they were to be seen as fitting in. Autistic participants in Hull et al.'s (2017) study also reported that they were motivated to mask to access and retain employment. They felt that if they were more visibly Autistic, this would reduce their employment opportunities. Others reported that masking was essential for safety reasons – they had experienced being physically and emotionally attacked or intentionally isolated and left out when they had not masked their Autistic features.

Research suggests Autistic people may learn to mask as children, learning masking tactics from reading fiction or analysing soap operas, and may repeat phrases from TV series or mimicking socially successful peers. They may use toys to figure out past situations and experiences and to understand neurotypical social events, or as practice for future neurotypical-dominant interactions regarding what to say or do. Therefore, they may appear 'less' Autistic at face value and appear more like neurotypical children, but their presentation mechanisms are very different from those of neurotypical children (Hull et al. 2017). Autistic people may learn to consciously be less noticeable or to keep more distance from others, or refrain from making personal comments about others, either from consciously modelling neurotypical behaviour to gain greater social acceptance or learning from past negative feedback (Lai et al. 2017).

Research has shown that masking can have a considerable negative effect on mental health. It involves high levels of cognitive effort and can be exhausting and lead to increased stress, burnout and mental health challenges such as depression and anxiety (Lai et al. 2017). Cage and Troxell-Whitman (2019) found that constant masking and intermittent masking had a high price in terms of stress and anxiety, with participants reporting high-stress symptoms and anxiety. In contrast, those who consistently engaged in no or low masking had a significantly lower level of stress symptoms and anxiety.

Masking has been linked to the extremely high rates of suicide seen in the

Autistic population (see the section on suicide and self-harm in 'Co-occurring mood disorders'). Cassidy et al. (2018) reported that what participants described as camouflaging was an independent risk factor for long-term suicidality in their Autistic participants, as were unmet support needs.

Autistic girls and other Autistic people with gender experiences that deviate from the stereotypical male presentation can show a variety of distinct ways of masking. They may be 'Jekyll and Hyde' – when out in the world, at school or in work, they are extremely quiet or in a constant role of imitation, but at the end of the day, when at home and in a safe environment, having held in their frustration all day, the confusion about neurotypical social situations, sensory overload or repressed anxieties comes flooding out and results in a meltdown or shutdown (Attwood et al. 2019). Research suggests the prevalence of masking is higher in Autistic women and girls compared to boys and men (South et al. 2021).

Lack of knowledge about masking in professionals can cause major problems for identifying autism. Diagnostic overshadowing is particularly prevalent in Autistic girls and women (South et al. 2021). Autistic women and girls without co-occurring intellectual disabilities tend to be identified as Autistic later than Autistic boys and men, as clinicians direct their focus away from Autistic features, focusing instead on the mask (South et al. 2021). Those who have not been identified as being Autistic in childhood due to high masking can be misdiagnosed with other psychiatric disorders and continue without adequate support or self-understanding (Hughes 2015). Girls' common diagnoses before autism include 'personality disorder', mood disorder, generalized anxiety disorder, sensory processing disorder, eating disorders, behavioural problems, bipolar disorder and anxiety (Hughes 2015). Recent international research exploring perception, cognition, intolerance of uncertainty and anxiety in a sample of 486 Autistic adults found Autistic women and non-binary+ participants reported higher levels of psychiatric diagnosis than Autistic men: 36 per cent of non-binary+ and 31 per cent of Autistic women compared to 18 per cent of men reported experiencing two or more psychiatric disorders (Doyle and Wilson 2020).

Mundy (2022) proposes that an alternative conceptualization of masking might be 'shielding', which represents a more active and protective choice to create a safe 'bubble' around oneself. Mundy (2022) suggests that shielding strategies may include building connections within the Autistic community as a protective space, describing shielding as a 'force field, a membrane by which I can (usually) decide what comes in and out of my inner world, this shield protects me'. They highlight that while their shield is protective, it also contains great joy, such as following interests, talking deeply about things and being unique (Mundy 2022).

Community and practice-based learning

Many Autistic people describe an 'imposter syndrome' that is borne out of masking and not having a clear sense of who they really are behind that mask, or that their true authentic self feels much younger than their actual age because it has been trapped behind the mask and unable to get out and explore and develop in the world.

Overall, there is a greater number of undiagnosed women, and many who are wrongly misdiagnosed. Many Autistic people mask. While masking may be particularly pertinent for anyone who is not the stereotypical cis male, it occurs across Autistic experience. Clinicians need to be aware of masking, and naming it during the assessment meetings can be valuable to clients. Masking has significant negative effects on mental health, and bullying experiences can intensify the 'need' for masking.

Autistic people learn to mask from an early age. This is typically achieved through mirroring others, especially during school, and is typically in full force by secondary school, when social challenges exceed their capabilities. Our experience has been that many Autistic people describe feeling 'like an alien' and finding the multiplicity of social challenges in each interaction so overwhelming that they default to a position of 'copying' the person in front of them. Professionals may find themselves perplexed by clients who describe themselves as most likely being Autistic, and yet show very little observable 'evidence' of this. At such times, it is very useful to consider masking.

We have found the Camouflaging Autistic Traits Questionnaire (CAT-Q) screener useful (Hull et al. 2019). While it is not diagnostic, it is a simple and easy way to explore the degree of masking a person may be engaging in. Conflict avoidance often abounds to the point of agreeing with others whom they really disagree with, laughing when they do not know why, or finding something amusing and generally adjusting their own behaviour and actions vis-à-vis mirroring others present in order to cope with social interactions and events.

While the overlap with social anxiety can be glaring, on investigation it often transpires that Autistic people do not share the same fear aspects akin to social anxiety, and nor do they always present with any predisposing or precipitating factors or events that often pre-date and underscore social anxiety. Rather, Autistic people often report confusion and not fear in social settings. The masking itself becomes so taxing that rather than enhance social engagement, it further exacerbates avoidance of this.

The Privilege of Being Unmasked

To live unmasked is a privilege and option that not all Autistic people have, regardless of how much they embrace their authentic Autistic self, and no matter how much they wish to live as openly neurodivergent. We can only be unmasked if it is safe to do this. Safety can be a key driver of masking. Masking can be an essential survival strategy, and to drop the mask, even slightly, can put us at great risk. This may be due to many situations. Masking may be one of the few survival strategies available to someone and to drop it, even fleetingly, may put the person at risk of both physical and emotional harm (e.g., in an abusive relationship, or for Black Autistic people living in a hostile country).

We need to consider intersectionality as it relates to masking. Autistic people may have multiple identities that each lead to masking, and these will cumulatively impact on how safe someone feels to be authentically themselves, or the more they must mask an element of the Self. We have heard from Black Autistic parents in the USA who explain that they have had no choice but to put their children in an ABA programme to teach them to mask, regardless of their personal beliefs about ABA, because their child would be in danger if they were to be their true Autistic self. Others have described **having** to mask in specific situations growing up, as they were physically at risk in their environment, for example having been assaulted for not making eye contact with those living on their estate, and therefore learning that it is not just emotionally unsafe to be themselves, but also physically unsafe.

Unmasking is a privilege. We must be mindful of this and pay due regard as to how safe it is for someone to drop their mask. It may put them at risk of both emotional and physical harm.

Taking these issues into consideration, it is very important that standard answers to autism assessment questions are not taken at superficial level, and instead, an open, explorative approach is adapted to explore what has been 'learned' and to differentiate this from what just 'is'. An Autistic person may describe themselves as good at making friends, but we must then tease out what that means for them, how they go about this and their history of friendship making. This often results in narratives describing early difficulties making friends, not knowing how, and figuring out how to mirror popular peers in school and getting into groups, although mainly on the edge and not actively participating. Other patterns include always having one single person as a friend at a time, that friendship being very intense, and then, when the other person makes a new friend, the Autistic person cannot manage this change and the friendship invariably dissolves. In relation to friendships ending, Autistic people often report histories of friendships ending but never knowing why – they often hear things like 'You know what you did or said' when in fact they do not. When they do find out, it is usually that they have told a secret or shared personal information about a friend, which itself is often the result of not readily reading the non-verbal cues that would tell a neurotypical person that what they are hearing is confidential. Other patterns include making friends in context, that is, school, college and work, but never maintaining these friendships when out of that specific context. This itself speaks to the use of masking and the often-transient nature of friendship making for Autistic people.

What we recommend

- Some Autistic people are so ingrained in masking that they may simply be unaware of it, or unable to drop the mask at all. The mask may be ever-present, even in an apparent available and welcoming space. Offering a 'safe' space is not by itself going to be sufficient for the mask to drop; it is an ongoing process. Be mindful of whether your client is engaging with the 'mask' or supporting and allowing their authentic Autistic Self to emerge.

- Remember that a lifetime of masking is not going to change in one session, no matter how warm and welcoming you are. Respect why the mask exists and honour that. It can be a long and very painful process to strip back the layers behind the mask. Do not push clients. Instead, provide power sharing in sessions, and be curious about your clients' sensory preferences and needs to hold space for them to begin to advocate for their authentic ways of being.

- It can be helpful to draw on a broad range of communication methods to support the Autistic person to engage in the process as their authentic self, for example, inviting them to write or share poetry or stories that reflect their experiences, use other creative means of expression, engage through music, or through sharing gifs, etc. that capture inner experience. Words are not the only means by which to communicate. Your job is to support communication in all its forms.

- Remember that unmasking is as much a systemic process as an individual one. The process of unmasking needs and prompts systemic change. We can only begin to drop the mask if our system witnesses, embraces and celebrates authentic ways of being.

- Seeking out Autistic spaces on social media (e.g., #ActuallyAutistic, #AskingAutistics) can be very helpful for non-autistic clinicians in understanding the breadth and depth of Autistic people's experiences. This must, of course, be done respectively and not voyeuristically. The non-autistic clinician is a guest in Autistic space, and must be mindful of respectfully engaging in it.

- Recognize masking as a survival strategy and the means by which Autistic people stay safe in a neurotypical world that often pathologizes, invalidates and traumatizes them.

- Recognize the possible damages masking may have caused.

- Be guided by the client's choices during the assessment session (e.g., not having the video on), providing an option to the client that may decrease their anxiety in relation to masking during the session.

- Screen for masking in mental health services – CAT-Q is something that could be considered.

- Masking may be so instinctual that someone's first response may be driven by the mask. Giving time to process and further exploration is important.

- Pay effortful attention to thinking 'Am I engaging the authentic self or the mask? Am I allowing space for the authentic self?'

- Your work is to welcome and find space for the authentic self, not for the Autistic person to show it.

- Be careful not to convey a sense of blame or shame that the Autistic person masks. There should not be a focus on clients needing to stop masking, that it is their fault they are masking (e.g., attributing this falsely to low self-esteem, confidence or feeling bad about themselves). Convey a message that society trains and encourages Autistic people to mask. Autistic people typically experience more positive response when they do mask (e.g., they avoid giving their natural preference for direct responses) compared to when they are authentically Autistic.

- Do not assume that Autistic people mask because they feel uncomfortable with who they are and wish to hide it. Masking is often not internally motivated but externally driven by society. Masking can be a survival strategy in a world that is invalidating and threatening to the Autistic experience.

- Masking may serve different purposes for different people, or indeed meet different needs across contexts within the same person. Do not make assumptions about the meaning of masking for each person, but rather explore the client's mask and the meaning and purpose that they ascribe to it.

- The emphasis of any work is not about dropping the mask, but about moving towards understanding and being able to be one's authentic Autistic Self. It is a constant process of discovery and learning across contexts and time, and becoming more consciously aware of when masking may be happening (e.g., if someone becomes aware they are stimming in a busy supermarket in order to calm themselves, being aware of a potential pull towards masking can support them in consciously not suppressing the stim, but allowing themselves to continue stimming because it is meeting their Autistic needs).

- We can make active choices around masking **if** we are informed about our needs and the process of masking. For example, we can choose (if we have the privilege to do so) to surround ourselves with other Autistic people with whom we feel safe and able to be our Authentic selves rather than spend time with neurotypical people with whom we feel far less safe and able to be our Authentic selves.

- Offer a comfortable, safe, and genuine assessment space to allow for people to be honest and to communicate about parts of themselves that they have kept hidden.

- Being clear and consistent in your communication with people helps set up this safe space. Asking people about their communication preferences, providing options to turn off a video camera, etc. can all help people feel more comfortable. Do not judge people for how they show up to a session, and genuinely invite people to be as they would like to be.

Later Years of Life

Research

Research is significantly lacking in understanding the Autistic experience in later years of life. Bishop-Fitzpatrick and Rubenstein (2019) found that older Autistic adults experience increased levels of physical and mental health conditions compared to the general population. Their study looked at 143 Autistic adults aged 40–88, and found that a range of physical and psychological health conditions (varying from immune conditions, heart disease, sleep conditions, gastrointestinal disorders, neurological conditions and psychiatric conditions) had a higher prevalence than in the general population, and they also found that prevalence of epilepsy was higher for those with co-occurring intellectual disability but that there was a lower prevalence of depression and anxiety for those who had a co-occurring intellectual disability (Bishop-Fitzpatrick and Rubenstein 2019). They suggest that while further research is needed to understand this prevalence better, it highlights the need for general physicians (e.g., GPs working in family medicine and later years of life services) to have increased awareness of the experiences of Autistic adults, and to be aware of the high incidence of mental and physical health conditions in Autistic adults in midlife and old age. Bishop-Fitzpatrick and Rubenstein (2019) note that Autistic people experience health inequalities, and that systemic changes are needed to address these inequalities and design supports that can be put into place in community settings.

Research by Mason et al. (2019a) found that older Autistic adults having the experience and severity of psychological conditions such as anxiety and depression are associated with reduced quality of life (QOL). They also discovered normative outcomes were not associated with QOL as they were for neurotypical adults, and those goals leading to QOL for neurotypical older adults, such as increasing socialization, independent living and employment, may not be as important or valuable for some older Autistic adults, and that an individualized approach to improve QOL in older Autistic adults is much better.

The limited studies into the Autistic experience in later years include exploring the benefits of assistive technology (AT). Zheng et al. (2021) suggest that AT can be helpful in several ways, such as keeping a sense of control in different contexts, managing sensory differences and as an aid for executive challenges with everyday tasks such as cleaning, shopping and cooking, and technologies such as noise-cancelling headphones, smart lighting and control over sound stimuli through reduction and control over the music. In their thematic analysis participants described how technologies helped older Autistic adults manage day-to-day life, and how they could help increase control over communication, with many indicating that they preferred text-based communication over telephone calls as texts gave them more time to consider the meaning rather than having to understand straightaway.

AT also increased their feelings of safety, for example, having a telephone with them or an alarm system that could notify others if they were to trip and fall. As well as the benefits of AT in providing cognitive support for challenges such as executive functioning, memory issues and cognitive overload, technologies could help reduce effort and cognition capabilities, such as by using Google maps for navigation or to-do lists and alarms to aid memory.

Participants also described how technology was useful in socializing and entertainment, highlighting how the internet provided so many opportunities to learn new things, how there were so many stations for entertainment on the TV, and that social media provided connection. Zheng et al. (2021) described a similar system to the raising of a child under Bronfenbrenner's ecological model in which to support an older Autistic adult, outlining interventions across three distinct levels: (1) individual level – control, predictability, sensory seeking and psychological regulation; (2) provision of services with more external needs provided by an outside person, such as those who prepare meals, help with executive functioning and medical services; and (3) systemic level – cultural, societal and political changes, such as increasing the understanding of the Autistic experience and Autistic expression communication. Similarly to research that found that AAC for older Autistic adults is challenging due to security and privacy issues, one of the five key barriers of technologies for older adults in Zheng et al.'s (2021) study was privacy concerns. Other barriers included accessibility and useability relating to the interface, barriers associated with learning curves and cost, and the unpredictability of making a change and introducing something new.

The experiences of older Autistic individuals living in geriatric care and residential settings is extremely limited. Crompton et al. (2020c) point out that we do not know if Autistic adults' needs in these settings are being met, so, as a start to understanding this Autistic experience, they set out to identify research priorities for older Autistic people in residential care from the perspective of family members, older Autistic adults themselves, service providers, medical professionals and researchers in the UK. They identified 10 key priorities for research and practice:

1. Managing transitions

2. Training about Autistic experiences and needs

3. Respecting Autistic differences

4. Supporting physical health

5. Sensory environment

6. Promoting autonomy and choice

7. Design principles

8. Creating community and belonging

9. Advocacy

10. Evaluation care quality.

Crompton et al. (2020c) emphasize that we must increase awareness and research into the experience of later life for Autistic people.

Community and practice-based learning

Autistic older adults can bring with them a huge legacy or trauma, especially from their contact with services and having had a lifetime of being misunderstood. They may have a huge sense of hopelessness of having reached this stage of life and only just having that understanding. Older adults attending assessments may also be encouraging their adult children to be assessed in light of their own identification of being Autistic.

What we recommend

- Keep emails to clients short and to the point.

- Be ready to call and support the person to log on to Zoom (for example), or use alternative software if this is tricky for them (or family members should be encouraged to set it up) (see Appendix 2).

- All written information, from intake forms to emails, should be prepared and put into the criteria document before meeting the client. This gives clear areas for exploration and is particularly useful if clients struggle to recall events or pertinent information.

- The first session meeting the client should be used to identify supports or needs, both for assessment and post outcome (who do they trust or not trust etc.).

- Older clients are often very reflective regarding being Autistic, and less focused on the future uses or impacts of formal identification of being Autistic.

- Clients may realize that their own parents may have been Autistic, and this can open wounds or lead to healing and understanding or forgiveness.

- Many older clients may have troubled dynamics with their adult children, often centring on fall-outs that can be explained through misunderstood Autistic communication, for example their children blaming them or addressing how, when or if their emotional needs were met. The assessment can be useful to explore understanding and being kinder to oneself as well as forming starting points for reaching out and reconnecting with family.

- A 90-minute session can be very taxing. It may be easier to schedule 60-minute sessions and three to five of these instead.

- Loneliness and isolation, especially when the client does not have a partner or children, should be explored to identify if any external family, community or health service supports can or need to be accessed.

- It is important to consider that previous diagnoses feature largely, especially 'borderline personality disorder' and bipolar, which are often glaringly incorrect and contextual to old practices in psychiatry, especially in relation to females. Please also be aware that there are a number of people who are both Bipolar and Autistic.

LGBTQIA+/Gender, Sexual and Relationship Diversities

Definition

Stonewall defines LGBTQIA+ as lesbian, gay, bi, trans, queer, questioning and asexual (ace), aromantic (aro), and other sexual and gender minority identities.[2]

> Most people will be familiar with the term LGBTQIA+, which encompasses lesbian, gay, bisexual, trans, intersex, asexual, pansexual, etc. However, this does not include other relationship diversities such as those in polyamorous relationships or people involved in BDSM/kink power exchange relationships.[3] In this section we are considering all forms of gender and relationship diversities and are therefore using GSRD. Where original studies use LGBTQIA+, we are keeping to the terms used by those authors.

2   See www.stonewall.org.uk
3   See www.pinktherapy.com

Research

Stonewall published a report in 2018, which, based on Office for National Statistics (ONS) research,[4] indicated that an estimated 2.2 per cent of the population aged over 16 identified themselves as lesbian, gay or bisexual (but note that the true figure is likely to be much higher). In new data from 2022, the ONS states that 'An estimated 3.1 per cent of the UK population aged 16 years and over identified as lesbian, gay or bisexual (LGB) in 2020, an increase from 2.7 per cent in 2019 and almost double the percentage from 2014 (1.6 per cent) (ONS 2020). Stonewall noted the lack of reliable evidence on the trans population, but estimated that 1 per cent of the UK population identified as trans, including non-binary.

In a large study of LGBTQIA+ people in Ireland (Higgins et al. 2016), it was 'noted that Ireland has evolved from being considered LGBTQIA+ oppressive to being a forerunner on equal civil rights for LGBTQIA+ people. The study found the majority of participants aged 26 and over reported good self-esteem, happiness and life satisfaction, while those under 25 did not experience the same levels of positive mental health.

Roe et al. (2020) point out that viewing LGBTQIA+ identity through a heteronormative lens can lead to an assumption of a common 'LGBTQIA+' experience, whereas a great deal of variation occurs across sexualities, gender identities and depending on other intersectionalities.

A higher percentage of Autistic people identify as LGBTQIA+ compared to the general population (George and Stokes 2018a). Pecora, Mesibov and Stokes (2016) reported that 15 to 35 per cent of Autistic people who do not have an intellectual disability identify as LGBTQIA+. Research also suggests Autistic people are more likely to be transgender compared to the general population (George and Stokes 2018a).

From a recent large online survey, Weir, Allison and Baron-Cohen (2021b) reported that Autistic people were more likely to identify as LGBTQIA+ than non-autistic people. Warrier et al. (2020) examined cross-sectional datasets of 641,860 individuals who completed information on gender, neurodevelopmental and psychiatric diagnoses and measures of traits related to autism (self-report measures of Autistic traits, empathy, systemizing and sensory sensitivity). Notwithstanding issues with those measures, they reported that transgender and gender-diverse people are more likely to be Autistic compared to cisgender people, stressing that

4   https://www.ons.gov.uk/peoplepopulationandcommunity/culturalidentity/sexuality/bulletins/
     sexualidentityuk/2018

undiagnosed autism may also be higher in transgender and gender-diverse people. From a systematic review, Attanasio et al. (2021) report that autism and asexuality appear related, but note a lack of research in this area.

Hillier et al. (2020) stress that there has been little exploration of the intersectionality between being Autistic and gender identity. Some participants described feeling they did not really 'fit' in either group, whereas others mentioned positive aspects of dual identities, namely having additional groups to identify with. Participants discussed connecting to multiple communities, although some described rejection from the LGBTQIA+ community because of their Autistic experiences, and from the Autistic community because of their sexuality and/or gender identity.

Miller, Nachman and Wynn (2020) explored how Autistic LGBTQIA+ college students made meaning of and expressed their multiple social identities. Students described the challenges of working out when one identity became more salient than another, or when they intermingled. Miller et al. (2020) report that students used context to prioritize which identity was more salient, and that how they interpreted their intersecting identities was influenced by their strength of connection with their own identities, having others who accepted their identities, and peers who possessed similar identities.

Clinicians should be mindful of how best to affirm and support LGBTQIA+ Autistic people while also paying due regard to other intersectionalities.

Community and practice-based learning

Gay and bisexual men and women may face a unique situation growing up due to prejudices about being Autistic and their sexual orientation. As such, many report a kind of 'double masking', where they are hiding two major aspects of the self, namely their sexuality and neurodiversity. When assessing gay men and women it is important to explore their backgrounds for overlaps between sexuality and neurodiversity. This can be done by tracking their life story, from childhood to adulthood, examining prejudice, ostracization, bullying and confusion about self and others. Many report that during adolescence their lives became extra complicated, and mental health difficulties often arise in response to these challenges, including depression, anxiety and even self-harm or suicide attempts.

While identification of being Autistic can often be experienced positively, it can give rise to unique aspects. This is a type of 'reverse' or 'in-house' discrimination among other gay men and women. Perfectionism, 'superficiality' and managing the hyper-social aspects of the gay community (online apps, gay pubs and clubs, pride parades, etc.) can pose extra challenges for Autistic gay men and women from a sensory-social perspective. In families, the combination of being Autistic and their sexuality can often result in additional side-lining, rejection and exclusion as well as a sense of being totally different, alien even, within one's own family of origin.

While in recent years society has moved forward in great leaps, it is important to contextualize the experiences of gay men and women historically, as many will have grown up in less accepting times, and these experiences, combined with the social-communication differences of Autistic people, will likely have placed them at increased risk of mental health challenges and even self-loathing. Indeed, may gay men and women report eating disorders and self-image challenges that pervade across the lifespan. The combination of these factors may lead to a misdiagnosis of 'borderline personality disorder', which may only add to a sense of alienation and difference that could perpetuate long-standing difficulties.

Autistic people have described the potential wrestle of negotiating how to be GRSD in Autistic spaces and Autistic in GRSD spaces, whether to privilege one identity over the other, or how to manage their intersectionality. They have described experiences of having their sexuality doubted by others **because** of being Autistic, which may compound and replicate other experiences of invalidation throughout their lives.

Polyamory

We have supported many Autistic people who are in polyamorous relationships, who frequently describe how professionals have little understanding about polyamory or its prevalence. Polyamory is a form of consensual non-monogamy that involves committed relationships between two or more people (which may be sexual, but not necessarily). Polyamorous relationships can involve rich connections, emotional intimacy, deep feelings and commitments between all partners. A recent study measured the prevalence of polyamory in the USA and estimated a point prevalence of 0.6–5 per cent and a lifetime prevalence of 2–23 per cent (Rubel and Burleigh 2020).

Cardoso, Pascoal and Maiochi (2021) reported that compared to those not in consensual non-monogamous relationships, those in polyamorous relationships were more likely to define polyamory in terms of interpersonal feelings, whereas those outside of polyamory tended to focus more on sex and being 'allowed to' have multiple relationship rather than respecting the meaningful nature of these relationships. People in polyamorous relationships stressed the non-central role of sex.

Many people in polyamorous relationships experience social stigma, with their relationships being perceived as less trusting or less committed (Cardoso et al. 2021). This chimes with the stories that Autistic people have told us about frequently being subjected to prejudice, stigma and judgement for being in polyamorous relationships, from healthcare professionals as well as wider society, friends and family. This can be particularly difficult for an Autistic person who is already experiencing invalidation and judgement for an Autistic way of being in the world. What is so often missed is the depth of connection, closeness and intimacy that may be shared in a polyamorous relationship.

Our position is that all relationships are valid and to be celebrated, and we have heard stories of great love, affection and mutual care by our clients who are in polyamorous relationships.

Kink/BDSM

Some people we have worked with describe how they enjoy kink/BDSM (bondage and discipline, domination and submission and sadomasochism). They report comfort and predictability within the negotiated scripting of play scenes, which can provide intense sensory input (or deprivation) to meet sensory needs within a safe consensual space. Kink/BDSM as a practice or lifestyle involves explicitly negotiated consent about desires, limits and relationship dynamics (e.g., Dominant, submissive, S/switch) either in relation to play scenes or 24/7 power exchange relationships that rarely exist outside kink/BDSM (Kink Guidelines 2019).

Non-kinky relationships are often full of implied limits and dynamics, whereas for example, an explicitly negotiated Dominant/submissive dynamic makes the nature of the relationship clear and explicit.

Others experience real challenges if their sensory needs are competing with their partner's, and conversations around adapting the experience so that they can both have their needs met are paramount. Of course, within all communities, including the Autistic community, there are those who have no desire to experience sexual pleasure.

What we recommend

- Attend to intersectionality during all aspects of your work with the individual, including GRSD clients.

- Be mindful of multiple experiences of invalidation, both having a person's Autistic self invalidated and doubted coupled with invalidation of their sexuality.

- Be aware of your own assumptions and experiences and how these impact on how you frame and respond to a person's sexuality.

- Acknowledge the client's past experiences of being judged and invalidated for disclosing their sexuality, and allow a space for them to name this if this happens during your work together, even if unintended.

Gender Variance

Definition

Gender variance is a 'broad umbrella that encompasses diverse forms of gender identity and expression. In short, people who are gender variant do not fall neatly in the socially constructed and categories of male and female, man and woman, with their accompanied presentations and expressions' (Kourti 2021, p.13). This includes those who identify as transgender, non-binary, genderqueer, gender fluid, etc.

Research

There is a growing evidence base indicating that there is an increased level of expressed gender variance among the Autistic community. Research indicates that there is a higher rate of gender variance among Autistic individuals (e.g., Cooper, Smith and Russell 2018; Dewinter, De Graaf and Begeer 2017; Janssen, Huang and Duncan 2016; Strang et al. 2018) and elevated numbers of Autistic people attending gender clinics (Shumer et al. 2016)

While gender diversity or expressing gender variance is not a mental health issue, people who express gender variance are more likely to experience mental health challenges than the cisgender population (Downing and Przedworski 2018), most commonly anxiety and depression (Dhejne et al. 2016). This is likely related to minority stress, and the experience of stigma, discrimination and being misgendered (McLemore 2018; Meyer 2015; Testa et al. 2015).

The social, communication and clinical challenges faced by the Autistic community and by those who express gender variance are exponentially increased when a person is both Autistic and expresses gender variance (Lehmann and Leavey 2017), which can lead to greater social isolation (Kaltiala-Heino et al. 2015). Furthermore, Autistic adults who express gender variance experience a range of health disparities more often than Autistic cisgender adults (Hall et al. 2020), and they also face additional challenges when trying to access specialist gender services (Lehmann and Leavey 2017). There is a distinct lack of specialist knowledge regarding how therapeutic interventions may be developed for this group of people (Lehmann and Leavey 2017), and there is evidence of significant barriers in accessing the limited assessment and therapeutic services that are available (Mason et al. 2019b). These barriers relate to stigma or stereotyping, healthcare providers' lack of awareness and lack of openness to different modes of communication, and lack of trust in professionals (Mason et al. 2019b).

Community and practice-based learning

The relationship between Autistic and gender identity is well recognized within the Autistic and LGBTQIA+ communities. There are many aspects to these simultaneously held identities that are constantly emerging and evolving, with new terminology and narratives being explored and coined, leading to greater recognition and understanding of experiences. Recognizing the intersectionality between neurodivergence and gender identity is of key importance to the community. Understanding the interconnected nature and the overlapping experiences of being Autistic and expressing gender variance gives a deeper understanding of the particular nuances of this group.

With the advent of social media, connections between Autistic and LGBTQIA+ groups and communities are strengthening, and exploration of terminology and experiences has become faster-paced and more accessible to researchers, academics and clinicians working with this population. Although this is very much an emerging area within an evolving community, the growth in connection, conversation and sharing of experiences has supported the development and emergence of a number of key considerations within the community. Of central importance to the community is that the experiences of Autistic gender-variant people need to be understood primarily from the perspectives of the individuals themselves. This means that Autistic trans or non-binary voices need to be present in research, they need to be sought out and supported in order to inform clinical practice, and individuals need to be given access to supports in pursuit of professional qualifications within the areas of assessment and clinical support. It is currently quite often the case that there are professionals who may have experience or expertise in autism or LGBTQIA+ areas, but mostly these are separate areas, with few people overlapping in their professional competencies. It is therefore difficult for Autistic gender-variant people to access appropriate assessment and integrated holistic support.

There are high numbers of Autistic people discovering they are gender-variant and gender-variant people discovering they are Autistic. Often, people discover that they are Autistic and gender-variant at the same time. However, a tendency to pathologize being Autistic can create a barrier to people exploring their gender identity. Further advocacy, education and real-world implementation of research findings is needed in order to remove the barriers that exist – if a person doesn't understand their inner experiences, how can they be expected to understand their outer experiences?

The relationship between Autistic identity and gender identity is unique and complex, and current conversations and evolving terminology within the community reflect this. The term 'Autigender' refers to when a person's understanding of their gender is fundamentally altered by being Autistic, that being Autistic impacts the way they perceive and feel about their gender. Autigender is used to explain how autism and non-binary identities overlap and influence each other and cannot be completely detangled from each other (Boren 2021).[5] Autigender is a somewhat controversial concept within the community, however, as it can be misinterpreted as people thinking 'Autism' is their gender, which is incorrect, as autism is not a gender but a neurotype (Lynch 2019).

Supporting Autistic gender-variant children and young people with exploring their identities is a key area of progression and continuous concern with the community. As stated previously, the pathologizing of Autistic identity and the impact of ableism play significant roles in terms of creating barriers to supporting young people with gender identity exploration. Accessing gender identity clinics for young Autistic people can and has been challenging for many, and litigious action has been taken in some jurisdictions in an effort to prevent access for Autistic people. This has led many to conceal their Autistic identity in order to access support with gender identity, a situation that leads to increased clinical, social and mental health distress and a fragmented sense of self.

The importance of language use within the Autistic and LGBTQIA+ communities

---

5   See also www.queerundefined.com/about

cannot be over-stated. Using the preferred language of the community being served indicates that a clinician is engaged with the community, listening to the community, and respectful of the preferences of the community. Using incorrect or outdated language indicates that a clinician is not engaged with the community they serve, it is disrespectful to the community and to the person, and it casts doubt over the clinician's skill and knowledge base. Within the LGBTQIA+ community, incorrect language use, being misgendered (mistakenly assuming an individual's gender based on their name or appearance) or misidentified demonstrates a lack of understanding or respect, and can and does result in increased minority stress and significant levels of repeated trauma for an individual.

It is our experience that there are a significant proportion of adults attending for an autism assessment (and those identifying as Autistic) who express gender variance. For clinicians engaging in autism assessments with adult populations, it is essential to be cognisant of the high incidence of gender variance among Autistic people. Awareness of this is not only necessary in terms of supporting a person in exploring their sense of self and identity, but is also essential in being aware of the additional challenges in accessing services and supports people face, who are both Autistic and who express gender variance.

For anyone engaging in autism assessments with adults expressing gender variance, it is vital that they work closely with the Autistic and LGBTQIA+ communities. Listening to and learning about the experiences of Autistic transgender, non-binary, gender-fluid people is essential in understanding the nuanced experiences within this population. This then allows the clinician to support an individual in exploring whether their experiences relate to those of the Autistic gender-variant community. Be extremely mindful of Neuro-Affirmative and Gender-Affirmative language and approaches within assessments and documentation – for example, offering resources in relation to the formative experiences of cisgendered Autistic women is not helpful to a transgender woman as their experiences will differ. Clinicians must also work to remove the known barriers that exist for multimarginalized groups in accessing autism assessments (e.g., mistrust of professionals due to difficult past experiences or not being believed, being misgendered or misidentified, lack of support available, stigma, lack of accessible communication, etc.).

Thinking again about how most Autistic people are adults, do not have a co-occurring intellectual disability and are likely to be undiagnosed (Berney 2020), and how, therefore, medical and clinical professionals may underestimate the number of Autistic clients already accessing their services (Zerbo et al. 2015), it can thus be assumed that physical and mental health services are already offering healthcare services to Autistic adults, often unknowingly. For clinicians working in gender clinics or in mental healthcare settings where adults and/or young people expressing gender variance may attend, it is important to be aware of the high incidence of autism among the gender-variant community, and to consider whether there are indicators of Autistic traits among those already attending services.

Clinicians need to be aware of experiences such as masking and camouflaging, and be mindful of not assuming that all of the distress a person may be experiencing is related to stress surrounding their gender identity experience. Clinicians also need to be aware of diagnostic overshadowing, and the tendency is for some not to question or explore the underlying factors that may be contributing to a person's mental health challenges. On countless occasions in our experience, people (both cisgender and those expressing gender variance) have attended for autism assessment where they have been previously 'diagnosed' with social anxiety, and in the vast majority of cases, clinicians have not gone a step further to consider what may be contributing to or underlying the observed anxiety. Always consider the possibility that a person might be Autistic if they express gender variance and are experiencing challenges in relation to their mental health or social experiences.

Within the context of an autism assessment process, it is essential for clinicians to ensure that language use is correct and affirming. Remember that words matter, both in what is spoken to a person and in what is written in a person's official documentation or health record. Stigmatizing language used in notes or reports can influence future clinicians and services working with a person in terms of their attitudes towards an individual and the supports offered to them, and bias can be propagated from one clinician or service to another (Goddu et al. 2018). Reading that a person has 'deficits', is 'manipulative', is 'rigid' or 'talks too much' creates a very different narrative about a person than reading about a person who 'perceives things differently to others', is a 'strong advocate', 'thrives within structure and certainty' and is 'passionate'. Gender-affirming language is an essential component of an assessment process and should be a core component in the operation of any service. Along with being asked about how they experience their gender, all people attending for assessment should be routinely asked for their preferred pronouns, and these should be used throughout the process and in written documentation.

What we recommend

- Be aware of the high incidence overlap between the Autistic and gender-variant communities.

- Use Autistic and gender-affirming language.

- Ask about clients' preferred pronouns in intake forms and use the preferred pronouns throughout.

- Ask for the client's preferred name and use this throughout.

- Check the preferred name the person wishes to be used in their documentation or report. It is often helpful to issue two sets of documentation – one in a person's legal name and one in their preferred name.

- Do not assume that all stress is associated with experiences of gender variance or mental health experiences. Be aware of the sometimes-subtle indicators of Autistic experiences within those expressing gender variance who are also likely to be experiencing mental health challenges.

- If engaging in autism assessments with those who express gender variance, it is essential to engage with the LGBTQIA+ Autistic community.

- Work to remove known barriers to accessing autism assessments for multimarginalized groups.

Trauma or Post-Traumatic Stress Disorder

Definition

Trauma is an emotional response to a significant event that is typically negative, such as an accident or a natural disaster (APA 2022). Following a traumatic event, a person may experience denial or shock in the immediate aftermath, but there can be longer-term reactions, including emotional distress, flashbacks, physical symptoms and an impact on relationships (APA 2022). The APA (2022) holds that post-traumatic stress disorder (PTSD) can occur following exposure to a traumatic event, and results in intense, disturbing thoughts and feelings related to the experience that last long after the traumatic event has ended. Some of the signs of PTSD are intrusive thoughts, avoidance, alterations in cognition and mood, and alterations in arousal and reactivity.

Research

Autistic people are unfortunately likely to have experienced high levels of trauma in their life. In a study of 687 Autistic adults, 72 per cent reported having experienced interpersonal trauma and 44 per cent met the criteria for PTSD and scored higher on measures of dissociation (Reuben, Stanzione and Singleton 2021). Zablotsky et al. (2014) found that in a sample of 1221 families of Autistic children, 63 per cent reported that their child had experienced victimization in their lifetime, with 38 per cent experiencing victimization in the last month.

While many people will have experienced significant events in their lives, whether or not the person experiences trauma or PTSD as a result is related to a number of objective and subjective factors (Weinberg and Gil 2016). Objective factors relate to the type of trauma a person has experienced and demographic characteristics. Subjective factors include proximity to the trauma, subjective experience of the trauma as a threat, personality traits and dissociative experiences. Other experiences may be traumatic that non-autistic people (or indeed clinicians) may simply not consider, for example, sensory trauma, chronic experiences of being shamed, chronically having Autistic needs invalidated, misunderstood or ignored.

Rumball, Happé and Grey (2020) studied the experiences of trauma and PTSD symptoms in a sample of 59 Autistic adults. Their findings indicated that Autistic adults described a wide range of life events as being experienced as traumatic and as increasing the risk of or acting as a catalyst for PTSD (including those that meet DSM-5 criteria for the definition of a traumatic event and those that do not). They hypothesized that possible non-DSM-5-defined traumas for Autistic people might include the diagnostic assessment process and experiences within therapy where neurotypical approaches may have been applied. The ICD-11 PTSD criteria (WHO 2019) define trauma in a more subjective way, which might allow for people who experience PTSD following a range of different events to be identified and supported appropriately.

Given the very high prevalence of trauma experiences and PTSD within the Autistic population, it follows that trauma should be considered a core possibility within an Autistic person's experience. It is therefore concerning that it does not seem to be the case that clinicians and services are considering this. A recent study in the USA suggests that only 10 per cent of autism services routinely screen for or assess trauma-related symptoms (Kerns, Rast and Shattuck 2020). It is likely that lack of awareness, understanding and knowledge among clinicians and services in relation to trauma experiences within Autistic people is a contributing factor to the lack of consideration, alongside a lack of availability of accessible, reliable and valid assessment measures and therapeutic supports for Autistic people experiencing trauma. It has been shown that within the general population, PTSD can go undetected if a person is not asked about the occurrence of specific traumas (Solomon and Davidson 1997). Autistic people, both speaking and Non-Speaking, need to be asked about their trauma experiences. Clinicians need to consider the wide range of experiences a person has as potentially being experienced as traumatic, and should be aware of the subjective experience of Autistic adults (Rumball et al. 2020).

There is a distinct lack of research in many areas associated with Autistic experiences of trauma. There is little in relation to investigating the risk factors for trauma among Autistic people, causes of trauma responses, how trauma presents or the psychological aftermath of trauma, and how best to support Autistic people who experience trauma or PTSD. The prevalence of many co-occurring conditions in Autistic people has been documented and researched, but trauma and PTSD is an area that appears to have been largely overlooked. It is known that events are experienced differently by Autistic people, and it is likely that aspects of trauma experiences present differently within Autistic people, but without research investigating these experiences, this is currently difficult to classify.

Content warning: The following two boxes, on sexual violence and interpersonal victimization, may be distressing for some readers.

Sexual Violence

We make it very clear here that the responsibility for sexual abuse and sexual violence lies entirely with the perpetrator. It is a damaging narrative to frame Autistic people as being more 'vulnerable' to sexual violence. It is always the responsibility of the perpetrator.

Mailhot Amborski et al. (2021) describe sexual violence as any sexual act that is committed or attempted by another person without freely given consent of the victim or against someone who is unable to consent or refuse. They explain that sexual violence includes forced or alcohol- or drug-facilitated penetration of a victim (rape), forced or alcohol- or drug-facilitated incidents in which the victim was made to penetrate a perpetrator or someone else (ordered rape), non-physically pressured unwanted penetration, unwanted sexual contact (e.g., having sexual body parts fondled or grabbed and being kissed in a sexual way), and non-contact and unwanted sexual experience.

Overall, Mailhot Amborski et al. (2021) report that disabled people of all ages are twice as likely to be the victim of sexual violence during their lifetime than the general population. It is problematic, however, to focus on risk factors located within the **victim**. This can shift responsibility away from the perpetrator and direct focus on to how the individual can stay safe

– whereas the focus **should** be at systemic levels and on the perpetrator's actions.

Overall, higher rates of childhood sexual abuse are reported by Autistic people, particularly by women and girls, as well as higher rates of sexual and physical violence, emotional and domestic abuse and victimization compared to non-autistic people (Stewart et al. 2022). Dike et al. (2022) conducted a systemic review of literature pertaining to sexual violence inflicted on Autistic people. Nine of the 22 included studies reported elevated rates of sexual violence inflicted on Autistic people compared to non-autistic peers, particularly in adulthood. From a cross-sectional survey, Gibbs et al. (2021) found that a higher proportion of Autistic adults than non-autistic adults reported sexual violence (and physical violence) during childhood. Autistic adults were more likely to report never having confided in anyone about these events.

Reuben et al. (2021) reported that 72 per cent of 687 self-identified Autistic adults completing an online survey had been sexually assaulted, or had other unwanted or uncomfortable sexual experiences or been physically assaulted. They reported that Autistic cisgender women and gender minorities were more likely to report sexual trauma compared to cisgender men. Similarly, Weiss and Fardella (2018) summarize research suggesting that Autistic students were twice as likely to have unwanted sexual contact compared to non-autistic peers (Brown, Peña and Rankin 2017).

Brown-Lavoie, Viecili, and Weiss (2014) found that 78 per cent of Autistic respondents reported at least one occurrence of sexual victimization compared to 47 per cent of non-autistic respondents. Their study used self-report and demonstrated that Autistic people were between two and three times more likely to experience sexual contact victimization, sexual coercion victimization and rape than non-autistic participants. This was the case for both male and female Autistic respondents.

Given the above, clinicians need to pay careful attention to the trauma of sexual violence during assessments, be mindful that the client may have never disclosed these experiences before, and ensure appropriate support and containment is in place given the limited assessment space.

Interpersonal Victimization

Many of our clients describe multiple instances of interpersonal victimization across different contexts, including in friendships and intimate relationships. The United Nations (UN) defines domestic abuse as a 'pattern of behaviour in any relationship that is used to gain or maintain power and control over an intimate partner. Abuse is physical, sexual, emotional, economic or psychological actions of threats of actions that influence another person' (United Nations n.d.).

This includes stalking and harassment, controlling and threatening behaviour. Domestic abuse is not only acts of violence but also psychological and/or emotional abuse. Domestic abuse can happen to anyone, is often hidden and may go unrecognized, both by the person themselves and others around them. It can occur insidiously and over time, such that it becomes very difficult to recognize as abuse.

In 2015, coercive control finally became a criminal offence in the UK, and is defined as a pattern of intimidation, degradation, isolation and control with the use or threat of physical or sexual violence. Coercive control may include use of technology (e.g., phone trackers, controlling social media use, barraging the person with text messages), sexual coercion, monitoring behaviour, isolation or threats of or actual physical violence. It is a pattern of behaviour aimed at dominating and controlling another person, designed to undermine their autonomy (Barlow and Walklate 2022).

In their *Policing Coercive Control Project Report*, Barlow and Whittle (2019) describe issues with police understanding, identification and attitudes towards coercive control. Participants reported that the police typically focused on physical abuse when responding to domestic abuse, which influenced their assessment of risk and likelihood of arrest. Participants also described negative responses from other agencies (e.g., being told to save money for when they 'want' to leave the relationship, having services refuse to hold meetings separate from past abusers, and being told to accept responsibility for the relationship 'breakdown').

Pearson, Rees and Forster (2022) point out that Autistic people's experience of interpersonal victimization remains understudied despite indications of disproportionately high prevalence rates. They suggest that between 49 and 80 per cent of Autistic adults have been victimized by someone known to them. In their qualitative study, many participants reported repeated acts of victimization, and while some went on to form good relationships, others internalized a view that they themselves were the 'problem'.

To be clear, our position is that all responsibility for interpersonal victimization or abuse lies with the perpetrator. It is flawed and fundamentally unhelpful to consider 'vulnerability' factors within the individual for being subjected to abuse. Drawing on narratives of deficit around 'vulnerability' of Autistic people shifts the onus away from the perpetrator's choice, and we do not condone such a position. As Pearson et al. (2022) explain, perception of 'vulnerability' can lead to interpersonal victimization being taken less seriously by the criminal justice system, and assumes that vulnerability is an innate characteristic at an individual level rather than an interaction between the person, environment and wider systemic factors.

Reflection Point

People are so often encouraged to 'reach out' for support from mental health services. What is less spoken about is the potential consequences of doing so. For survivors of sexual violence, abuse or other interpersonal victimization, these consequences are often being disbelieved or doubted, having distress and experiences invalidated, with people being told that their very essence is deficient and disordered. So often, people have been subjected to abuse and trauma, and instead of the care and compassion that they **should** receive, they are subjected to further abuses of power by the actions of mental health services and told that **they** are the problem.

Too often we have heard from people who describe having entrusted their story to services only to find that they do not listen. Instead, services focus on the distress and despair, and often pronounce the person to have a 'personality disorder'. At this point survivors may find their words recast, rearranged into a meaning that bears little relation to the one they gave.

Many survivors of domestic abuse will describe constantly being on 'eggshells', needing to be hypervigilant for any signs that the abuser might 'blow', and constantly having to monitor their own behaviour and emotional expressions. Tragically, we hear many stories about how people learn to be hypervigilant in how they express distress within clinical settings, monitoring themselves to show just the 'right' amount of distress, and expressing themselves with great caution. In short, people may have to do with mental health services exactly what they had to do in the abusive situation.

A perpetrator will often twist and manipulate words until they bear little resemblance to what was actually said or intended. For example, if the person makes a neutral comment that 'the ironing board is broken', the perpetrator may take this as evidence of provocation, and launch a physical or verbal attack. During contact with mental health services, survivors may find that, yet again, their words are reshaped and manipulated to fit the diagnostic frame that clinicians have chosen to impose.

Many survivors of domestic abuse describe how mental health services have turned a blind eye to the abuse, or recast it as 'tension', 'disagreements' or a 'rocky patch'. This is unacceptable and inexcusable. Too often services are quick to explain away domestic abuse and minimize what is happening. In other words, they mirror what may have happened (or may still be happening) if the person tries to talk to the perpetrator about their behaviour. For many people, their experience of domestic abuse and intimidation is one of being silent, learning to keep quiet, to refrain from any comment about mistreatment, and always treading carefully lest they say the 'wrong thing' in the eyes of the perpetrator and trigger a tsunami of rage. They may be constantly trying to read moods and adapt their behaviour accordingly, and learn that challenging the status quo is never wise and always leads to negative consequences. Sadly, mental health services often re-enact this double bind, leading to devastating consequences for the person concerned.

Too often, survivors must 'read the room' to decide if a professional is someone who can hear their story without their emotions and opinions becoming recast and weaponized against them in the form of pathologizing diagnoses and narratives of blame (e.g., 'Why didn't you just leave?', 'You must have provoked him', 'You're vulnerable to exploitation'). They must be careful to present just the right amount of intensity or 'muchness', which means being sufficiently emotional so as not to be cast as cut-off, 'detached' and 'empty', yet simultaneously not so emotional that they are judged 'labile', 'dysregulated' and 'overly sensitive'. Many of our clients learn from their time with mental health services that professionals will misinterpret and filter all action and distress through their distorting lenses. They learn to be careful in every encounter about how they speak and what they speak about in case any issues are further pathologized.

These shadows will be lurking in your assessment space. Name them, welcome them, be mindful of your relationship with them. Heeded or not, the shadows of domestic abuse are long and need careful support and care.

The Trauma of Medical Model Autism Assessments

We saw in Chapter 9 how traumatic medical model autism assessments can be. This approach can feel demeaning, infantilizing and invalidating, with many feeling that the clinician simply did not listen. Clinicians need to be acutely aware of the great emotional risks that people take in entrusting them with their stories and experiences, and that while they may not intend to leave their clients feeling invalidated, unheard and traumatized by their approach, they can inflict this on people by taking a deficit-based stance or simply not listening. Clinicians must always be mindful that they are afforded a great privilege in hearing their clients' stories, and it is their fundamental duty to ensure that those stories are heard, held gently and explored collaboratively and respectfully within a Neuro-Affirmative lens.

Community and practice-based learning

There is currently no evidence-based practice for therapeutic support in relation to trauma for Autistic people (Stack and Lucyshyn 2019). This is the case despite there being awareness and acknowledgement of the very high rates of trauma experiences (e.g., bullying, abuse, assault and neglect) experienced by Autistic people, alongside the complex trauma associated with growing up within neurotypical environments with neurotypical expectations in relation to communication, interaction and regulation. Autistic people are more vulnerable to being targets for abuse and assault, and consistently demonstrate higher levels of distress, mental health challenges and rates of suicide. Autistic people report that they experience trauma from chronic exposure to sensory overwhelm or intolerances, constant societal expectations around masking, and being denied access to opportunities to engage in stimming. Constantly being misunderstood and the burden of adapting to a neurotypical society being placed on Autistic people is causing high levels of trauma within the community. Many Autistic people experience ongoing trauma from being shamed for showing Autistic responses, such as stimming.

There is deep and valid concern within the Autistic community that the trauma experiences of Autistic people are poorly understood, with research and understanding in relation to trauma being in its absolute infancy from an academic perspective. There is very little knowledge and understanding among professionals in recognizing trauma within Autistic people and about what approaches may be helpful. As one Autistic professional and advocate notes, 'We don't know what it looks like, we don't know how to treat it, and we are told by behaviourists that a quiet child means a happy child' (Memmott 2019). Memmott (2019) hypothesizes that there is a deeply problematic core belief in society that Autistic distress is a 'problem behaviour' to be trained out of a person. Many behavioural approaches target trauma distress indicators (e.g., anger, aggression, panic, hypervigilance, etc.) as aspects of a person's functioning that they should be trained out of. Memmott (2019) notes that there is often a reward offered to an Autistic person to make their 'internal terror invisible to outsiders'. There is valid concern within the community that if a child or adult learns not to show their distress, the intervention is deemed as having worked. However, the risk of this is that by not encouraging Autistic children to show how they feel, or by not asking them about their experiences, we are promoting the internalization of trauma, which leads to worse outcomes in the longer term. This is of major concern to the Autistic community, for Autistic people of all ages and of all communication preferences, that is, both speaking and non-speaking.

There is clarity within the Autistic community as to what is required in furthering the knowledge base, the evidence base, and access to support for Autistic people who have experienced trauma. This includes research and training led by Autistic people; a reduction in behaviours of distress being seen as 'Autistic behaviour' or 'challenging behaviour'; recognition that quietness is not an indicator of therapeutic success; acknowledgement of chronic lack of sensory regulation as traumatizing; asking Autistic people about their actual experiences via spoken and no-spoken methods with Autistic specialists as interpreters; not merely asking others around a person about their observations of that person; funding for Autistic-led and Autistic-informed therapies; and finally, a move away from blaming Autistic people for their behaviours or calling their behaviours 'deficits', and instead acknowledging the potential for trauma to be underlying their distress responses (Memmott 2019).

In clinical practice, the overwhelming majority of those attending for an adult autism assessment report having experienced trauma in their lives. Common trauma experiences include abuse, bullying, exclusion and being misunderstood by family, friends and society. Many report that they have been diagnosed as experiencing PTSD or complex PTSD, and while most agree that these fit with their experiences, many have also experienced various clinicians and/or services misunderstanding their experiences as purely trauma-related, without considering the possibility that the person is also Autistic, or wrongly assuming that their experiences are only attributable to trauma. Many report finding it intensely distressing that their Autistic experiences pre-date their experience of trauma, but this is not then given due consideration within an assessment process, and all of their experiences are attributed to trauma or PTSD. This often leads to people being gaslighted by clinicians, with the validity of their own lived experience not being accounted for. This can, for many, subsequently add an additional trauma experience.

Within an assessment process, it is vital that consideration is given to the person's trauma experiences, that each person is asked about their experiences and offered a choice in terms of how they communicate about them. Communicating about previous traumas within the context of an assessment piece can be extremely challenging for a person, as the communication is occurring outside the context of a supportive therapeutic relationship and within the confines of a brief assessment piece. Appropriate support needs to be provided as well as awareness of secondary distress in communicating in relation to trauma.

Clinicians undertaking an adult autism assessment need to have a deep understanding of the trauma experiences of Autistic adults. There needs to be acknowledgment of the likely longer exposure to potentially traumatic experiences that often date back to childhood, and the experience of a cumulative effect of chronic exposure. The impact of trauma on physical health and chronic pain conditions also needs to be kept in mind.

It is of vital importance that an individual is trusted as an expert on their own experience. It is essential to listen to each person in terms of how they understand their own narrative and what makes sense to them in terms of how they know themselves. Most people seeking an autism assessment have carried out their own extensive research and have listened to and are informed by a variety of other Autistic voices in considering their own trauma experiences. It is quite often the case that a person describes being told by other clinicians that, due to the presence of trauma, the presence of autism cannot be determined. Most people describe this as deeply invalidating, and that it doesn't make sense to them in how they understand their own experiences. It is helpful throughout an assessment process to check with the person whether the information being gathered and formulations being arrived at make sense to them, and if not, why not. It is also essential to know that it is not an 'either/or' determination, and that both autism and trauma can (and most often) co-occur. Autistic experiences and trauma experiences need to be understood in the context of each other so that the person can have a full understanding of their sense of identity.

For many clinicians, differentiating between Autistic and trauma experiences within adult autism assessments can be challenging. This is partly related to the lack of informed research within the area of Autistic trauma experiences. Although it is known that there are very high rates of trauma and autism co-occurring, and high rates of diagnostic overshadowing in relation to trauma and autism, it also has to be stated that for some people attending for autism assessment for the first time as an adult, their experiences might actually be best understood through a trauma lens and do not fit within an Autistic framework. Some of the indicators of trauma can overlap with Autistic experiences, and consideration needs to be given to how a person's experiences make sense from a holistic perspective. In differentiating between Autistic and trauma experiences within an assessment context, it is important to work collaboratively with the person as an expert on their own experiences, and to consider the presence of Autistic strengths, the timeline of traumatic events, the presence of Autistic experiences that would not be an expected outcome of trauma experiences and the possibility of the presence of both.

What we recommend

- When undertaking an Autistic assessment with an adult, due regard must be given to the person's experiences of trauma in their life.

- It is important that any clinician or service undertaking autism assessments with adults routinely enquires about trauma and the person's trauma experiences.

- Due consideration must be given to the two types of trauma that a person may have experienced:

  - Trauma relating to specific distressing events that may have occurred, e.g., abuse, assault, illness, parental separation or distress, natural disaster, etc.

  - Trauma resulting from being misunderstood, e.g., chronic exposure to having to adapt to the expectations of a neurotypical society, being denied access to stimming or regulation needs, previous experience of being misunderstood in assessments or within therapeutic contexts, chronic expectations from society around masking, etc.

- It is important to hold in mind, and acknowledge openly, that many people have had difficult encounters with mental health services previously in which they have been fundamentally misunderstood, unheard or indeed experienced services replicating the dynamics of previously experienced relational trauma. Do not refrain from naming this openly – this is an important piece in supporting the person to feel safer in the assessment process, showing that this can be heard and tolerated within the space. This also opens up the conversation about how to manage in the session if you misunderstand or cannot truly understand Autistic experience. Without naming it, it will remain there unheeded, but fundamentally impacting on the work.

- Be aware of the power held in meeting with someone for an assessment. Even if you do not seek to wield the power, it is nonetheless ever-present, and how it is managed and addressed will impact on discussion of trauma, particularly relational trauma.

- Be mindful of the challenges for people in communicating about trauma experiences within a brief assessment process. Ensure additional support is offered where necessary.

- Consider the possibility of trauma and autism co-occurring. Work collaboratively with each person as an expert on their own experience in determining the best understanding of their identity.

'Borderline Personality Disorder'

Definition

According to NICE guidelines, 'borderline personality disorder' is characterized by:

> Significant instability of interpersonal relationships, self-image and mood, and impulsive behaviour. There is a pattern of sometimes rapid fluctuation from periods of confidence to despair, with fear of abandonment and rejection, and a strong tendency towards suicidal thinking and self-harm. Transient psychotic symptoms, including brief delusions and hallucinations, may also be present. It is also associated with substantial impairment of social, psychological and occupational functioning and quality of life. People with borderline personality disorder are particularly at risk of suicide.

The prevalence of 'borderline personality disorder' is just under 1 per cent of the population, and is most common in early adulthood, with women presenting to services more often than men. Its course is variable, and although many people recover over time, some people may continue to experience social and interpersonal difficulties.

Research

Lack of knowledge by professionals about masking can present challenges in the identification of autism. Diagnostic overshadowing is particularly prevalent in Autistic girls and women (Espadas et al. 2020). Autistic women and girls without co-occurring intellectual disabilities tend to be identified as Autistic later than Autistic boys and men (Begeer et al. 2013). Professionals who don't know about masking may find their attention diverted from recognizing Autistic features (South et al. 2021). Those who have not been identified as being Autistic in childhood due to high masking can be misdiagnosed with other psychiatric disorders, and continue without adequate support or self-understanding (Hughes 2015). A common misdiagnosis is 'borderline personality disorder' (also referred to as 'emotionally unstable personality disorder', but we refer to it here as 'borderline personality disorder', for consistency).

Any discussion of 'borderline personality disorder' must start from a point of acknowledging the real and justifiable concerns about this construct within the Mad community of those assigned this diagnosis. The community write eloquently, evocatively and powerfully about the iatrogenic harm perpetuated by mental health services to those given this diagnosis. Iatrogenic harm refers to the harm caused by the process of 'treatment'. There are so many heart-breaking accounts of people given this diagnosis who die by suicide while in the care of mental health services, and many narratives of how this 'care' ended up re-enacting previous abusive and neglectful experiences.

This diagnosis is overwhelmingly given to women with a complex history of trauma and those who express intense distress. Mental health services may, and do, end up re-enacting those experiences. We must bear witness to the accounts of those who have been exposed to abuse and degradation during their contact with services, and rather than being met with compassion and care, are told that their very essence is 'disordered'. We need to sit with that. We must heed the profound distress caused by a system that adds another layer to the shame those experiences may engender.

As Berger (2014, p.2) writes, a personality disorder diagnosis (rooted in a system of classifying people into typologies of deficit) 'declares the deficit to be a fundamental feature of a person rather than a transient state'. Such a diagnosis defines the perceived 'deficiency' as a fundamental quality of the Self. Nicki (2016, p.218) argues that giving this diagnosis to female survivors of chronic childhood trauma 'pathologizes their life experiences, behaviour, and survival strategies'. We can find this littered across the personal stories of survivors of childhood trauma.

Reflection Point

We must name and acknowledge the iatrogenic harm perpetuated by mental health services towards those given a 'personality disorder' diagnosis. Professionals need to be aware of the power that they wield, even if they do not intend to, and must think critically about the entire construct of 'personality disorder' and the damage inflicted by viewing people through this lens. Welcome this into the assessment space, give it a voice, and pay heed to the damage that this diagnosis may cause.

I performed my mental illness and trauma in a way which was easier for you to understand and cope with, laughed off times you left me to die. But you never noticed. Reading my notes, without meeting me, a person would be forgiven for believing I am some kind of hell child. My thanks, praise, compliments, patience, kindness, understanding, humour, flexibility, the nice conversations, the thank you cards, they never happened because they have not been documented...

The power you have had over me is immense. You have taken my soul, torn it to shreds to examine the pieces, and yet all you have seen is your own reflection. You have never listened to me; I don't think you have ever really even seen me. I exist in your world as a reflection of your negative expectations. I am nothing but a stack of paper to you. A pile of words you invented. You have labelled me, lied to and about me, assassinated my character, discredited my words, belittled and rewritten my experiences, deliberately my words and actions, assumed the worst in me, pushed me into corners, ignored me, refused all my requests for appropriate support while telling me it was OK for me to choose to die you have made me feel utterly and completely worthless, to the point that it has been hard to keep living. (WrenAves 2022)[6]

Autistic adults are commonly 'misdiagnosed' with 'borderline personality disorder' (and we again note the considerable criticisms of this as a valid diagnosis or construct). Authors have noted that it has considerable overlap with other conditions and neurodivergencies (Arkowitz and Lilienfeld 2017). Many 'borderline personality disorder' features and Autistic experiences can appear similar at a surface level, but on analysis, can have very different foundations. For example, one diagnostic criteria for 'borderline personality disorder' is consistent and significant disturbance in self-identity and image (APA 2013). Autistic masking can either be mistaken for an unstable self-image or lead to an unstable self-image due to

---

6   Quoted with permission.

continued use. Fitzgerald (2020, p.2) notes that 'there is so much overlap between personality traits and so-called personality disorders that the idea of a valid personality type is absurd.'

It is women who primarily receive a diagnosis of 'borderline personality disorder' (75 per cent of those diagnosed in the USA). Berger (2014) points out that diagnosis of 'borderline personality disorder' is based on self-reported symptoms and subjective interpretation of someone in authority. The diagnosis of 'borderline personality disorder' holds a lot of power. Additionally, many people assigned this diagnosis end up with the diagnosis based on the 'gut feeling' of a psychiatrist rather than a detailed formal assessment (e.g., the Millon Clinical Multiaxial Inventory – Third Edition (MCMI-III), or the 'structured clinical interview' for the DSM-5). And, of course, while these structured assessments can provide a formal means by which to explore a person's needs, they do not confer validity on the construct of 'personality disorder', and any resulting information should be thoughtfully incorporated into a psychological formulation and not be relied on slavishly without taking a critical perspective. The lived experience of those given this diagnosis tells us it is often given to people 'psychiatrists don't like', those who are deemed 'complex', who challenge patriarchal assumptions, or who raise concerns about their care.

A diagnosis of 'borderline personality disorder' pronounces a deficit within the person rather than a temporary state, and pronounces the person as defective at a fundamental level. Many people given this diagnosis will have a history of trauma and abuse, and yet this diagnosis gives a message that rather than those experiences being the 'disordered' or problematic issue, it is the person's personality and very self that is disordered. How can this be acceptable? What is determined 'pathological' depends greatly on cultural values (Berger 2014).

Another criterion of 'borderline personality disorder' is recurring suicidal ideation and actions, threats, gestures or self injurious behaviour (APA 2013). Some types of self-harm that serve society, such as overworking at work to the point of burnout, are not seen as self-harm as they echo societal values (Berger 2014). In terms of autism, hiding one's authentic self to the point of psychological disorder or suicide to fit in with social expectations is not considered pathological. At the same time, other types of self-harm that are not linked to cultural values are considered pathological (Berger 2014).

Other 'borderline personality disorder' criteria include intense or misdirected anger and issues with anger management, and impulsivity relating to two or more areas that is self-damaging (such as substance use, sexual activity, binge eating, speeding, spending) (APA 2013). Shaw and Proctor (2005) suggest that a diagnosis of 'borderline personality disorder' can be used as a form of social control to silence women, for example those who do not behave to culturally valued gendered roles and display aggression, anger or sexual behaviours not considered stereotypically feminine, or women who overly adhere to gender roles and internalize their feelings of anger, leading to depression expression through self-focused actions such as self-harm.

There is clear evidence of increased variation in gender experience in the Autistic population (Warrier et al. 2020). There is also evidence that Autistic women tend to experience more internalizing challenges such as somatic symptoms, anxiety and depression than Autistic men (Solomon et al. 2012), and that they connect less with stereotypical female roles. Kourti and MacLeod's (2019) research found that participants described not identifying with normative gender roles, feeling more like a tomboy or wanting to be a boy. Participants described how they felt pressure to mask their external identified gender role as children, but began to resist societal expectations around gender as they grew older.

Another 'borderline personality disorder' diagnostic criterion is anguished efforts to avoid genuine or imagined abandonment (APA 2013). Clinicians are more likely to give a diagnosis of 'borderline personality disorder' when women have experienced sexual abuse and severe disorganized attachment (van Dijke, Hopman and Ford 2018). Childhood trauma and abuse can often result in fear of 'abandonment' (Milot et al. 2010) and understandable feelings of reduced safety. There is evidence that Autistic people may be at a higher risk of traumatic life events (Fuld 2018) and at a higher risk of adverse childhood events (ACEs) (Berg et al. 2016). The trauma of invalidation is caused by the social context (Harvey 2012). Many Autistic people experience invalidation of their authentic self when they feel pressured by a neurotypically dominant society to change who they are in order to be accepted and included or face isolation and ostracism from mainstream society. This contributes to chronic psychological stress and the experience of trauma.

While there are apparent overlaps between the 'borderline personality disorder' construct and being Autistic, the focus is too often placed on whether they **overlap** rather than whether 'borderline personality disorder' reflects unidentified Autism. 'Borderline personality disorder' is a deeply problematic concept, and may reflect social control and power dynamics and the multimarginalization effects of being identified as a woman and being Autistic. People are too often given this problematic diagnosis rather than clinicians thoughtfully and curiously considering whether they are supporting someone who is, in fact, Autistic. Careful clinical assessment can unpick and understand that which has been labelled 'borderline personality disorder'.

Community and practice-based learning

For many, identification of being Autistic negates a 'borderline personality disorder' diagnosis. There is a great deal of justifiable negativity and distrust of this diagnosis in the first place.

Reflection Point

Being labelled with 'borderline personality disorder' can have a devastating impact on both the Self, and on someone's experience within mental health services. Once given a 'borderline personality disorder' diagnosis, people can find that all staff interactions become delivered through one rigid lens that fundamentally misunderstands the person and their needs. It can and has had tragic and catastrophic consequences. Out of respect we will not name those who have died by suicide, but there are many heart-breaking stories where Autistic people have been given an additional label of 'borderline personality disorder', and it is through this lens that all care has been delivered rather than working to understand their needs as an Autistic person.

Autistic people (as any person would) want their experiences documented correctly, and in a way that matches their own perspective and experiences. Having one's story mislabelled and misunderstood in medical records is deeply traumatic and invalidating, and replicates wider experiences within society of being fundamentally misunderstood. Imagine sharing your story, only to have it rewritten in such a way that the meaning is fundamentally changed, where the lead character becomes the one to bear the shame of the events that happened to them at the hands of another.

Many people coming for assessment are distressed by a diagnosis of 'borderline personality disorder' and understandably want it expunged. It is difficult if that diagnosis remains on someone's medical notes unquestioned, and can be intensely distressing. In our experience, for a vast majority of people a 'borderline personality disorder' diagnosis is not a helpful account of someone's needs and they do not meet diagnostic criteria (we acknowledge here that the concept of 'personality disorder' itself is problematic). All people diagnosed with 'borderline personality disorder' need for an Autistic identity to be considered as a better fit. People may often be accessing mental health services for many years and be seen as 'not responding' to treatment, and yet the possibility that they are Autistic is not considered.

Too often, if a person does not 'respond' to standard treatment approaches, the responsibility is assigned to them (e.g., they 'aren't trying', 'they want someone else to do the work', 'they aren't taking responsibility for their recovery'), rather than clinicians reflecting whether the treatment approach itself was inappropriate or did not meet the person's needs. If a treatment approach is not working, clinicians should not blame the client but should instead take responsibility for curiously attending to that and exploring why. Find a wavelength together; do not expect the client to tune to yours. Many of our clients have been misdiagnosed with 'borderline personality disorder', which can undermine their Autistic experiences and leave them even more confused as they describe experiencing things and the world differently. However, many find the process of working through the criteria for 'borderline personality disorder' validating in order to explore whether this is a helpful framework within which to understand their experiences and needs. This can be done after the identification of being Autistic, to determine that this alternative explanation does not make sense. It is an important part of the process.

Very often, sensory experiences are not taken into consideration when 'borderline personality disorder' is diagnosed. Some clients receive dialectical behaviour therapy (DBT) intervention for 'borderline personality disorder', and despite the diagnosis not being a good fit, they have nonetheless found DBT skills helpful. Clients often start to question the diagnosis, finding it does not reflect their experiences and needs. Often people have been told they have 'traits' of 'borderline personality disorder'. Although there has been no formal assessment or diagnosis, professionals act 'as if' someone **does** have this diagnosis, and this subsequently drives all treatment. It is very hard and disempowering for people to do anything about this as typically services maintain there is no formal diagnosis. Multiple recent inquests have documented the risks associated with this. In addition, many clients have the distressing experience of discovering that a diagnosis of 'borderline personality disorder' was given covertly by professionals, yet never shared with them (e.g., when requesting their medical records).

In our clinical experience, the narrative becomes based around the 'borderline personality disorder' diagnosis in their families, driving how they are thought about, viewed and responded to within relationships. This can be traumatic, intensely invaliding and disempowering.

What we recommend

- Adopt a critical stance towards this diagnosis, familiarizing yourself with the critiques of this construct, and immersing yourself in the testimony of those suffering harm due to this label. This may be uncomfortable for those who are accustomed to accepting this diagnosis as a valid construct, and we invite you to sit with the discomfort. It offers a point of learning and should be fostered.

- As part of the identification process, support clients in collaboratively making sense of previous diagnoses and how Autistic experience can be misunderstood or misinterpreted.

- Be aware of the level of masking that could unconsciously happen during the session.

- Ask people whether a former diagnosis of 'borderline personality disorder' makes sense to them.

- Collaboratively work through the diagnostic criteria with clients to explore whether these make sense to them or not. This is a process of power sharing, and you need to be very mindful that in previous interactions, where the person was told that they 'have' a borderline personality diagnosis, there is likely to have been no power sharing, and clients may understandably be anxious and sceptical about discussing diagnostic criteria. It must be done sensitively and collaboratively, with a clear sense that you are not seeking to confirm the diagnosis.

- In our experience, a 'borderline personality disorder' is typically neither an accurate nor helpful explanation of a person's difficulties, and should be expunged. This can be a highly therapeutic part of the assessment process.

- It is very important to clarify issues around diagnosis moving forward and ensuring that this is clearly communicated within the person's system, for example, attempting to work with previous professionals to share the new formulation that the person's needs are most helpfully understood as reflecting Autistic identity.

- Following identification of Autistic identity, both an individual and systemic shift in understanding needs to take place for the person to start living as their authentic Autistic selves. How can a person thrive authentically as an Autistic person if the system around them continues to mislabel, misinterpret and invalidate their Autistic needs by continuing to filter all their needs through a distorting and unhelpful lens of 'personality disorder'?

Intellectual Disability

Definition

Intelligence is the general mental capacity that involves reasoning, planning, solving problems, thinking abstractly, comprehending complex ideas, learning efficiently and learning from experience (AAIDD 2010). There are two core aspects to determining the presence of intellectual disability: intelligence (as measured by standardized measures) of two standard deviations below the mean of 100 in the population (IQ score of below 70), and significant challenges in adaptive skills, that is, conceptual, social and practical skills that are learned and performed by people in their everyday lives (AAIDD 2010). There are different classification systems for intellectual disability – the American Association on Intellectual and Developmental Disabilities (AAIDD) (2010), the DSM-5 and the ICD-11 – all of which encompass the above two core aspects, with each system also stating that onset must be within the developmental period, within childhood, or prior to adulthood. Within the different classification systems, there is also a greater shift towards recognizing the importance of individual support needs in relation to determining the level of a person's intellectual disability.

Research

Research limitations must be acknowledged when considering research into Autistic people with co-occurring intellectual disabilities (ID). There is a lack of sufficiently validated research instruments and measures for use with Autistic people and those with ID. Many measures used in such research are found to be inaccessible to Autistic people, leading to issues with the reliability of results (Nicolaidis et al. 2020). Nicolaidis et al. (2020) suggest that to fully adapt research instruments to be valid and reliable for Autistic and ID populations, they must be co-designed with Autistic and ID people who hold equal power throughout all research stages.

A 2020 systematic review found that there was a lack of sufficiently reliable screening and diagnostic tools for Autistic people with co-occurring ID (Metcalfe et al. 2020). It was thought previously that ID co-occurred within 50 to 70 per cent of Autistic people (Fombonne 2003). However, current research suggests that co-occurrence is considerably less, at an estimated 20 per cent (Rydzewska et al. 2019).

The validity of the measurement of Autistic intelligence has been questioned. Measurements used to test Autistic intelligence, such as the Wechsler Intelligence

Scales, require the use of spoken language, and are therefore unlikely to fully measure intelligence in Autistic people who use a diversity of communication (Ostrolenk and Bertone 2016). Measurements such as Raven's Progressive Matrices may be a more valid measure of intelligence in Autistic people, as they do not require spoken language ability (Ostrolenk and Bertone, 2016). Assessment of autism in adults with ID is tricky. Diagnostic overshadowing is an issue, as is obtaining family and childhood history. Many adults with ID may have grown up in institutions or lost contact with families over time, so gaining complete records can sometimes be impossible. There is also a lack of evidence-based metrics available for this population (Sappok et al. 2013). Research into the use of the Autism Diagnostic Observation Schedule (ADOS) found it to have low specificity and high sensitivity (Sappok et al. 2013) within an ID population. The Autism Diagnostic Interview – Revised (ADI-R) had high sensitivity and specificity, but was only feasible for 37 per cent of participants (Sappok et al. 2013).

In a study of American Autistic adults aged 40–88, in receipt of Medicaid, with co-occurring ID compared to those without co-occurring ID, results found higher health issues such as sleep, cardiovascular, gastro, neurological, immune and mental health conditions than the general population. They also found higher rates of epilepsy but lower rates of depression and anxiety in those with co-occurring ID (Bishop-Fitzpatrick and Rubenstein 2019).

In terms of the treatment of mental health conditions in Autistic people with co-occurring conditions, studies have found alarming rates of symptom-specific, unmonitored, off-label, psychotropic drug prescriptions (Houghton, Liu and Bolognani 2017). Research from Spain shows high preclearance of polypharmacy treatment. In 83 Autistic adults with co-occurring ID, they found 253 co-occurring conditions between all 83 participants, with a median of three co-occurring physical and serious mental health conditions per participant. Results showed high rates of polypharmacy with a median of four prescriptions per participant; 13 per cent of participants were given a higher than recommended dose (Espadas et al. 2020). In terms of psychiatric treatment specifically, 33 per cent of participants had a co-occurring psychiatric condition, and the most prevalent drug type to be prescribed was antipsychotics, notably risperidone, followed by olanzapine and quetiapine, prescribed at a higher than recommended daily dose. Benzodiazepines such as clonazepam, clorazepate and diazepam were also prescribed at high rates, with clonazepam accounting for most of the higher than recommended daily dose (Espadas et al. 2020).

STOMP (Stopping the overmedication of people with an intellectual disability, autism or both) note that antipsychotics are often used as a treatment for Autistic people who are communicating distress in atypical ways, to either calm or sedate the person, and while used initially as a short-term multidisciplinary team-led intervention, lead to long-term unmonitored use (Branford et al. 2019). However, there is evidence that the long-term use of antipsychotics is inappropriate in such instances. They are often prescribed based on treating symptoms rather than understanding the reasons for the roots of the distress (Glover et al. 2014). Antipsychotic use has also been linked to increased obesity (De Hert et al. 2011).

In studies of Autistic children, higher rates of being overweight and obesity have been found compared to the general population. There is evidence that Autistic people with co-occurring ID have a higher prevalence of cardiovascular disease and diabetes than the general population (Flygare Wallén et al. 2018; Tromans et al. 2021). Antipsychotic-induced weight gain is a significant issue in treating co-occurring mental health conditions and symptoms for Autistic people with co-occurring ID. It can further increase the risk of cardiovascular and diabetic diseases (Barton et al. 2020), and can lead to a decrease in the quality of life for Autistic people with co-occurring ID over time.

Community and practice-based learning

There is a common misperception that the neurodiversity movement only encompasses neurodivergent people who do not have an ID. This is a total myth. As Bailin (2019) states, just because neurological differences are valued, this does not mean the reality of disabilities is being denied. Bailin (2019) noted that the neurodiversity movement holds that people with neurological differences are not 'flawed', that having a disability does not lessen personhood, or take away human rights, and that disabled people can live rich, meaningful lives. Variation is a vital part of humanity and every person is valuable. Bailin (2019) also noted that disability is often defined more by the expectations of society rather than anyone's individual experience.

The neurodiversity movement does not deny that challenges exist, and that some challenges can continue to be present even when accommodations are made. The community perspective holds that behavioural, social, learning and functional differences are not always problems. Bailin (2019) gives the example of how not wanting to socialize is different from wanting to participate and not being able to – one requires acceptance, the other requires assistance.

It is vitally important to the community that there is a broader understanding of what a meaningful life is. The neurodiversity movement advocates for the inclusion and respect of all individuals whose brains function in different ways, regardless of the level of disability they might experience. Those with disabilities advocate for their lives to be seen as meaningful and important and to challenge the perspective of society in terms of what is valued in life. Taylor (2004) describes how society values a person's ability to be independent and to support themselves financially. Is a disabled person's lifestyle less meaningful if it does not lead to financial support? Disability continues to be seen by society as something to pity and a burden, which makes it very challenging for disabled people to be viewed as having meaningful existences (Taylor 2004).

Our culture has a limited concept of what being a meaningful member of society is, but for meaningful change to happen, it must be understood that a person's worth and meaning can be beyond the monetary, and needs to incorporate personal empowerment. Our own personal experiences limit our understanding of what a meaningful life is, with each of us having a different definition of what that is. Advocacy within the community progresses the view that those with profound disabilities still have a right to self-determination, and to determine their own goals within self-determination. We do not have a right to project our own personal views on what a meaningful life is onto others. Subjecting Autistic intellectually disabled children and adults to therapies that teach them not to behave in ways that are comfortable, not to engage with activities they enjoy, and to be more compliant with the demands of others not only diminishes their human rights and their 'personhood', but also places those in the community at increased risk of abuse.

Reflection Point

Clinicians need to consciously attend to the likelihood that professionals or non-autistic people may have very different views of what a 'good life' looks like. This is important in the suggested focus of support offered by services. For example, professionals may see an adult or child's life as 'small' and 'limited', but that's not how the adult or child experiences it.

Our ability to fully assess and understand intelligence, learning capacity and learning ability within Autistic people is significantly limited by a lack of appropriate assessment tools that have been developed with the Autistic community and standardized with Autistic populations. We do not have reliable methods of measuring intelligence within Autistic populations, and instead, neurotypical standards, norms and expectations are applied. This leads to gross misunderstanding of intelligence and learning ability within Autistic people, with many identified as having an ID in accordance with neurotypical measures of intelligence. It leads to assumptions that Non-Speaking Autistic people are not 'intelligent' (as per neurotypical standards), do not understand what is being said to or around them, and do not have the potential to experience a meaningful life and to contribute to society.

There is a belief among society that Autistic people with ID cannot learn, when there is a clear lack of understanding of the trajectory of learning ability and the supports required to access learning within this population. We know from many Non-Speaking Autistic self-advocates (e.g., Carly Fleischmann, Ido Kedar and Naoki Higashida) that a person's inability to respond in spoken language does not mean an inability to comprehend. What is reflected is society's inability to understand different communication preferences, needs and choices. We need to call ourselves out on privileging spoken communication, and acknowledge that **all** forms of communication are just as valid and meaningful as spoken language. All voices have a place at the table, no matter how they express themselves.

It is a human right for all people to have their needs understood, acknowledged and met. This is much less likely in situations where a person's experience of the world is not fully understood. The first step in understanding a person's experience is considering whether there is a possibility that they may be Autistic, which may indicate whether further, more comprehensive, assessment is warranted or not. The NICE guidelines in relation to carrying out an autism assessment with an adult with co-occurring ID (last updated in June 2021) suggest that a brief initial assessment should be considered to ascertain whether there are specific indicators of Autistic experiences. The behaviours suggested by the diagnostic guidelines (including the NICE guidelines) can be reviewed, and re-framed to a Neuro-Affirmative framework, as follows:

Traditional medical model examples of behaviours used in diagnostic manuals	Re-framed within a Neuro-Affirmative perspective
Difficulties with reciprocal social interaction, e.g.:	Preference to be by themselves and not to be around others
• Limited interaction with others (e.g., being indifferent, aloof or unusual) • Interactions fulfil needs only • Interactions are one-sided or naive	Interaction with others in order to have needs met, but content not to engage with others outside of this Preference to engage with others in relation to own interests
The individual shows a lack of responsiveness to others	Preference to engage with own interests away from others Preference for others not to disturb, unless help required or particular needs arise
Little or no changes are observed in behaviour in response to various social situations	Engages with others in the same way across a variety of different situations

cont.

Traditional medical model examples of behaviours used in diagnostic manuals	Re-framed within a Neuro-Affirmative perspective
Shows a limited social demonstration of empathy	Demonstration of empathy in different ways to neurotypical expectations, e.g., may demonstrate distress themselves, may move away, may continue with own preferred activities, etc.
Rigidly sticks to routines and is resistant to change	Preference for particular routines and ways of doing things Preference for things to be the same or to happen in the same way Preference for certainty and predictability
Displays clear repetitive activities (e.g., hand or finger flicking or rocking), especially when stressed or expressing emotion	Observation of hand, finger or body movements that the person appears to find calming, or that they engage in when excited or stressed

The NICE guidelines state that if two or more of the above categories of behaviour are present, a comprehensive assessment for autism is warranted.

All the same principles of a Neuro-Affirmative approach apply when undertaking an autism assessment with an adult with co-occurring ID. There should be an exploration of the person's strengths, preferences and experiences, and the challenges they encounter. The process by which this information is gathered needs careful consideration. The person's expression of their experiences should hold a central position in the assessment process. The way they may communicate their preferences and experiences might be via spoken communication, non-spoken communication (e.g., AAC), or within behavioural communication.

In addition to understanding the person's own communication of their experiences, supplementary information from caregivers can add additional insights into the person's preferences across different aspects of their lives. While obtaining additional information from others in a person's life can be helpful to the process, it is vital to keep the person undertaking the assessment at the centre of the process, and not to default to others in providing the information.

It is extremely important to be aware of diagnostic overshadowing within the ID community in relation to considering Autistic experiences. For people with more significant levels of support needs in relation to their ID, establishing the presence of their Autistic identity is profoundly important, as the focus of understanding their needs can move towards gaining better insight into their sensory processing needs. The sensory processing experience of adults with co-occurring ID can be very poorly understood, with significant consequences for the individual, including trauma, pain, discomfort, PTSD, mental health challenges, inappropriate use of pharmacological interventions, and barriers to education, occupation and support. Carefully considering the need for and subsequently undertaking a comprehensive autism assessment with an adult with co-occurring ID can have a profoundly positive impact on their lives, as those around the adult develop a better understanding of their experiences and needs.

What we recommend

- Be aware that an adult autism assessment may be indicated and required for those within the adult ID population.

- It is important to be aware of what to consider and what to investigate in determining whether a more comprehensive autism assessment is indicated.

- It can be of profound importance to identify the Autistic experiences of those within the ID population with more significant support needs (i.e., those who have been identified as experiencing severe-profound ID).

- A Neuro-Affirmative approach to an autism assessment with an adult with co-occurring ID is essential and should be applied with adaptations to accommodate a person's preferences and experiences at the centre of the process.

Anxiety

Definition

The American Psychological Association (2022) defines anxiety as an emotion characterized by feelings of tension, worried thoughts and physical changes, such as increased blood pressure. Those who experience anxiety often have intrusive thoughts or concerns and may avoid certain situations due to worry. Anxiety can be thought of as an uncomfortable state of hyperalertness due to fear. It is a typical human emotion and is a helpful response in situations of actual threat, with physical changes being a typical part of the anxiety response.

Anxiety becomes a clinical response when a person experiences excessive anxiety in response to routine situations where there is a perceived threat, but no actual threat. There are different types of clinical anxiety (American Psychological Association 2022):

- Generalized anxiety: Persistent and excessive worry that interferes with daily activities.

- Panic disorder: Recurrent panic attacks consisting of an overwhelming combination of physical and psychological distress.

- Phobia: An excessive and persistent fear of a specific object, situation or activity that is generally not harmful.

- Agoraphobia: The fear of being in situations where escape may be difficult or embarrassing, or help might not be available in the event of panic symptoms.

- Social anxiety: Significant anxiety and discomfort about being embarrassed, humiliated, rejected or looked down on in social interactions. People with social anxiety will try to avoid the situation, or endure it with great distress.

- Separation anxiety: Excessive fear or anxiety about separation from those with whom a person is attached.

Research

Autistic people are more likely than non-autistic people to experience anxiety. From a large population-based study in Sweden, Nimmo-Smith et al. (2020) found that Autistic adults were over two-and-a-half times more likely to have a diagnosis of an anxiety disorder compared to non-autistic people, particularly diagnoses of OCD and phobic anxiety disorders.

Less is generally known about the prevalence of anxiety disorders in Autistic adults compared to Autistic children and adolescents (in whom anxiety disorders are known to be common). Nimmo-Smith et al. (2020) point out that various methodological issues in extant research means that existing evidence about prevalence rates is difficult to generalize, and may be subject to confounding and selection bias. Estimates vary from between 28 and 77 per cent of prevalence of anxiety.

Hollocks et al. (2019) conducted a systemic review and meta-analysis to examine rates of anxiety in Autistic adults, reporting that the pooled estimated of current and lifetime prevalence was 27 per cent and 42 per cent respectively. They stress the lack of appropriate measures that are validated for use with Autistic people, which means there should be caution around accepting the validation of findings. Notwithstanding this, their review indicates considerably higher rates of anxiety among Autistic adults compared to the estimated 1–12 per cent of the general population. Their review indicates the following prevalence rates: social anxiety (estimated current prevalence 29 per cent, lifetime prevalence 20 per cent); OCD (estimated current prevalence 24 per cent, lifetime prevalence 22 per cent); generalized anxiety (estimated current prevalence 18 per cent, lifetime prevalence 26 per cent); panic or agoraphobia (estimated current prevalence 15 per cent, lifetime prevalence 18 per cent); PTSD (estimated current prevalence 1 per cent, lifetime prevalence 5 per cent); and specific phobia (estimated current prevalence 6 per cent, lifetime prevalence 31 per cent).

A significant issue that merits attention is diagnostic overshadowing, which can mean the research literature does not accurately reflect true rates of anxiety among Autistic people. Either Autistic experience is misattributed to anxiety, or anxiety is conceptualized as a fundamental part of the Autistic experience and is not formally assessed, diagnosed or given support. Social differences in Autistic people may be mislabelled as anxious avoidance of social situations and attributed to social phobia, and compulsive behaviours in OCD may be falsely attributed to the strong need for routine and sameness in Autistic people. Prevalence rates must be considered with this in mind. Hollocks et al. (2019) also point out that the current literature fails to consider how variability in alexithymia may influence reported emotional experiences and anxiety.

Focus on Obsessive-Compulsive Disorder

Obsessions are recurring thoughts, impulses or images that cause anxiety distress, are intrusive and unwanted, and result in actions taken to mitigate these thoughts (e.g., through certain behaviours or thought processes). Compulsive behaviours are typically repetitive covert or overt actions that aim to reduce the anxiety related to the obsession. Not carrying out the compulsion can lead to acute anxiety.

The average length for OCD treatment is over 10 years as it is often misunderstood and unrecognized. For example, Ziegler et al. (2021) report a mean duration of 12.78 years between symptom onset and diagnosis, pointing out that studies show that it can take up to 17 years from the onset of the first symptoms of OCD to the start of adequate therapy. Often OCD is not correctly recognized, and people may receive a wrong diagnosis or treatment. Individuals may also conceal their OCD-related experiences due to shame and/or fear of being stigmatized, which can delay help-seeking or correct identification.

During this time, those with OCD remain unsupported and unable to access the appropriate support, and may be subjected to such additional stressors as unnecessary safeguarding referrals, which reflect professionals' lack of knowledge rather than real risk. This can, of course, still happen, even when someone has been correctly diagnosed. There is little risk that someone with OCD will act on their intrusive thoughts, but unfortunately, some health and social care professionals continue to make unnecessary and potential harmful child safeguarding referrals (Gupta and Kiran 2019). Gupta and Kiran (2019) explain that the most common reasons underlying a safeguarding referral are clinicians' lack of awareness about OCD, inability to do a proper risk assessment before referral, or a risk-averse attitude.

Without careful assessment and detailed knowledge of both OCD and autism, there is a real risk of OCD being missed in Autistic people. This is despite the considerable co-occurrence of OCD in Autistic people. Stone and Chen (2015) explain that there are widely differing estimates of co-occurrence of OCD in Autistic people, but that the rate of 3 to 7 per cent is 6 to 14 times the rate of the general population. Either Autistic experiences become incorrectly viewed through an OCD lens (e.g., needing to walk over drain covers being viewed as a compulsion to relieve anxiety rather than it being part of Autistic routine) **or** are attributed to being Autistic and the OCD is missed (e.g., needing to walk over drain covers because otherwise someone will die).

Clearly, distinguishing between Autistic experience and possible OCD needs careful assessment and collaborative formulation, resisting the temptation to make assumptions about a person's experience and being curious about exploring **why** someone does a particular thing. We also need to hold in mind the same behaviour may serve different purposes at the same time. For example, cleaning the floor with wipes before getting started with any other part of the day could represent Autistic routine, and that it is distressing not to engage in this behaviour because is **the** morning routine, and disruption to that is very unnerving. It may also provide proprioceptive input, be alerting and a necessary part of getting ready to be in the world.

Equally, it could represent the anxiety of OCD, with the factor driving the cleaning being managing perceived risk. For example, the person may experience such thoughts as 'If I don't clean the floor, X, Y and Z will happen', 'It's too dangerous not to clean the floor, X, Y and Z', 'If I don't clean the floor immediately, it means I don't care that I'm responsible for X, Y and Z happening'.

These may simultaneously be true for the Autistic person. The same behaviour may serve different needs on different occasions, or equally, may be appeasing both OCD and Autistic needs at the same time. Assuming that only one of these experiences underlies a behaviour means that the clinician misses the underlying reason and may misinterpret whether this is an area of concern for the person.

When working within a cognitive behavioural framework using exposure and response prevention, clinicians need to pay careful attention to building up the client's energy reserves and attending to the person's wider Autistic needs as the starting point in therapy. Not doing so sets the person up to fail.

The initial assessment piece needs to support the person to attend to and meet their sensory needs, manage their energy reserves, etc. so that they are in the best possible place to tackle exposure and response-prevention tasks. It is essential that clinicians providing therapy around OCD have both expert knowledge of OCD **and** about Autistic experience, and that they dedicate time to careful exploration with the person about their Autistic needs as part of the collaborative formulation. Not doing so runs the risk of blaming the client when therapy is not helpful, instead of recognizing that the approach did not fit the client's needs. Our job as clinicians is to find a mutual wavelength together, not impose our wavelength on the person we are working with. This will take additional effort and attention if you are a non-autistic clinician as you will need to suspend notions of your own wavelength and consciously attune to Autistic experience.

Community and practice-based learning

> In its simplest form...
> Autistic routine gives me spoons. OCD takes spoons. (Anonymous)

Too often clinicians fall into the trap of assuming that anxiety is a fundamental part of the Autistic experience. This assumption often drives Autistic people's exclusion from mental health services and from receiving the support they need. Often Autistic people achieve identification of being Autistic only to be discharged from mental health services as unknowledgeable clinicians begin to frame previously supported anxiety, etc. as 'only' being part of being Autistic, and therefore not meriting treatment or being something that that they can or will support.

It is echoed in the experiences of both adults and children. Time and time again we hear stories that CAMHS (Child and Adolescent Mental Health Services) are 'not commissioned' to provide support to Autistic children and young people. This is discriminatory and reflects a systemic lack of understanding of the Autistic experience and how best to support Autistic people.

Or, if mental health services are deemed to offer therapeutic support, what they offer too often fails to take into account Autistic people's way of being in the world. They may be offered 'standard' CBT for anxiety, understandable given the evidence base and current NICE guidelines supporting its use. However, they are either offered CBT that is delivered with no recognition of Autistic experiences and needs **or** they are offered 'adapted' CBT based on the assumptions of what non-autistic clinicians **think** they need. This is often driven from a deficit-based understanding of Autistic experience, and can end up feeling more unhelpful than having received no support, given the profound mismatch between the therapist's conceptualization of Autistic needs and the lived experience of being Autistic.

What is needed is therapeutic support that holds both our strengths and needs, attends to our sensory and processing needs, and uses them as a fundamental part of the therapeutic process. Non-autistic clinicians need to enter **our** world, our ways of being, of thinking and feeling, and embed these robustly across the whole piece. Non-autistic clinicians need to seek out the Autistic community, learn from it, and ask us what we need. Non-autistic clinicians need to monitor their own responses to the work and be mindful of what assumptions they bring to the therapeutic space (e.g., that people intuitively recognize and understand bodily signals of anxiety and are able to name them). In a time of stretched resources, there may be little time to do this piece. But it is essential. Services need to be flexible in respecting and meeting our needs.

Within clinical practice, the vast and overwhelming majority of people seeking an adult autism assessment have previous experience of anxiety, at both clinical and sub-clinical levels. Those who do not experience anxiety are likely to be already self-identifying as Autistic, have fully embraced their identity, and have chosen or developed work or an occupation to fit their neurology. For many, the anxiety they experience mostly relates to social anxiety, and most often this diagnosis makes sense to the person in the context of their experiences. However, while a diagnosis of social anxiety might make sense to a person in terms of some of their experiences, quite often they feel as though it doesn't account for many other aspects of their experience. For most people attending for autism assessment who experience any form of anxiety, it is typically the case that previously involved clinicians have not questioned or explored what underlying factors might be present that a person's experience of anxiety may relate to. There is a high co-occurrence rate of anxiety in Autistic people and a person will often meet criteria for both, but an Autistic framework occasionally offers a better account of a person's overall experience, including their anxiety experiences.

In terms of differentiating between anxiety (typically social anxiety) and being Autistic, there is much overlap between anxiety experiences and Autistic experiences. In determining whether autism is an underlying factor to an individual's anxiety, it is helpful to consider whether a person's strengths align with Autistic strengths, whether they experience sensory processing differences, and whether they engage in Autistic regulatory self-stimulatory behaviours ('stimming'). Exploring with a person their experiences of these areas will assist in determining whether they are Autistic alongside their experience of anxiety, as these would not typically be expected experiences for a non-autistic person who experiences social or other types of anxiety.

Anxiety is a highly prevalent experience for Autistic people. However, it is extremely important that the causal foundations of anxiety within the context of being Autistic are recognized as being entirely different to the causal foundations of non-autistic anxiety experiences. Anxiety within an Autistic framework is understood in a different way, and therefore requires a different approach in terms of management and support. When a person accesses support for anxiety and it is not understood that they are Autistic, the traditional approach of gradual exposure and working on anxiety management within the moment is experienced as highly stress-inducing for the person, and can be considered as cruel and very exposing. Autistic people have experience of their needs in this regard being poorly understood, and of being labelled 'avoidant'. Careful formulation must take into account Autistic needs and experiences.

Within an Autistic framework of anxiety, the impact of all the demands and expectations of a neurotypical environment needs to be considered and understood. Society is currently designed with the needs of the majority neurotype in mind, with all other neurotypes being expected to adapt. The impact of developing, growing, learning, working, living, communicating, interacting and functioning within an environment that does not accommodate one's neurotype cannot be understated. For Autistic people, the unpredictability and uncertainty, the sensory demands and the expectations around communication all serve to encourage and maintain the experience of anxiety.

Within a non-autistic framework, the approach to anxiety is to learn to tolerate the uncertainty and to be gradually exposed to anxiety-inducing scenarios in an effort to reduce anxiety. Relaxation and deep-breathing techniques are often employed. For Autistic people, approaching anxiety in these ways will likely increase the experience rather than reduce it. Understanding the environmental influence and the impact of living in a society that does not cater for a particular neurotype is key to managing anxiety for Autistic people. Understanding a person's sensory experiences and adjusting the environment to reduce sensory demands can serve to decrease anxiety. Understanding that there are sensory experiences associated with traditional relaxation, mindfulness and breathing techniques that are often intolerable for Autistic individuals, and adapting these approaches to better suit the person's sensory system, is supportive and helpful. Accommodating communication and interaction preferences and recognizing the need for predictability from the perspective of sensory perception can serve to decrease anxiety. If the people and the environment around an Autistic person are changed, anxiety can reduce.

A key component in supporting an Autistic person with anxiety is in identifying or recognizing that they are Autistic. If autism has not yet been considered, then the process of undertaking the assessment and supporting the person to better understand their identity can greatly support them to better understand their anxiety experience, and to learn about what contributes to it and what helps to reduce it. It can also help for the person to gain insight into the role of the environment and society in maintaining their anxiety experience, which can significantly help in reducing the self-blame and associated reduced self-esteem that can accompany anxiety, which does not respond to traditional therapeutic approaches. In considering the double empathy problem, and applying it to the experience of social anxiety within Autistic experiences, the burden of adapting to societal expectations has always been on the Autistic individual, which has led to widespread experiences of very high levels of anxiety among the Autistic population.

What we recommend

- The process of undertaking an autism assessment is often carried out from a neurotypical perspective, with neurotypical expectations in relation to communication and engagement.

- Within our clinical practice, significantly reduced anxiety has been observed when communication and interaction preferences are accommodated. For the vast majority of people, providing detailed advanced information about clinicians (including pictures and videos so that the person can see and hear how a clinician moves and speaks) and about the assessment process (including how many sessions there will be, what will happen in each session, and what will be asked) is extremely helpful in reducing anxiety.

- In order to further support the reduction of anxiety, it is vital that clinicians leave their position of authority or their 'expert' position to the side and approach the process collaboratively. The collaborative nature of the assessment process helps to reduce anxiety, as even if there is a level of uncertainty in relation to determining the outcome, there is trust that both clinicians and clients are working on things together.

- Also consider that most Autistic people like detailed information and explanations in relation to their experiences, and it is therefore important not to overly simplify the formulation of their experiences. The outcome of approaching things in this way is that a person experiences a deeper level of safety and trust with a clinician, and is therefore better able to engage with the assessment process, leading to a more reliable outcome.

Co-Occurring Mood Disorders

Definition

Co-occurrence in a mental health context can be understood and described when a person experiences two or more mental health conditions. The conditions can occur at the same time, or one right after the other.

Research

Research has found co-occurrence of psychiatric disorders in Autistic people is higher than in the general population (Nicolaidis et al. 2020), with some studies suggesting 45 per cent of Autistic people have a co-occurring psychiatric disorder. Research shows that many Autistic people are less likely to agree with co-occurring psychiatric diagnosis, stating that health professionals often confused Autistic features with mental health conditions and have insufficient of autism awareness (Au-Yeung et al. 2019). Mood disorders are one of the most prevalent types of psychiatric conditions that co-occur in Autistic people (Skokauskas and Gallagher 2010). It remains unclear whether these rates are due to misinformation about autism or reflected through co-occurrence (Crane et al. 2021; Skokauskas and Frodl 2015). Research has found rates of co-occurring mood disorder to be significantly higher in the Autistic population than in the neurotypical population (Oakley, Loth and Murphy 2021), with a prevalence rate ranging from 70–80 per cent of Autistic individuals having mental health difficulties (Lever and Geurts 2016), and from 0–56.9 per cent for the co-occurrence of autism and bipolar affective disorder (Skokauskas and Frodl 2015).

Depression features can overlap in observed external presentations of autism, such as reduced facial expressions, 'monotonous' tone of voice (Skokauskas and Frodl 2015), sleep disturbance or social withdrawal (Crane et al. 2021). It remains unclear whether co-occurrence between autism and mood disorder reflects a real or artificial co-occurrence (South et al. 2021). Misinterpretation of Autistic behaviour can occur when diverse communication is not considered. In a society that does not tolerate or accommodate various communication styles, differences in communication and expression may be judged as disruptive. Communicating distress may be judged as challenging behaviour. Restlessness, excitement or aggression can be interpreted as features of a mood disorder instead of Autistic features in a mismatched world. Equally, the trauma and psychological stress of living in an ableist world (one in which Autistic people are often stigmatized and ostracized, have their needs unmet due to society's restrictive design, or have to mask their authentic self) can lead to isolation, loneliness, depression and suicide (Cassidy et al. 2018).

Research shows that there is a familial link between autism and mood disorders, with studies showing high rates of both bipolar and unipolar depression in relatives of Autistic people (Sullivan et al. 2012). There is a lack of Autistic-specific tools to identify co-occurring mood disorders in Autistic people, and psychological interventions have not been validated Autistic people and are based on research with a neurotypical population (Oakley et al. 2021).

In terms of pharmacological intervention, while rates of off-label trial-and-error psychotropic medication use in Autistic people are high (Haker et al. 2016), there remains little research into its effectiveness for Autistic people. Research in the UK found that in contrast to 6.5 per cent of the neurotypical population, a third of Autistic people were prescribed a psychotropic drug (Murray et al. 2014), with 10 per cent being prescribed more than one. Autistic men are 26 per cent less likely to be prescribed a psychotropic drug than Autistic women (Houghton et al. 2018). There is often a mismatch between drug treatment and identified co-occurring conditions (Murray et al. 2014), with the suggestion that clinicians often treat per symptom rather than investigating a diagnosis (Titman 2018).

Suicide and Self-Harm

Camm-Crosbie et al. (2019) note that while Autistic people are at high risk of self-harm and suicidality, there has been little exploration of their experiences of treatment and support around this. In a Special Issue of *Journal of Autism and Developmental Disorders* dedicated to self-harm and suicidality, it was highlighted that early research suggested that not only had 66 per cent of Autistic people contemplated suicide, with 35 per cent planning or attempting suicide (Cassidy et al. 2014), but also that large-scale population studies have demonstrated that Autistic people are more likely to die by self-harm and suicide compared to non-autistic people.

Cassidy et al. (2014) explain that lifetime prevalence of suicidal ideation in Autistic adults ranges between 19.7 and 66 per cent, and suicide attempts between 1.8 and 36 per cent (Haddock and Hagopian 2020), with highest prevalence rates in late-identified adults (Cassidy et al. 2014). Kõlves et al. (2021) conducted a national retrospective study in Denmark of 6,559,266 people aged over 10. They reported that Autistic people were overall over three times more likely to attempt suicide compared to non-autistic people (particularly women, where Autistic women were more than eight times more likely to attempt suicide compared to non-autistic women, with Autistic men being 1.93 times more likely to attempt suicide than non-autistic men). Kõlves et al. (2021) also report that, alarmingly, Autistic people were overall nearly four times more likely to die by suicide compared to non-autistic people (this broke down as Autistic women being 2.63 times more likely to die by suicide, and Autistic men being over three times more likely to die by suicide compared to their non-autistic counterparts). They reported that more than 90 per cent of Autistic people who attempted or died by suicide had a psychiatric co-occurring condition, positing that the social isolation and poor access to healthcare might explain the link between being Autistic and suicide risk. The authors note that results may not necessarily be able to be generalized outside of Denmark. Cassidy et al. (2022) recently examined Coroner's inquest requests of 372 people who died by suicide and interviewed family members, exploring possible autism. They found that 10 per cent of those who died by suicide were likely to be unidentified Autistic people.

Cassidy et al. (2021) stressed that while research has demonstrated that there are higher rates of suicide and self-harm in Autistic people, little research has focused on understanding **why** this is and what the Autistic community's priorities are for support around risk. They reported that what participants described as camouflaging was an independent risk factor for long-term suicidality in their Autistic participants, as were unmet support needs. Costa, Loor and Steffgen (2020) reported that high levels of alexithymia in those with 'high levels of Autistic traits' were associated with increased risk of suicidality, as was use of antidepressants and depression. They stress the importance of considering alexithymia when managing risk in Autistic people. Cassidy et al. (2021) posit that an increased tendency to perseverate on specific thoughts or behaviour, and difficulty imagining alternatives, may increase a sense of being trapped in Autistic people, meaning that suicide is perceived as the only possible means of escape (see, for example, Arwert and Sizoo 2020).

Cassidy et al. (2021) report the Autistic community's 10 priorities for research around suicide and self-harm as being:

1. Exploring the barriers so often encountered by Autistic people when attempting to obtain help and support. These additional barriers can increase suicide risk (and we have often heard in our clinical practice of how difficult it is to get Autistic needs met in crisis).

2. Research on suicide-related risk and protective factors for Autistic people of all ages.

3. Looking at how often Autistic people have their severity of their distress misunderstood or disbelieved when seeking help (and we have heard in our clinical practice how neurotypical clinicians 'misread' Autistic distress and therefore underestimate risk).

4. Research how suicidality across all ages of Autistic people can develop independently of mental health needs.

5. Focus on how best to conduct risk assessment of suicidal thoughts and behaviour in Autistic people in practice and research.

6. Explore adaptations to interventions to ensure they more adequately meet Autistic needs.

7. Examine how Autistic people experience suicidality, and whether this is similar to or different to non-autistic people.

8. Explore Autistic ways of seeking help in crisis (and we hear in clinical practice about the many systemic barriers that exist to obtaining help, e.g., many ways of seeking help in a crisis rely on the ability to make phone calls).

9. Research whether current models that seek to explain suicide in non-autistic people capture Autistic experiences.

10. Research the contribution of poor sleep to Autistic people's risk of suicide.

Community and practice-based learning

Many Autistic people are given a mood disorder diagnosis when they are, in fact, in Autistic burnout. Given many professionals have little understanding of what burnout is, they typically do not consider this as an explanation. In burnout an Autistic person may:

- Have increased sensitivity to sensory input.

- Have more meltdowns or shutdowns.

- Feel more irritable.

- Have more issues with executive functioning.

- Be less able to communicate needs.

- Feel more anxious.

- Feel overwhelmed more easily.

- Have problems sleeping.

- Experience brain fog or forgetfulness.

- Find it hard to manage distressing emotions.

In our experience nearly every client has been diagnosed with one (or more) mental health condition. Anxiety is also commonly experienced linked to Autistic needs and experiences but may occur in addition to this. The risk of services ascribing anxiety as an inevitable part of being Autistic is that Autistic young people and adults may be excluded from services because their anxiety is conceptualized as an inevitable part of being Autistic rather than additional to this. If someone is not responding to standard treatments, it is important that Autism is considered as an explanation. It is important to work on a sensory profile with each person at intake.

What we recommend

- Discuss with clients if autism makes more sense for them rather than another diagnosis.

- A follow-up meeting can assist clients to make more sense of their Autistic experience, which will open up the possibility of reviewing previous diagnoses.

- Undertake a sensory profile at intake to mental health services.

- Autism should be considered at intake.

Eating Disorders

Definition

Beat (n.d.) describes eating disorders as:

> ...serious mental illness affecting people of all ages, gender, ethnicities and backgrounds. People with eating disorders use disordered eating behaviour as a way of coping with difficult situations or feelings. This behaviour can include limiting the amount of food eaten, eating very large quantities of food at once, getting rid of food eaten through unhealthy means (e.g., making themselves laugh, misusing laxatives, fasting or excessive exercise of a combination of these behaviours).

Eating disorders include anorexia nervosa, binge eating disorder, bulimia nervosa, avoidant/restrictive food intake disorder (ARFID) and other specified feeding or eating disorders (OSFED).

Research

Research looking at the relationship between anorexia nervosa and being Autistic provides evidence that one in four of those with anorexia nervosa are also Autistic (Kinnaird et al. 2019), while other research reports a range of 4 to 52.5 per cent of those with anorexia nervosa meet the clinical cut-off for autism (Kerr-Gaffney et al. 2020). When exploring the occurrence between Autistic adults and those with anorexia nervosa, studies suggest that poor self-esteem and social worries mediate the connection between eating disorders and Autistic traits (Kerr Gaffney et al. 2020). Research also suggests that there is a similarity in features and characteristics of both those with the Autistic experience and those with an eating disorder experience, such as challenges with recognizing emotions, as seen in alexithymia, social anxiety, differences in what is considered salient information and social environments as well as similar cognitive patterns such as increased attention to detail and diversity in executive functioning (Kerr-Gaffney et al. 2020).

Kinnaird et al. (2019) suggest that often those who have co-occurring eating disorders and are also Autistic are not picked up as being Autistic prior to having an eating disorder.

Kinnaird et al. (2019) conducted a thematic analysis of the experience of 13 Autistic women with anorexia nervosa in treatment. They identified three themes: problems with adaptions in treatment, the relationship between anorexia and being Autistic, and a common experience being that Autistic styles of thinking (e.g., reluctance for change, preference for sameness) was associated and contributed towards the development of fixed schedules and rituals around food that were difficult to alter. Participants also explained how traditional beliefs about anorexia, such as low self-confidence, body image and desire to lose weight, were less important for them in the development of their eating disorders. They identified issues that were important in the development and trajectory of their eating disorders as including a need for control, sensory differences, dealing with social confusion, executive functioning (e.g., cooking and shopping for food) and eating as a special interest. Many participants identified that the typical treatment timeframe was insufficient for them accessing treatment.

An additional barrier to treatment was sensory differences around food and the issues this presented in re-feeding programmes that did not accommodate for these sensory differences. The women also described a lack of understanding and consideration of the connection between being Autistic and eating behaviours, explaining how challenging it was when a focus was placed on changing what **appeared** to be 'eating disorder behaviours' but which were actually Autistic features. Many felt misunderstood by treatment teams who did not understand Autistic needs, and reported that confusion around meltdowns had led these to be conceptualized as anxiety or indicative of 'borderline personality disorder'.

Participants suggested a range of treatment adaptions that could help, for example, greater flexibility and individualized approaches. The study highlighted the importance of clinicians recognizing and being able to identify autism, which offered greater insight, development of self-awareness and exploration of the connection between being Autistic and having an eating disorder. This also gave participants more confidence to describe their own experience to the clinicians, with this, in turn, being linked to a more positive treatment outcome. Participants also noted the importance of identifying autism when it came to recovery. They explained that while food restriction related to a need for control, it was also connected to being Autistic. Participants expressed doubt about fully recovering since they identified that some eating behaviours reflected their Autistic needs rather than being an eating disorder. Some also stated that the focus should be more on improving good quality of life rather than limiting or eliminating all food-related behaviours.

Other research outlines other barriers to treatment of anorexia nervosa in Autistic individuals, such as the role of context and the characteristics of treatment settings, which are often overloading for Autistic people (e.g., an inpatient setting can often be very sensory overloading). Tchanturia et al. (2020) report coproduced research between professional and Autistic patients that explored adaptions that made a positive difference. These included replacing the colour scheme with neutral colours, making alterations on weekends when many patients went home, decreasing disruptions, de-cluttering of ward spaces, noise reduction adaptions, and supporting sensory differences and control-related anxiety through menu changes that were co-created by patients and dieticians to meet sensory needs (e.g., keeping choices bland, predictable and supported by photographs) as well as being nutritional (Tchanturia et al. 2020).

Community and practice-based learning

There is considerable frustration that clinicians working in eating disorder services do not have expert knowledge about Autistic experience, and similarly, the teams supporting Autistic people do not have specific knowledge about eating disorders. Services are fractured and it is easy to 'fall between the gaps'. While PEACE (Pathway for Eating disorders and Autism developed from Clinical Experience) is a welcome move towards adapting eating disorder treatment for Autistic people, and does well at recognizing sensory issues impacting on eating (e.g., texture, smell, eating environment), it does, however, have a deficit-based formulation of Autistic experience, and describes autism problematically. Viewing Autistic experience like this provides fertile grounds in which an eating disorder can flourish as it centres on the Self as being deficient.

PEACE does not do well looking at interoceptive differences. It assumes we can make sense of our body signals to work out how we feel. Despite the considerable overlap between being Autistic and eating disorders, standard treatment approaches do not often take into account the specific needs of Autistic people (sensory differences, the need for 'sameness', interoceptive differences and disconnection with one's body). Eating disorder treatment protocols do not consider the challenges that interoceptive differences pose in recovery from an eating disorder. We cannot regulate what we cannot recognize, and this applies to both emotional and physical needs. Eating disorder services are also often unaware of how interoceptive differences contribute to the experience of an eating disorder (e.g., not intuitively recognizing hunger, how distressing fullness can be, etc.). They do not often understand eating disorders as embodied experiences and the sensory distress caused when beginning to eat more, for example.

Eating disorder treatment needs to focus to a greater extent on helping individuals develop an understanding of their bodily signals, regardless of neurotype, as this underpins the ability to identify and regulate emotions as well as understand physical state. Without interoceptive awareness, it is very difficult to feel connected to both the self and others.

Standardized protocols, such as MANTRA (Maudsley Model of Anorexia Nervosa Treatment for Adults), posit socio-emotional domain differences related to avoidance of emotions as key to anorexia nervosa, but do not consider how this might be related to Autistic people, and whether this is more an inability to identify emotions due to interoceptive differences.

Many eating disorder services deliver treatment in a group-based format, and this is challenging for Autistic people for many reasons. Services or inpatient staff can easily misunderstand or misinterpret attempts to meet Autistic needs as representing 'eating disorder behaviour'. For example, an Autistic person may feel intensely distressed after eating on the ward and seek proprioceptive input by pacing to help themselves regulate. Staff will typically view this as an attempt to burn off calories and respond 'punitively'. This is, of course, an excellent example of the double empathy problem in action, and demonstrates the need for careful and collaborative formulation.

Reflection Point

- Be mindful that standard treatment protocols need skilful adaption to meet the needs of Autistic clients.

- Do not assume that Autistic people can intuitively identify and name emotions or body signals. What may appear to be 'avoidance' of emotions may reflect interoceptive differences.

- 'Feeling fat' may reflect interoceptive discomfort.

- Formulating Autistic experience using deficit-based language (as in PEACE) reinforces to the person that they are 'deficient' and 'impaired'. It is in that space that an eating disorder can easily flourish. It promotes disconnection from the Self, as the Self as seen as less than, or a problem.

- However, a Neuro-Affirmative approach honours and embraces Autistic differences. The Self is not seen as 'deficient' or less, but as authentically Autistic. This approach supports connection to the Self, and in that space an eating disorder is far less able to flourish.

- Adopting a medical, deficit-based approach closes the door to hope. A Neuro-Affirmative approach is hopeful, and props open that door for the person even if they cannot yet see the potential way forward.

Many Autistic clients describe eating disorders, frequently stressing the contribution of sensory needs to the eating disorder as well as body image issues. They often describe the need for predictability around eating 'same' foods. Standard eating disorder protocols need to be adapted to meet these needs. Addressing an eating disorder means working towards change, and this can be distressing for an Autistic person in itself, let alone when they are so deeply entangled in an eating disorder. It is a change that is painful and uncomfortable to make in terms of addressing eating disorder behaviour, let alone coupled with a need for routine and consistency to meet Autistic needs.

Clients often describe an increase in restrictive eating when life becomes more unpredictable. Restricting may be related to sensory seeking and liking the sensation of hunger. Interoceptive differences can compound eating difficulties due to difficulties in recognizing, understanding and responding to body signals of hunger. There is often an assumption by clinicians that eating disorders centre round a need for control. However, while a (restrictive) eating disorder **may** initially offer a sense of control, this is merely an illusion of control. It does not take long for the eating disorder to become the 'puppet master', creating a vicious cycle as the person feels even more out of control and at the mercy of the eating disorder.

What we recommend

- There should be proper screening for possible eating disorders in all clients.

- If it is known that a client has an eating disorder, then explore the reasons driving eating disorder behaviours, and resist assuming it is driven only by body image concerns.

- Ask about the client's dietary habits as a younger child.

- Give a detailed focus on sensory perception, including taste, smell, interoception, proprioception, etc., including recognition and understanding of hunger signals etc.

- Focus on an individual's life outside of the eating disorder as well.

Attention-Deficit Hyperactivity Disorder

Definition

The DSM-5-TR describes attention-deficit hyperactivity disorder (ADHD) as a persistent pattern of inattention and/or hyperactivity that interferes with a person's functioning or development. It is associated with:

- Inattentiveness (e.g., not giving close attention to detail, difficulty remembering where things were put or needing to spend a lot of time on the details of a task to ensure they are not forgotten, challenges sustaining attention during tedious tasks, difficulty following task instructions, being distractible, problems organizing tasks or activities, procrastination, misjudging how long it takes to complete tasks, ceaseless mental activity, difficulty in filtering and/or selecting information).

- Impulsivity (e.g., difficulty in waiting in turn, being very decisive and making rapid decisions, contributing to conversations before others have finished speaking).

- Hyperactivity (e.g., fidgeting, being physically or mentally restless, particularly when waiting, subjectively always needing to be 'on the go', may be talkative, very active lifestyle, restless sleep).

These may be experienced as a 'combined' type, predominantly 'inattentive' or 'hyperactive-impulsive'.

DSM-5 criteria for adult ADHD include:

- Five or more symptoms of inattention or hyperactivity/impulsivity.

- Several symptoms present by the age of 12.

- Several symptoms present in two or more settings.

- Symptoms interfering with or reducing quality of social, educational or occupational functioning.

- Symptoms are not better explained by another condition, such as mood disorder.

The 18 core symptoms of ADHD are described in the DSM-5. For a diagnosis to be given, an adult requires five symptoms (rather than six, as for a child) of either inattention or hyperactivity/impulsivity (or both, for the combined type). DSM-5 requires that 'several' of these must be present prior to the age of 12 across two or more settings. While ADHD children may appear physically hyperactive, ADHD adults may describe more mental restlessness with very active thought processes. This may be experienced as having thoughts on the go all the time, thoughts jumping from one topic to another, or having multiple lines of thought at the same time. ADHD adults may feel very restless, experience low self-esteem, have difficulty concentrating, often feel overwhelmed, and be distractible.

Research

Faraone et al. (2015) explain that ADHD affects 5 per cent of children and 2.5 per cent of adults worldwide. In children and young people, more males than females have ADHD, but by adulthood this discrepancy almost disappears, which Faraone et al. (2015) suggest may be due to referral biases or sex-specific effects over the course of ADHD. Typically, girls show less hyperactivity/impulsivity than boys, with boys showing more externalizing behaviours (see, for example, Mowlem et al. 2019). Research suggests that 1–2 per cent of adults may have so-called onset of ADHD after the age of 12 (Asherson and Agnew-Blais 2019).

Polanczyk, Casella and Jaffee (2019) suggest that one explanation may be that in adolescence or young adulthood the environmental scaffolds that support a person and provide a buffer are no longer available, and so their needs become fully apparent. They also suggest that those who are ADHD may show as different 'symptoms' earlier in life.

Describing the overlap between other neurodivergencies and specific learning difficulties with ADHD, UKAAN (the UK Adult ADHD Network) cite figures of 41 per cent of Autistic people, 30 per cent of Dyslexic people and 50 per cent of Dyspraxic people. ADHD is a common co-occurring condition in people with ID (around 15 per cent in adults). The previous diagnostic criteria of the DSM-IV did not allow for ADHD to be formally identified in Autistic people, and while there is a body of research regarding the considerable overlap between ADHD and Autistic children (40–70 per cent), there remains relatively little regarding ADHD in Autistic adults (Pehlivandis et al. 2020).

From a qualitative study exploring experiences of identification of ADHD as an adult, Hansson Halleröd et al. (2015) report that adults described having an explanation for a previously inexplicable life history as providing self-knowledge and increased value, but that it could also lead to devaluation and concern about identity. All but one interviewee described identification of ADHD as a positive experience. Participants also highlighted the positives of ADHD, including creativity, passion, quickness and productivity.

Community and practice-based learning

Many people who attend for assessment suspect that they may be both Autistic and ADHD. Where this is the case, there is a significant need for clarity around both diagnoses and whether a person meets the criteria for both. Autistic experiences overlap considerably with ADHD experiences, and from an identity perspective, it is extremely important that a person has clarity around their self-understanding. There are also key differences between Autistic and ADHD experiences, and understanding potentially competing inner urges (e.g., a hyperfocus on one task or topic for an extended period versus attention switching rapidly between different ideas or tasks) is not only vital in terms of identity cultivation, but also essential in terms of managing self-regulation and identifying strategies of support.

A major consideration for the Autistic ADHD community is the potential use of medication in supporting their needs. Medication is not warranted in Autistic people per se, but it can help support executive functioning challenges related to ADHD, if the person experiences these. Accessing medication can be challenging for people whose assessment was carried out by a psychologist and not a psychiatrist. If a person has been assessed by a psychologist, they will need to access a GP (if the GP is willing to prescribe medication) or a psychiatrist to access medication. Quite often, the prescribing clinician will understandably seek to carry out their own assessment prior to prescribing, which can mean a repeat assessment for the person, and the potential additional stress associated with it. Not all people wish to consider medication, with many managing their ADHD-related needs through developing a better understanding of how their nervous system works, and implementing regulation and organizational support strategies. However, where a person wants to consider medication, it is advisable that their assessment takes place with a clinician who can prescribe medication if warranted.

Within the umbrella of neurodivergencies, the ADHD community is one of the largest from a prevalence perspective, with estimates of prevalence varying between 2–7 per cent of the child population, and an average of 5 per cent (Sayal et al. 2018). It is likely that this is an under-estimate, however, as work is undertaken to better understand and identify broader ADHD experiences, for example, the ADHD experiences of girls and woman. Despite being one of the larger identified neurotypes, the advancement of the neurodiversity movement within the ADHD community appears to have been at a slower pace than it has within the Autistic community.

An example of this is illustrated in the language and terminology used within ADHD. 'Attention-deficit hyperactivity disorder' conflicts hugely with the premise of the neurodiversity movement as it implies that ADHD brains are 'disordered'. However, those who experience ADHD are not 'disordered'; rather, they have a unique nervous system that regulates attention and emotions in different ways to non-ADHD people (Dodson 2022). Dodson (2022) states that most ADHD people would prefer not to use the term 'ADHD', as it describes the opposite of their everyday experiences of not having a damaged or defective nervous system, but one that works well according to its own set of rules. The vast majority of ADHD adults are not outwardly hyperactive, but experience internal hyperactivity. ADHD does not mean a shortage of attention, but too much attention being paid and inconsistent attention. Neurotypical brains are not 'better' or 'normal'; rather, their neurology is endorsed and accepted by the world. Dodson (2022) noted that there is a tendency to view ADHD as coming from a defective or deficit-based nervous system, whereas it actually stems from a nervous system that works perfectly well, but according to a different set of rules. Unfortunately, however, the rules it works by are not generally taught or encouraged in the neurotypical world.

From the community perspective, trying to turn those who experience ADHD into neurotypical people should not be the goal of support. Dodson (2022) talks about two approaches that are helpful: (1) level the neurological playing field with medication so that an individual has the attention span, impulse control and ability to calm on the inside; and (2) stop applying neurotypical strategies in approaching tasks and consider the circumstances in which an individual 'gets in the zone' and thrives in their lives. Are they motivated by intrigue or competitiveness? Do they need urgency within a task? Moving the focus from where an individual falls short to how they achieve is more helpful in moving forward, and is reflective of what the ADHD community want to see happening.

Considering ADHD as a neurotype brings up the question about how to refer to people who experience ADHD. Currently, there is no clear distinction within the community about preferred terminology. Does an individual 'have ADHD', or do we say that they 'are ADHD', in the same way we might refer to an individual as 'being

Autistic', and not 'having autism'? For people who are both Autistic and experience ADHD, this lack of clarity on terminology has implications in terms of identity.

In approaching a Neuro-Affirmative assessment with a person whereby the aspects being explored might include both autism and ADHD, there are challenges in maintaining a Neuro-Affirmative approach to the ADHD aspects of the assessment alongside a Neuro-Affirmative autism assessment. If you are a clinician who is carrying out both aspects of the assessment (i.e., both the autism assessment and the ADHD assessment), then maintaining the Neuro-Affirmative framework is a little easier. However, if the individual is undertaking the ADHD part of the assessment with a different clinician in a different service, then it is currently likely that they will move from a Neuro-Affirmative approach within their autism assessment to a medicalized approach to their ADHD assessment. This can be challenging for the person to experience and can feel invalidating. It is therefore important to raise this possibility with the person prior to referral for the ADHD assessment, in order to allow them time to prepare for this, and to recognize the differences in approaches.

A further challenge in maintaining a Neuro-Affirmative approach to ADHD assessment lies in the terminology and language associated with ADHD. As mentioned previously, the word 'disorder' is included in the title, and this needs to be addressed and explained to the individual from a Neuro-Affirmative framework (i.e., that an ADHD nervous system is not 'disordered' but working perfectly, according to a different set of rules). The diagnostic classification systems (DSM-5 and ICD-11) are both medicalized in their approach to defining the criteria for ADHD, with all of the same problems and gaps as there are for autism criteria. In particular, the criteria are very old and primarily based on the experiences of boys, with a distinct lack of understanding and acknowledgement of the experiences of girls and women. Adult ADHD assessment tools that are used and accepted within support services (e.g., the Diagnostic Interview for ADHD in Adults – the DIVA-5) are also primarily deficit-based in their approach. This can be extremely challenging for both clinicians and individuals in undertaking a Neuro-Affirmative approach to assessment.

In undertaking an ADHD assessment alongside an autism assessment with an individual, it is our experience that the different 'traits' associated with ADHD need to be re-framed within a different framework, with a more balanced approach to understanding how an individual's experiences manifest. Re-framing ADHD within a Neuro-Affirmative framework is not just about viewing traits as strengths; it is about recognizing the importance of context, and noting that a particular trait can be a strength or a challenge, depending on the context. For example, 'impulsivity' can be viewed from the perspective of how it helps an individual (e.g., by helping a person to generate lots of ideas and motivating them to try them out), but it can also be viewed as something that might hinder a person (e.g., by making it more difficult to plan the execution of ideas).

In understanding autism and ADHD as different and distinct neurotypes with experiences individual to both, where they both co-occur, there are many unique experiences associated with experiencing both. The co-occurrence rate of ADHD and autism is very high, with approximately 28–44 per cent of Autistic adults also meeting ADHD criteria (Lai et al. 2019). In our practice we wonder about the future possibility of co-occurring autism and ADHD being considered as a neurotype in its own right.

In approaching an assessment relating to both autism and ADHD, it is important to consider the needs and preferences of the individual in gathering information relevant to the assessment. Be aware of different ways to gather information, and recognize that there may be challenges with gathering information in typical formats, such as completing lengthy forms. Difficulties in relation to executive functioning are likely required for those experiencing ADHD, but they are often also present for Autistic individuals, and should therefore not be dismissed as part of an ADHD experience and should be considered for both.

What we recommend

- In undertaking an autism assessment, ADHD should also be considered as a matter of course, and screening should take place routinely.

- Be aware of the need to consider different methods of gathering information as part of an assessment where a person may also experience ADHD.

- Be mindful that ADHD may not show itself in a clinical setting due to the novelty of the situation etc.

- In terms of cultivating identity from a Neuro-Affirmative framework, it is important to support clients to re-frame their experiences to consider the benefits and challenges of particular ADHD traits.

- Where an individual is accessing an ADHD assessment within a different service, support and prepare the person for the likelihood that their ADHD assessment experience may not be Neuro-Affirmative in its approach.

- If an assessment is going to encompass both autism and ADHD from a

Neuro-Affirmative framework, the same principles in re-framing autism to a Neuro-Affirmative framework can be applied to ADHD in terms of classification systems, information gathering, assessment tools and identity cultivation.

Alexithymia

Definition

Alexithymia is a challenge with recognizing what emotions we are feeling (Fletcher-Watson and Happé 2019). It is characterized by difficulties in recognizing emotions from internal bodily states, and is linked to interoceptive difficulties.

Research

Extensive research has shown that emotional processing variations observed in autism are due to alexithymia (Kinnaird, Stewart and Tchanturia 2020). The prevalence of alexithymia is considered higher in the Autistic population. Meta-analysis by Kinnaird et al. (2020), which reviewed 15 studies of self-reported alexithymia using the Toronto Alexithymia Scale, found prevalence rates ranging from 33.3 to 63 per cent in autism. The level of alexithymia is also thought to be elevated in the Autistic population compared to the neurotypical population (Berthoz and Hill 2005), but it is not universal in autism. Rather, it is thought to be a prevalent co-occurring condition common in a subgroup of Autistic people (Kinnaird et al. 2020). Research suggests that alexithymia is a significant contributory **factor** to the development of mental illness (Leweke et al. 2012).

Rates of mental illness, particularly anxiety and depression, are alarmingly high in the Autistic population. A recent systematic review of co-occurring depression and anxiety in Autistic people found that 27 per cent currently have a depressive disorder and 37 per cent will have a depressive disorder throughout their lives (Hollocks et al. 2019). There is limited evidence suggesting that Autistic traits are not directly connected to depressive symptoms but mediated through alexithymia, a more significant risk factor for the high rates of depression in autism (Fietz, Valencia and Silani 2018).

However, a major limitation of findings linking alexithymia to autism is that much research fails to control for co-occurring depression and anxiety, which is related to alexithymia, and is highly prevalent in the Autistic population (Bloch et al. 2021). There is a high degree of co-occurring alexithymia in the Autistic population.

However, the mechanisms behind Autistic alexithymia need further research. What is clear is that prevalence is high. There may be a need for specific understanding and support for the subgroup of Autistic people presenting with co-occurring alexithymia. Consideration needs to be given in the form of alexithymia screening for all Autistic people in clinical settings to recognize and provide support to those with co-occurring alexithymia, who may be at risk of developing further co-occurring mental health conditions related to alexithymia (Kinnaird et al. 2020). Programmes have also been developed to help people with alexithymia better interpret emotional processing, such as therapy designed to reinterpret situations emotionally (Gross 2015), and treatments designed to promote interoceptive awareness (Gaigg, Cornell and Bird 2018). There is recognition of the need for Autistic-tailored solutions that understand the Autistic experience and Autistic perception, and embrace this in the development of support systems. Neuro-Affirmative creative therapies – such as music, art and bodily expression that do not rely on the medium of speech – can address alexithymia (Poquérusse et al. 2018).

Community and practice-based learning

Alexithymia can make it difficult for a person to interpret body changes as emotional responses (e.g., someone may have trouble linking a racing heart to excitement or fear while still being able to acknowledge that they are experiencing some kind of physiological response). It can make it difficult to both recognize feelings and communicate how they feel to others. This can lead to misunderstanding and confusion, as it is very difficult to share, be understood and receive support if they cannot put words to their feelings. Emotions may be identified in a general sense of being 'positive' or 'negative', but it may also feel that so many emotions are being experienced at once that it feels overwhelming and impossible to identify what is being felt and why.

It can be very difficult, invalidating and traumatic when other people do not understand or comprehend individual ways of expressing different emotions. Clinicians need to explore how each person expresses emotions, not assume they have a lexicon, and find a way to communicate about emotions together. A potential roadblock in therapy is clinicians not understanding that someone simply does not know how they feel, let alone being able to support their client with this.

Mahler and Vermeulen (2021) point out that we need to understand mental states in **ourselves** before we can know what others feel, and that we need to nurture our ability to understand ourselves. They refer to this as 'theory of own mind'. We have seen how interoception is the foundation of feeling and understanding our emotions. It is our body that gives us crucial information about our emotional state and gives meaning to emotion words. We cannot regulate what we cannot recognize. We also need to be able to recognize our body state within **context**. For example, the clues that our stomach sensations are giving us vary according to context (e.g., we might not have eaten so are hungry, we might be in a new situation so feel anxious), and this alters what actions we take so that we can regulate ourselves. Research has shown that people with good interoceptive awareness are better at 'reading' other people's emotions as well as their own. So boosting our interoceptive awareness not only helps us understand ourselves better, but also other people. For example, using fMRI (functional magnetic resonance imaging), Bird et al. (2010) reported that people with reduced interoception reflected in high levels of alexithymia showed reduced activation in insular cortices while reflecting on both emotions and empathizing with others who were feeling pain.

What we recommend

- Recognize that for some clients describing emotions and feelings can be more difficult.

- Do not assume that all clients have an emotional language. It is the clinician's responsibility to check out with a client that they recognize body signals linked to emotions.

- Check out that you and your client have a shared understanding of what 'anxiety' etc. means. Your experience of anxiety and how your body feels it may be different to your client's.

Reflection Point

Clinicians often assume that if someone **uses** an emotion word, they **know** the feeling. However, there is a difference between **labelling** a feeling, **knowing** how it actually feels and **recognizing** that feeling in our body. For example, a child might say they feel 'very sad' every bedtime, but it may be that they actually feel completely exhausted (i.e., misinterpreting **and** mislabelling sensations). We need to know both the **semantics** of complex emotions as well as the **embodied experience** of them.

It is the clinician's job to explore what their client's understanding and experience of different emotions is **for them**: one person's embodied experience of anxiety, for example, will be very different to someone else's. There is no one way of experiencing an emotion. Non-autistic clinicians will need to pay extra attention to make sure they are not placing neurotypical assumptions onto the recognition, understanding and causes of different emotional states in their Autistic clients.

Assisting Communication/Non-Speaking Autistic People

Definition

Any method that involves supporting a disabled person to point to a letterboard or to type on a tablet or keyboard can be considered 'assisted communication'. One form of assisted communication is known as facilitated communication. This involves a support person providing various degrees of physical support, which is slowly faded. The goal is the most independence possible.

RPM (Rapid Prompting Method) and S2C (Spelling to Communicate) begin with large letter boards, which transition eventually to a keyboard. In the RPM and S2C methods, there is no physical guidance or touch at all with the person. Goals are as much independence as possible. These methods are all based on a principal of presumed competence.

People with motor difficulties can also have difficulties with speech, as speech is a motor skill. However, just because someone cannot speak it should not be assumed that they have cognitive impairments so significant that they cannot understand or communicate. The inability to use speech has traditionally been linked with a presumed reduction in cognitive functioning.

Research

AAC technologies have been used to support Autistic people's communication since the 1980s (Hines, Balandin and Togher 2011). However, AAC is often designed only for Non-Speaking Autistic children, and only to address functional communication (Zisk and Dalton 2019), and there remains a strong need for AAC to be designed for Autistic children and Autistic adults who experience intermittent speaking, or find they need other methods to accompany their use of the spoken language (Kudryashov 2021). These people are often not considered in AAC research design or provision.

AAC technologies range from basic low technology tools (e.g., communication cards and picture boards) to more high-tech technologies (e.g., smartphone and tablet apps) as well as specific variables, sign and gesture languages. Research into AAC for intermittent-speaking Autistic adults is under-researched, and recent research has shown that for Autistic adults, AAC can have a positive effect on wellbeing and access to things such as social participation, education, healthcare and employment.

From participatory research with five Autistic adults, Kudryashov (2021) identified that social stigma was a big challenge to accessing and productive use of AAC. The effect of social stigma had a negative impact on Autistic individuals' sense of agency. Research has identified that security and privacy are essential features of AAC technology, but despite this, they are often lacking.

Participants in Kudryashov's research identified 27 elements that were important in AAC technology, with privacy being the top priority, especially in contexts such as healthcare, and professional and employment settings such as for Autistic lawyers who use AAC. Participants also highlighted the importance that security and data control were accessible and under the control of the AAC user, not the professionals or guardian or app manufactures. Kudryashov (2021) suggests that this is why participants preferred dedicated and reliable devices for AAC such as wearables rather than an app on a smartphone, as this meant they had more control over its security.

Other essential elements identified included saving specific phrases and choosing between multiple languages and more intuitive interfaces. Not relying on an internet connection or dealing with a low battery was also highlighted. A way to individualize tones to express emotions, predictive text and including words to talk about abuse and vocabulary that was more relevant to adults was also noted as essential elements.

Participatory research by Donaldson et al. (2021) identified the importance of access to AAC for everyone, not just as a final option for children who do not meet neurotypical-defined milestones concerning spoken communication or as a device solely to address functional speech, but to ensure equality of communication and access for all Autistic adults, to develop not only functional communication but also rich dialects without stigma. Many of Donaldson et al.'s (2021) participants highlighted that AAC was something that they found as adults and that they used spoken languages as children, as access to AAC was often restricted. Donaldson et al. (2021) explain this as a loss of choice and a force of communication towards speaking rather than exploring the benefits of AAC. Participants reported that they had very little accessibility to forms of communication that were not the spoken language, and that AAC was often only offered as a last resort.

Participants in Donaldson et al.'s (2021) study also described how it would be good if AAC was available to all Autistic individuals regardless of their use of speech, and that increased accessibility and considering diverse forms of communication as valid and vital would be a significant positive paradigm shift from seeing AAC as unfavourable or something to be wary of or avoided. It would be a positive empowering change to recognize AAC as valid and as accepted as spoken communication. This would increase accessibility and increase agency for those who may have been discouraged from using AAC in the past.

Community and practice-based learning

There are huge numbers of non-identified Non-Speaking or minimally speaking Autistic people who have lived a life of trauma and unmet needs, with multiple and repeated experiences of being presumed incompetent. We need to acknowledge how ableist assumptions about people who do not use mouth words as a primary form of communication drive the services that they receive. For example, GPs may deny them a referral for an autism assessment, questioning what difference identification of Autistic identity might make when they already receive services.

Clinicians working with someone who uses any form of AAC, paper-based or speech-generating, need to see that as a body part. It is part of the person's communication toolkit so that they can autonomously communicate using words or the AAC. For an AAC user, this is part of who they are, part of their identity, part of their body, and so must be respected as such. Too often, professionals will look over the person's shoulder while they are generating a sentence, which is very off-putting. There is an etiquette. If the person is typing a sentence on an AAC app or text, their communication partner should not look over their shoulder or anticipate the end of the person's sentences. Clinicians also need to respect the additional cognitive and physical labour that it takes to produce an utterance on AAC. The amount of time to deliver the intended message is significantly increased, meaning that therapy and assessment time could be doubled. Fatigue involved in communicating using AAC needs to be factored in.

Some people are part-time AAC users and will use text messages and speech assistant as tools to help express when they cannot access mouth words. There are many adults who would benefit from knowing about this technology, so they do not always have to labour to produce mouth words when it is simply not an option available to them. It is important to explore this option with clients, and explain that it is entirely valid to use mixed modes of communication at different times.

One of the biggest myths and preconceptions to debunk is that being non-speaking means non-thinking. If you are working with a client who has multiple disabilities, such as someone with cerebral palsy who is coming for an autism assessment and is not able to produce speech easily, this does not mean they are not capable of intelligent thought. Do not infantilize them.

It can be extremely liberating to realize that mouth words do not need to be the only means by which to communicate. There are many other ways. If an Autistic person has many responsibilities, and perhaps little support with those, they may feel on the verge of a meltdown and struggle to produce speech. Recommending part-time AAC use to all people is very helpful, and there are many apps available to support this.

There is a long history of people with communication differences being presumed incompetent and treated like a child, with an associated lifetime of trauma and being misunderstood. Sometimes AAC may have been introduced later in their life, and they may experience stigma associated with its use, or trauma in relation to how communication partners respond to AAC use. If a Non-Speaking or minimally speaking person attends for a health appointment with AAC, the most important aspect is the relationship between the clinician and the client being respectful and based on trust. An AAC user is unlikely to risk using their AAC with someone they do not trust or feel safe with.

Clinicians should respect the AAC as an integral part of the person. AAC is part of a full multimodal communication toolkit, and can be used when the person needs or wants to be an autonomous communicator. When interacting with an AAC user, the other person should look at both the person and the AAC to value both. Do not touch the AAC without being asked or given permission (consider rules about touching another's body to apply to the AAC). It is important to remember that some AAC devices have mechanical sounding voices; this is outside the control of the AAC user, and it is rude and insulting to complain about this. AAC cannot produce tone, so misinterpretations may occur. Interpret communication literally, and seek clarification if necessary.

Medical Issues

Research

Research has shown that Autistic individuals experience an increased level of co-occurring medical conditions compared to the general population. Epilepsy is common in the Autistic population. Research suggests that there is a diversity in brain development when comparing Autistic individuals to the general population. Research relying mainly on Autistic male children has found that there are structural and connectivity differences in the Autistic population, such as diversity in cortical thickness and hippocampal volumes, the amount of cerebrospinal fluid (CSF), grey matter volume and developmental trajectories of neurobiological processes often lasting longer into adulthood and being less fixed (Braden et al. 2017; McAlonan 2004; Raznahan et al. 2010).

Epilepsy is a condition of the central nervous system. Abnormalities in brain activity are thought to cause epileptic seizures. In their systematic review, Liu et al. (2021) provided evidence that epilepsy is more prevalent in the Autistic population than in the general population. They also found that rates of epilepsy were higher among Autistic adults than Autistic children. They found that 1 in 10 Autistic individuals has epilepsy, and that epilepsy increases with age, gender (increasing for females) and co-occurring ID.

Another common medical condition that co-occurs with autism at higher rates than the general population is Ehlers-Danos syndrome (EDS) and hypermobile Ehlers-Danos syndrome (hEDS). EDS and hEDS can affect proprioception, resulting in such symptoms as increased fatigue and pain. Research into children with EDS and hEDS have found it to co-occur at a higher rate in children with ADHD and children who are Autistic (Kindgren, Quiñones Perez and Knez 2021). In Kindgren et al.'s study (2021), they found that three times more than the expected rate of those with hEDS and EDS had co-occurring ADHD and an estimated twice the expected rate were Autistic. Autistic children and ADHD children with co-occurring hEDS also experienced increased symptoms, such as high rates of fatigue, urinary tract problems and sleep disorders. Kindgren et al. (2021) did, however, find that Autistic and ADHD children with co-occurring h/EDS did not have more pain.

Similarly to a diagnosis of autism in birth-identified females, Kindgren et al. (2021) found that a large number of girls in their study did not seek out medical care until after puberty, and that boys as compared to girls were diagnosed on average two years earlier. They found that the peak age of diagnosis for males was 5 to 9 years, while for girls it was 15 to 19 years (Kindgren et al. 2021). In a national Swedish population-based study looking at EDS and hEDS, those with different neurodivergencies and psychiatric conditions, they found that Autistic individuals, individuals with bipolar, ADHD and schizophrenia had an increased risk ratio of having co-occurring EDS and hypermobility syndrome (Cederlöf et al. 2016). Casanova et al. (2018) found that Autistic women have increased rates of co-occurring generalized joint hypermobility and EDS. In their study they explored Autistic women's experience of immune system and endocrinology symptoms as well as experience of pain and history of seizures. Their study showed that Autistic women with generalized hypermobility experienced more immune system and endocrinology conditions compared to those who did not have generalized joint hypermobility.

Casanova et al. (2020) suggest that hEDS, similar to autism, may be related to proprioceptive diversity, leading to differences in coordination and posture, but also in the acquisition of spoken communication, and this may point to a distinct subtype of autism or of Autistic presentation that is a presentation of those with co-occurring hEDS who are Non-Speaking. They also point out that autism and EDS/hEDS share similarities as they are both on a spectrum and share similar co-occurring neurological psychiatric and neurobehavioral co-occurrences such as mood disorders, anxiety, proprioception differences and ADHD as well as eating disorders, epilepsy and similar neurobiological brain differences, which, taken together, may represent a subtype of autism. Further research is needed to understand more.

Specific Learning Difficulties: Dyslexia

Definition

The British Dyslexia Association (BDA) draws on the definition of Dyslexia as described in the Rose (2009) report, *Identifying and Teaching Children and Young People with Dyslexia and Literacy Difficulties*, as a learning difficulty that affects skills involved in accurate and fluent word reading and spelling, phonological awareness, verbal memory and verbal processing speed. It can occur across a range of intellectual abilities and is best thought of as a continuum. The BDA also notes that Dyslexia can potentially be accompanied with differences in aspects of language, motor coordination, concentration and organization.

Made by Dyslexia is a Dyslexic-led organization aimed at redefining and promoting understanding and strengths of Dyslexia. They suggest an alternative definition of Dyslexia as being:

> a genetic difference in an individual's ability to learn and process information. As a result, Dyslexic individuals have differing abilities, with strengths in creative, problem-solving and communication skills and challenges with spelling, reading and memorising facts (Made by Dyslexia 2021).

Research

Around 20 per cent of people are Dyslexic (Shaywitz, Shaywitz and Shaywitz 2021). There is little detailed research exploring the connection between autism and Dyslexia. Common overlaps include differences in communication. Extant research is mixed regarding rates of Autistic individuals meeting diagnostic criteria for Dyslexia.

Intriago, Rodríguez and Cevallos (2021) suggest that Autistic children are no more likely to be Dyslexic compared to their non-autistic peers, but note it may be harder to pick up Dyslexia for a variety of reasons. Huang et al. (2020) explains that a gene (DOCK4) is shared between autism and Dyslexia. Brimo et al. (2021) summarize research regarding the overlap between Dyslexia and other neurodivergencies, citing between 25 and 40 per cent of ADHDers as also being Dyslexic, but note that the relationship between autism and Dyslexia is more complex. They explain that around 12 per cent of Dyslexic children are also Autistic, but note the wide range of reading skills in Autistic children. Many adults may have learned to 'get around' any challenges with reading, etc., and clinicians should be mindful that those attending assessment appointments might have undetected Dyslexia.

What we recommend

- As Dyslexia relates to information-processing differences and can impact on organization skills, be mindful of how best to support a Dyslexic person during assessments, for example, ensuring all written material, including formal assessment measures, are accessible to them and that adjustments are made as required to support processing of information.

- Clearly, all individuals will have a different pattern of strengths and needs related to their Dyslexia. It is helpful to support individuals to identify their unique pattern of strengths (e.g., strong visual and creative skills, ability to approach problems from a different perspective).

- The interested reader may wish to read *The Value of Dyslexia* report (2019) for a strengths-based description of Dyslexia.

Specific Learning Difficulties: Dyscalculia

Definition

Dyscalculia is classified as a specific learning difficulty in the DSM-5 (APA 2013), and is described as difficulty with producing, understanding quantity, mathematical symbols or operations (e.g., addition, subtraction) that would be otherwise unexpected (e.g., due to a person's age or educational experience).

The BDA describes Dyscalculia as: 'A specific and persistent difficulty in understanding numbers which can lead to a diverse range of difficulties with mathematics. It will be unexpected in relation to age, level of education and experience and occurs across all ages and abilities' (n.d.).

Research

There has been less research and fewer resources focused on Dyscalculia compared to Dyslexia, but it is estimated that between 3 to 7 per cent of children and adults have Dyscalculia (Haberstroh and Schulte-Körne 2019). The Dyslexia-SpLD Trust note that there are no figures related specifically to adults. They also point out that many adults and children go undiagnosed due to limited understanding of Dyscalculia. Dyscalculia can impact on multiple areas of daily life, including managing money, following a diary and keeping track of time. Unrecognized and unsupported it can result in difficult educational experiences and challenges in daily life.

Dyscalculia often occurs with other forms of neurodivergency. Soares and Patel (2015) explain that between 17 and 70 per cent of children with Dyscalculia have Dyslexia, and that 11 per cent are ADHD. Haberstroh and Schulte-Körne (2019) also cite the overlap between Dyslexia (30–40 per cent) and ADHD (10–20 per cent). From a study of 2241 primary school children, Morsanyi et al. (2018) identified 5.7 per cent as having a profile of specific learning difficulties related to maths, with about half of these having a language or communication difficulty, noting that some of these children were Autistic or had ADHD.

What we recommend

- Overall, however, while the literature makes reference to the overlap between Autistic experience and Dyscalculia, it is hard to find any specific figures to illustrate this relationship further. Be vigilant to the possibility of co-occurring Dyscalculia, and do not assume that lack of diagnosis means lack of difficulty in this area, particularly given the overall relative lack of recognition and understanding of Dyscalculia.

Specific Learning Difficulties: Developmental Co-Ordination Disorder (Dyspraxia)

Definition

The DSM-5 (APA 2013) diagnostic criteria for Developmental Co-Ordination Disorder (DCD) includes motor performance that is substantially below the expected level, causing a 'disturbance', which, without accommodations, significantly and persistently interferes with activities of daily living or academic achievement. 'Symptoms' must start in the early developmental period. Motor skill 'deficits' need not to be better explained by ID or visual impairment, and not be attributed to a neurological condition affecting movement.

Movement Matters is a group formed in the UK in 2011 to represent several organizations (including DCD-UK, the Dyspraxia Foundation and the National Handwriting Association). They produced a consensus statement describing DCD as a common disorder that affects fine and/or gross motor coordination in children and adults, formally recognized by international organizations. They describe it as distinct from other motor disorders such as cerebral palsy, and note that the range of intellectual ability is in line with the general population. Dyspraxic traits can vary and may change over time, depending on environmental demands and life experiences. Dyspraxia persists into adulthood. Social emotional difficulties can be present, as well as difficulties with time management, planning and organization, which can impact education and employment.[7]

To balance the difficulties highlighted in these definitions, it is helpful to consider the strengths of those with DCD, as explained in *Teaching for Neurodiversity: A Guide to Specific Learning Difficulties* report (Dyspraxia Foundation 2016), which include being tenacious, creative, empathetic, kind, sensitive and often good at drama, singing or creative activities.

Research

It is estimated that 5 to 6 per cent of children have DCD (Rainer et al. 2019). DCD can lead to significant challenges in activities of daily living or school. Adults may often report issues with executive functioning, attention, anxiety and depression, and low self-esteem (Rainer et al. 2019).

Lachambre et al. (2021) explain that ADHD frequently co-occurs with DCD (co-occurring in approximately 50 per cent of children), and autism is also common (30 to 50 per cent concomitance). Over 79 per cent of Autistic children have movement difficulties, which is consistent with DCD (Rosenblum et al. 2019), although many of these may not have had a full clinical assessment. Bhat (2020) notes the importance of motor screening, assessment and intervention for children following a formal autism diagnosis, given that 86.9 per cent of children in the SPARK study fell into the 'at risk for motor challenges' category on the screening measure used, yet only a third were receiving any physical therapy sessions. This study relied on a parent-completed screening measure rather than clinical assessment, but does indicate the large proportion of Autistic children who also

---

7   UK DCD Consensus Meetings, 28 October 2011 and 19 January 2012.

have motor challenges. Another report from the SPARK study (Best 2020) states that of 10,234 Autistic children aged between 5 and 15, 85 per cent had DCD questionnaire scores consistent with being 'at risk for DCD' while only 14 per cent had a formal diagnosis. High rates are reported by Miller et al. (2021), who retrospectively reviewed standardized assessments and parent reports of 43 Autistic children, finding that over 90 per cent met diagnostic criteria for co-occurring DCD.

Camden et al. (2022) conducted a systematic review of articles published between 2013 and 2019, including studies involving Autistic children with and without DCD, comparing autism and DCD, or providing specific recommendations on seeking DCD diagnosis in Autistic children with motor difficulties. From the 11 studies they included, they found that few recommendations were included giving guidance about seeking a DCD diagnosis for children with motor challenges. They concluded that more research is needed to inform guidelines for clinical practice about pursuing a DCD diagnosis in clinical practice in Autistic children, and highlight the need to be needs-based, not diagnostic-driven.

What we recommend

- Motor challenges are common in Autistic children and adults, but it is not clear how many would reach diagnostic criteria given many may not have been given the opportunity for formal assessment. There is the risk of diagnostic overshadowing such that motor challenges are attributed to autism without proper consideration and assessment. Clinicians assessing adults or children need to be mindful not to simply attribute motor challenges to autism in the absence of proper clinical assessment by appropriate professionals.

- Growing up as the child who is 'clumsy', 'accident prone' or the one needing additional help with tasks that others complete seemingly with ease can leave a lasting legacy, and counter-balancing that narrative needs careful attention during assessment and subsequent support.

11

How to Make Your Assessment Accessible

Accessing an assessment in a timely and supportive manner is of critical importance to people who are wondering if, or who are relatively certain that, they are Autistic. While self-identification is generally wholeheartedly accepted within the Autistic community, some would prefer, for personal or practical reasons, to seek a formal assessment. For this cohort of people, a formal assessment can bring significant clarity, self-understanding, validation, relief, liberation and self-compassion. It can give access to supports, accommodations and therapies that might otherwise be inaccessible without a formal assessment.

For those who are working with a therapist or other clinician, and where it is the professional they are working with who identifies and raises the possibility that they may be Autistic, having access to an assessment that can clarify whether this is the case or not is extremely important. It can be intensely stressful for many to tolerate the uncertainty of the raised possibility of whether they are Autistic or not, especially if they do not intuitively know the answer themselves.

For many people, establishing and processing the likelihood that they require an assessment can take some time and support. When they have determined that an assessment is required and have worked through the next stage of establishing that they wish to pursue one, the third stage of sourcing, accessing and waiting for an assessment can be highly challenging and stressful for many, for multiple reasons. In most countries, there are two pathways to assessment – via the public health system or via private services. In some countries, there is no access to assessment via the public health system, and private pathways are the only option. This is an unacceptable situation and needs to be addressed so that everyone has the opportunity to access timely assessments, as delays to identification can lead to worse mental health outcomes for Autistic people.

Each pathway (public or private) unfortunately has its own challenges in terms of accessibility. Some of the challenges relate to system challenges and some to there being a lack of accommodations in place to make assessments accessible. There are also financial considerations and challenges to overcome in relation to the availability of appropriate and Neuro-Affirmative expertise. As practitioners, it is imperative to be aware of what the barriers to accessing assessment are, and to establish what can be adjusted in order to improve equity of access.

Barriers to Accessing Assessment

It is clear that Autistic people encounter many more barriers in accessing physical and mental health care than neurotypical individuals (Doherty et al. 2022; Mason et al. 2019b). This typically leads to worse outcomes for Autistic people in terms of most medical conditions, co-occurring mental health conditions (Croen et al. 2015; Cashin et al. 2018) and suicidality (Lever and Geurts 2016) when compared to the general population. These outcomes are likely even more significant for those who are unaware they are Autistic or who have found accessing a formal assessment prohibitive.

In clinical practice it is clearly often the case that many of the challenges many adults experience before being identified as Autistic improve over time once they are identified as Autistic and are supported in learning about their Autistic identity. It is therefore vital that the barriers to accessing assessments are better understood and a process is put in place to reduce and/or remove them.

The most common areas in which benefits to identification as Autistic are noted include a person's sense of identity, accessing appropriate mental health supports within an Autistic framework, accessing accommodations within educational and workplace settings, enhancement of family relationships and access to financial supports. Access to appropriate, tailored support can empower people, increase autonomy and facilitate inclusion in social networks and wider society, leading to a more hopeful future.

In considering the barriers people encounter when trying to access assessments, there are three areas to explore. The first relates to factors within the system(s) in which a service provider is operating, the second relates to factors associated with the service providers themselves, and the third relates to specific barriers associated with individual preferences in relation to communication and interaction not being understood and/or supported (the double empathy problem, see Chapter 4).

System factors

Most Autistic people are adults, do not have a co-occurring ID, and are likely to be undiagnosed (Berney 2020), and so one of the most significant barriers to being identified as Autistic is the underestimation by medical and clinical professionals of the number of Autistic clients already accessing physical and mental health services (Zerbo et al. 2015). There is repeated anecdotal evidence of individuals accessing mental health services, and sometimes physical health services, with co-occurring mental and physical health needs, and the possibility of the person being Autistic is not considered by the service. This is despite there often being a high likelihood that an individual is Autistic, and that knowing this offers a different framework for understanding and addressing many co-occurring mental and physical health needs. In both The Adult Autism Practice and in Thriving Autistic, this is something that is reported exceptionally frequently, with many clients having engaged with several different services and having seen a variety of different professionals, and the possibility of them being Autistic has not been noticed or explored. Frequently, it is the individuals themselves who realize the possibility and begin to explore it.

Within many countries, there is no dedicated public service pathway to access an assessment. For countries that do have a public pathway to access assessments, the waiting times are often so long that they are prohibitive. The complexity of navigating the public and private systems within any country can be extremely challenging. Accessing a public assessment often requires a formal GP referral, which can be difficult to obtain for various reasons, such as challenges liaising with medical personnel and a lack of knowledge or awareness among medical personnel about Autistic experiences and the need for further assessment. Where there is no public route to assessment, or where the waiting time is significant, individuals have the option of a private assessment. However, the cost of undertaking a private assessment is often significant and unaffordable for many, and geographical factors in accessing an assessment can also create challenges where an in-person assessment is the only option available.

It is important to be mindful that public services for adults are unlikely to be well coordinated. It is therefore possible for individuals to be 'passed around' from one service to another, and to fall between services, particularly for adults who do not have co-occurring ID or significant mental health issues, as they may be denied access to supports offered by disability and general mental health services. It is also often the case that individuals with mental health issues experience challenges in accessing Autistic supports, due to diagnostic overshadowing and lack of consideration being given to Autistic experiences when a mental health diagnosis is already present.

Service provider factors

Sourcing and accessing professionals with the necessary skillset and understanding of Autistic experiences can be hugely challenging for many people seeking an assessment and seeking support following self-identification or formal identification. It can be even more challenging to source and access professionals with good understanding and knowledge of Autistic experiences in multimarginalized groups, for example the LGBTQIA+ community, racial ethnicities, etc. Training courses are often outdated or a professional possibly hasn't undertaken any further training since their initial training.

There is a particular challenge in sourcing and accessing neurodivergent professionals, as there are many barriers to neurodivergent people pursuing professional training, and for those who are currently working professionally, there are many barriers in disclosing their neurodivergence. This is a core aspect of why Thriving Autistic was founded – to cultivate a supportive space for neurodivergent professionals to practice in an environment where they would not be subjected to prejudice, to connect self-identified or formally assessed neurodivergent adults with support service professionals who truly understand their needs from an insider perspective of shared experience, and to educate and train mental health professionals on how to adapt clinical offerings to better serve the neurodivergent community.

Many people have unfortunately had the experience of being misdiagnosed and misunderstood in their past encounters with professionals and services, which frequently leads to a trauma experience, an understandable mistrust of professionals, and a potential risk of re-traumatization in exposing themselves to further professionals who may not have the necessary expertise to understand and recognize their Autistic experiences. A fear of not being believed or of not being listened to in relation to their experiences is the most frequently cited and most significant barrier to accessing an assessment for most individuals (Lewis 2017). Related to this, many people also describe having spent all of their lives masking Autistic traits and being perceived by others as 'coping', when they are, in fact, internally really struggling. As a result, many report their concern about being Autistic and their Autistic traits not being 'observed' by a professional – a valid concern if observation-based assessment tools are primarily being relied on by the clinician (see the section on 'masking and camouflaging' in Chapter 10).

Many people have had negative experiences with mental health services and have encountered a lack of knowledge about Autistic experiences and misdiagnoses, and have been hugely misunderstood by non-autistic professionals. The lack of knowledge and misdiagnoses are mostly borne from a double empathy problem where the individual's experiences are framed from the perspective of the service and are located as 'problems' within the individual as opposed to a mismatch between different neurotypes (see Chapter 4). This double empathy issue may also contribute to why so many Autistic people feel that a safe connection with clinicians during assessment processes is not established, and can feel misunderstood and disregarded by many non-autistic professionals.

When accommodations are not provided

Many services continue to hold the expectation that a person must approach and engage with the service via mostly neurotypical methods of communicating and engaging, without providing appropriate accommodations for Autistic communication and engagement or choice for people in relation to how they most comfortably communicate and engage. The level of accommodation and provision by services of different options for communicating and engaging is extremely poor. One study found that only 25 per cent of primary healthcare providers reported high confidence in communicating with Autistic adults or in identifying and making necessary accommodations to support Autistic people to access their services (Nicolaidis et al. 2020). Most health and mental health care settings are organized with the prevailing needs of neurotypical people in mind, including many of those that offer assessments and services to Autistic adults.

Many clinical settings expect there to be spoken communication ability to arrange appointments via phone calls, to communicate during appointments and to infer meaning that might only be implied during spoken consultations (Lehmann and Leavey 2017), and there is blatant disregard for the fact that a significant number of people find spoken communication extremely challenging.

It is imperative when engaging in assessment work with potentially Autistic adults that Autistic communication is valued and held at the core of the assessment process. Some Autistic people experience auditory processing differences and executive functioning challenges, both of which can make spoken communication (either by phone or in conversation) significantly challenging and unpredictable. Some Autistic people experience visual processing differences, which can make written communication more challenging. Differences in perception and communication can make phone calls unpredictable. It can also be significantly challenging for a person to advocate for their own communication needs where they may not be aware of what their needs are after a lifetime of becoming used to having to adapt to neurotypical preferences.

There is a distinct lack of research exploring the need for diversity within communication and engagement methods provided by healthcare services, the dominant view within the literature appearing to suggest that

Autistic communication in broader society is less valued than neurotypical communication (Lehmann and Leavey 2017), with this pattern appearing to be similar in healthcare settings. This does not mean that diversity within communication is not needed; it means that it is not being valued. There is a double empathy issue here, which interferes with individuals being able to access assessments. It is a double empathy problem that Autistic communication is not valued, understood or accommodated by services in supporting individuals to access assessments, and providing only neurotypical methods for communicating and engaging is prohibiting access. In this scenario, the person cannot engage with the service and the service cannot engage with the person.

Although for some, not being able to access an assessment in a timely manner can be intensely distressing, there are many people who experience significant anxiety in relation to proceeding with the assessment process. Anecdotal feedback suggests that even after they have identified a service they would like to progress with, many people take some time after this before they feel comfortable enough to approach the service and commence the process. For a significant proportion, this anxiety remains until after the assessment process begins, and for some it continues throughout the process and beyond. Many people experience significant difficulty in describing their experiences through spoken communication, with a new person, and in a strange environment, while many others experience difficulty in communicating about their experiences via written communication, for example, text or email. An Autistic person may experience alexithymia where they find it challenging to identify and describe their emotional experience. Many will have had repeated experiences of encountering professionals who have no understanding of interoceptive differences and alexithymia.

Autistic people frequently encounter barriers in relation to the communication methods offered by different services. Or rather, the barrier lies within the lack of variety of communication methods offered, with the methods that are offered typically favouring neurotypical individuals, that is, expectations around spoken communication with others and around immediate processing of information, and a lack of consideration being given to auditory, visual and sensory processing difficulties, etc. Due consideration needs to be given to removing communication barriers and providing access to choice in relation to other communication methods, for example, written communication, voice note communication, synchronous and asynchronous options. Consideration also needs to be given to barriers that are created by the sensory elements of an assessment space, neurotypical methods of interaction (e.g., expectations around 'small talk'), and also differences in perception (e.g., additional perceiving of all elements of an interaction, which requires more processing time and can make encounters with others particularly overloading).

How to Make Your Assessment Accessible

Given this high-risk situation in relation to outcomes, it is imperative that the possible barriers to assessment for Autistic individuals are recognized and removed so that people have the opportunity to deepen their self-understanding and sense of identity, and so that they can access what they need in terms of supports and accommodations. The following are recommended to clinicians and services in making their assessments accessible:

1. **Consider the barriers within your own service:** Prior to offering an Autistic assessment service to adults, clinicians and services need to be aware of and give consideration to the potential barriers to those within their community in accessing an assessment with their service. It is essential for a service audit to be undertaken to ensure that it is accessible to everyone, and that Autistic communication, Autistic engagement and the impact of sensory perception in the environment where assessments will be offered are considered. If there isn't an Autistic professional already within the service, then services need to consult with one in relation to carrying out the audit. Not having a neurodivergent team member is a distinct disadvantage to any service that proposes to serve the Autistic community. There is a clear need to foster trust and facilitate open communication (which may be either spoken or non-spoken) with clients, particularly where an individual has previously been involved with multiple professionals, and where potential misdiagnoses are a factor.

2. **Self-identification:** If a person already self-identifies as being Autistic, and is seeking to access formal identification, this should be thoroughly and respectfully explored in a collaborative approach with the person via open discussion, for example, 'Tell me more about your self-identification', 'What led to your understanding of yourself as being Autistic?', etc.

3. **Be aware of how your communication may be interpreted:** Neurotypical clinicians need to be aware of their body language, the tone of their spoken and written communication, and how they articulate what they are saying, as the person they are working with might have a different interpretation of these cues than a neurotypical person, or they may find it challenging to interpret them at all.

4. **Universal accommodations:** Consider what universal accommodations can be implemented to ensure that all communication preferences are accommodated regardless of a person's neurotype. An example of this would be to offer all clients the option of engaging with a service in written format as well as through spoken language.

5. **Ask about communication preferences:** Ask potential clients what their preferences are in communicating with others. When asked, most people can identify what works best for them in terms of communicating with others and what communication methods they find uncomfortable. When a person has indicated what their preference is, for example, written communication, email communication, phone, voice notes, video-call, in-person communication, movement while communicating, etc., it is vitally important to facilitate this.

6. **Provide information in advance on what to expect during a session:** As a result of sensory perception differences and perceiving uncertainty, most people find written, visual or spoken information in advance of an assessment session helpful (provided it is matched with their preferred communication style), as it reduces uncertainty and surprise, and helps them to understand what to expect. This information should outline what will be discussed during the session, any questions they might be asked during the session and any information they will need to provide. This gives the person the opportunity to prepare what they would like to communicate in advance of the session. An outline of what to expect in relation to the interaction element of an assessment session with a person should also be given, even if the session is online. Spoken language (communication styles, tone of voice, use of words, etc.) and non-spoken communication (body language, eye contact, facial expressions, etc.) can be experienced as very demanding and, indeed, stressful, by some Autistic people. It is important to communicate in advance to a person that eye contact is not expected during sessions, that they are free to have pets (if the session is remote or online), calming objects or stim toys with them, and that they are free to move about if needed. For some, choosing to keep their camera off during a video call session is much more comfortable. It is also extremely helpful to provide a short introductory video of the particular clinician a person will meet. This only needs to be a few seconds long, but gives the person advanced information about how the clinician sounds, the way they move, how they gesticulate, etc. when engaging with others, which allows a person time to process this information in advance of meeting with the clinician. Doing each of these things brings more certainty to the meeting for the person seeking assessment, which creates a safer and more relaxed environment for them. The above is common practice within The Adult Autism Practice and Thriving Autistic, and feedback from clients indicates that it makes the process much more comfortable and supportive, and they feel valued and respected, which results in a more meaningful engagement with a better outcome.

7. **Communication preferences vary and may change:** It is essential to offer people engaging with an assessment to confirm their neurology as Autistic

a variety of options in terms of how they would prefer to communicate information to the professional as part of the process. Professionals need to also be aware that a person's preferred method might change over the course of the assessment as the professional becomes more familiar to the person. Some people find written communication (e.g., email or text) their preferred method, and are extraordinarily articulate in writing about their experiences. Others are more comfortable talking about their experiences, reading from notes they have prepared, or monologuing about their experiences, which can be a very reflective process. If engaging in a remote session, some people are comfortable being viewed on camera and some find this intolerable. Some prefer open-ended questions, while others need very specific and clear questions. Ensure that regular feedback is sought from the person in their stated communication preference about how they feel the process is progressing, and whether they feel anything needs to be changed.

8. **Gather information using a person's preferred communication method:** Respecting a person's communication preferences is extremely important in gathering meaningful and reliable information during the course of an assessment. For many people, spoken communication is their preference, and where this is the case, this should be accommodated for them. However, it is important to understand that neurotypical spoken communication and Autistic spoken communication are different. In neurotypical spoken communication, there might be regular back-and-forth in conversation, whereas within Autistic spoken communication there is often a preference for monologuing, or a person might talk through music, or explain something through sound or even singing. The person might need to listen to music while talking or prefer to speak via voice notes. For those who prefer spoken communication, written communication can be highly stressful. For many others, spoken communication is highly stressful, and if it is the only option available, this significantly limits the person's ability to engage with the process as it reduces the amount of information the person provides. If it is their preference to communicate via written formats, this can be done via completing forms that ask specific questions about their experiences, clarification on the information can be sought by email, further questions can be sent by email, a person can use the 'chat' function on video calls to type their answers, etc. Using a less comfortable communication method for a person can be very demanding for them. It promotes masking and directly impacts the person's ability to concentrate, pay attention and respond within a face-to-face interaction, even if it is via video call. Engaging via Autistic communication methods, either spoken or non-spoken, is less demanding, and can generate less anxiety for a

person for whom neurotypical social interactions can be difficult. It can therefore be much easier and more comfortable for many people to provide information about their experiences as part of an assessment process via their own preferred communication method. The uncertainty of whether spoken or non-spoken communication will be expected can often cause huge stress for people when contemplating booking an assessment. When an Autistic person can access their preferred choice of communication method during an assessment process, they typically provide extraordinarily detailed, expressive, articulate and rich accounts of their experiences in their preferred format.

9. **Allow time for processing information:** Due to differences in sensory perception and executive functioning, having additional time in advance of meeting with a professional in order to process information is vital and hugely important to those seeking assessment. If a person is comfortable with and if they prefer written communication, text and email are very efficient ways for a person to relate to information, process it and respond to it in their own way. If the person has a preference for spoken communication, then information can be voice recorded and shared in advance of sessions. This provides the person who is seeking an assessment time to think through, write or speak about and relate to their own information in a way that might be more valid for them.

10. **Provide a summary following a session:** Following a session, it is helpful to provide a summary of the information gathered. This should be offered to the person in a communication style of their choice (e.g., written, video or voice recording). This allows a person time to review the information they have shared, to clarify anything that may have been misinterpreted, and to add any information a person feels they may have left out.

11. **Transparency in relation to being neurodiversity- and gender-affirming:** In creating an open and accessible assessment space for adults, it is hugely important that professionals determine their own personal ethos, values and approach to assessment, and to communicate these to those who will potentially engage with an assessment with them. This will allow those who are considering an assessment to evaluate whether the professional's values align with theirs, and whether it is likely that they will feel safe and comfortable in working with them. Of central importance to this, it is essential for professionals to outline their position in relation to neurodiversity and that their approach to assessment will be Neuro-Affirmative, collaborative and respectful. This means that they view being Autistic as a neurotype that doesn't require 'fixing' or changing, but requires

understanding and accommodating. It is also important for professionals to reflect on and communicate their position in relation to whether their approach is gender-affirming. Although the exact prevalence rate is not yet fully known, there are many studies that demonstrate increased rates of gender diversity in Autistic children (Hisle-Gorman et al. 2019) and adults (George and Stokes 2018b), and it is therefore highly likely that all professionals will meet with LGBTQIA+ adults during assessments to identify Autistic experiences. It is essential that professionals ask those engaging with their service what pronouns they would like to be used, and that these preferences are adhered to throughout the process.

12. **Remote assessments:** For most adults seeking an assessment, anxiety in relation to the assessment process and uncertainty about the outcome are significant factors. It is hugely stressful for many Autistic adults to meet with an unfamiliar person and to communicate in relation to potentially difficult experiences that they have had. It is therefore critical that the different options available as to how the process is undertaken are considered, with the goal being to establish a safe and comfortable assessment space for the person to collaborate with a clinician within. There is increasing evidence to suggest that telehealth approaches to assessment can be beneficial. Potential benefits include increased access to services (Reese et al. 2015) and a decrease in costs (Gros et al. 2013) including travel time, transport expenses, missed work, personal energy, etc. Adopting a remote approach to assessments with adults who are seeking to explore Autistic experiences has many potential benefits. Of primary importance is the anecdotal feedback received regarding the personal benefits a person experiences of being in their own surroundings when engaging in a process that has a high potential to be significantly stressful. Many people have reported that they have found it helpful to have access to their own stimming objects, their own items used for sensory regulation, access to their pets and even being able to choose the most comfortable area in their own surroundings within which to engage in an assessment session. It is also helpful to have access to these things immediately following a session. Many Autistic people find engaging with unfamiliar people in unfamiliar places to be highly stressful. Supporting an Autistic person to communicate through a method of their choice from the comfort of their own home or safe space reduces stress and supports them in engaging in the process. Given that the primary focus of this assessment process is not on 'observing' a person's communication and engagement but is about working collaboratively with the person to support them in making sense of their own experiences and whether these experiences align with Autistic experiences, it is imperative that both parties feel comfortable meeting and engaging with each other.

12

How to Conduct a Neuro-Affirmative Assessment

Introduction

It is important to state at the outset that the steps outlined in this chapter are those involved in a Neuro-Affirmative approach to an assessment exploring Autistic identity with an adult without an intellectual disability (ID). Many of these steps are also relevant in the assessment of Autistic identity with adults with co-occurring ID, but some adaptations are required when engaging in Neuro-Affirmative Autistic identity assessments with this community. Prior to engaging in a Neuro-Affirmative approach to the assessment process, such as that outlined below, it is essential for clinicians to have a solid understanding of the foundations of a Neuro-Affirmative approach to the assessment and confirmation of a person's neurology as Autistic as well as the history of the neurodiversity movement. This gives a robust platform from which to reflect on previous assessment approaches, and to build a new assessment approach where necessary. For these reasons, it is imperative that the earlier chapters of this book should be read prior to engaging with this chapter.

There is a wealth of information in the earlier chapters of this book relating to different areas that need to be considered prior to undertaking an exploration of Autistic identity with a person attending for assessment. Considerations in relation to gender identity, ID, ADHD, co-occurring conditions, trauma, etc. need to be fully understood and explored (as appropriate) during the process. What follows in this chapter needs to be adapted depending on the individual experiences of the person.

Reflection Point

It is important at the outset of this chapter to note that the assessment process is constantly evolving. This is not only due to our understanding of Autistic experiences advancing, but also relates to the collaborative nature of the assessment process, and the need for it to be tailored specifically to suit the needs of the person.

The Importance of Autistic and Neurodivergent Professionals Being an Integral Part of the Team

The Adult Autism Practice is a mixed team of neurotypical and Autistic professionals, while Thriving Autistic is made up solely of Autistic and/or otherwise neurodivergent professionals. The reflections, insight and professional growth that have occurred within The Adult Autism Practice would not have been possible without our Autistic and otherwise neurodivergent colleagues, and at Thriving Autistic, clients continually tell us of the relief and safety they feel in finally working with a professional who truly understands their experiences. For professionals currently working on teams that have no meaningful input from Autistic professionals or the Autistic community, this is a vital goal going forward. This is about providing the best service you can to the people you are trying to serve. It is the only way to provide assessments, which, from the very start (i.e., first contact) are accessible and designed for a broad range of neurodivergence. It is the only way that teams can develop their knowledge enough to provide best practice assessments, truly understand their clients and provide the best recommendations and support for clients following assessment.

Assessment as a Therapeutic Process

Although the process of supporting an individual to determine whether they are Autistic or not is termed an 'assessment', it could more appropriately be described as a 'therapeutic exploration of identity'. A core central component of the process relates to supporting a person to make sense of their inner experiences (i.e., to begin the process of discovering their true sense of identity), and to integrate a person's inner experience with how they relate to others and with the world. In other words, the process involves moving towards integrating a person's inner self with their outer self in order to develop a complete and authentic self.

Throughout the course of engaging with a person, a process of reviewing, describing, bearing witness to and documenting their inner experiences takes place. This process allows the person to make sense of their experiences and to establish whether their experiences align with Autistic experiences or not. Many people who engage with this process have spent a significant amount of time in their lives believing there is 'something wrong' with them, or that they are 'lesser than' other people because they may have done things differently to others, moved their bodies differently to others, have not understood things in the same way as others, or engaged with tasks or activities differently to others. Not being as good as others may have been communicated to them directly by those in their family or acquaintance circles, or it might be a conclusion they have arrived at themselves as they have noticed that their instincts, needs, preferences and urges might appear to differ to those around them.

Working through the process of identity exploration gives the person an opportunity to re-frame their past beliefs about themselves and also how they previously knew and understood their identity. It creates an opportunity for them to establish connections between their inner experience and what is relayed outwardly, so that they can begin to move towards an understanding that there are many others who experience the world in the same ways they do, and that there is nothing 'wrong' with different ways of thinking and experiencing the world. There are, in fact, many advantages, and the human race benefits. Within the process, there is much for a person to discover and many connections to be established, where previous experiences might now make sense through an Autistic lens.

Recognizing the presence of Autistic strengths in a person's experiences can be a powerful and meaningful therapeutic experience for many. This can often lead to the identification and realization of how being Autistic has helped a person in many areas of their lives. There have been many cases within The Adult Autism Practice where the confirmation that a person is Autistic centres round the clear evidence of the presence of their Autistic strengths as opposed to the evidence coming from the challenges experienced. A person does not have to be experiencing significant challenges or crises in order to be identified as being Autistic, and many Autistic people are not experiencing challenges or crises. Indeed, the proliferation of the notion that being identified as Autistic is underpinned by 'deficits' has itself led to swathes of individuals not being taken seriously by professionals and services when seeking to explore Autistic identity that best captures their lived experience. This highlights the 'expert–patient' dyad that has thus excluded many Autistic people from discovering their true selves.

Such realizations strongly support the need for a more collaborative dyad between the individual seeking assessment and the professional providing one. The therapeutic components of an assessment process that centre round identity exploration, identifying Autistic strengths, integrating all aspects of the self (inner and outer), establishing connections and re-framing past experiences create a base from which a person can begin or continue to cultivate a different sense of identity that is based on their authentic and whole self.

People are Collaborative Partners within the Assessment Process

Before contemplating the procedural aspects of an assessment of Autistic identity, the nature of what is being 'assessed' needs consideration. Traditionally, within the area of clinical assessment it is broadly considered that the professional is 'assessing' the person who is attending a service, and the professional's observations, clinical judgement and clinical opinions hold a central position in determining what the outcome of the assessment is. Within a framework for exploring Autistic identity with adults using a Neuro-Affirmative approach, the idea of a professional holding the majority share of the responsibility for determining the outcome of the assessment is not supported.

Reflection Point

For all professionals engaging in clinical work with adults (regardless of discipline), we encourage you to reflect on your practice as a whole. Consider the power share within your work currently, and reflect on whether there is a true collaborative approach within your engagement with others, both in terms of Autistic exploration processes and also in relation to other clinical work. While it is vital that an exploration of Autistic identity is carried out in a collaborative way with a person, with both parties holding shared responsibility and contribution in terms of the conclusion, it is also important that all clinical work is approached in this way. Within professional conversations, we often hear of thought processes raised by professionals of 'needing to be sure' before they can 'give a diagnosis'. This frame of mind suggests a power imbalance that is biased towards the professional, which leads to misdiagnosis and missed diagnosis, along with higher likelihood of trauma for the person and higher emotional and financial cost. Working in a truly collaborative way with people results in a more meaningful process for the person, a safer engagement for them, and a far more reliable outcome.

A central principle within a Neuro-Affirmative approach to assessment is that a person attending for assessment is viewed as an equal partner in the process, and what is being jointly assessed by both parties is a person's experiences, their strengths, their needs and preferences in relation to communication and engagement, and the challenges that have arisen. Although they can help to inform aspects of the process, a professional's observations of the person themselves are not central to the process, and can often be highly misleading within a collaborative exploration of Autistic identity with an adult.

The 'assessment' process within a Neuro-Affirmative assessment of Autistic identity is a highly collaborative process of identity exploration between a professional and a person. The person attending for assessment is considered the expert on their own experiences and their internal processes, and the 'assessment' cannot progress without this expertise. Professionals bring an understanding of an Autistic neurotype from a Neuro-Affirmative perspective and knowledge of the criteria used to identify Autistic experiences, and together, both parties share information in order to support a person to make sense of their experiences, and to establish whether their experiences align with Autistic experiences. This then leads to a shared understanding on whether a person is Autistic or not, with this understanding being arrived at jointly and collaboratively between both parties.

It is not the role of the professional to cast doubt on a person's experiences, to question their experiences or to seek outside confirmation or validation of a person's inner experiences, unless the person concerned specifically requests this or communicates that they require additional support in order to express their experiences. The professional also does not need to 'observe' a person's Autistic experiences, as relying on this method will most often result in there being little to 'observe' within a short session where a person has likely become skilled at masking Autistic characteristics over the course of their lives. Placing a higher value on 'observable' traits or Autistic characteristics than on a person's description of their inner experience is felt by Autistic people to be invalidating and dismissive, and will very often lead to the wrong conclusion. Rather, it is crucially important as a professional within the assessment partnership to listen and to explore a person's internal experiences with them. Working collaboratively in partnership with people helps to avoid making significant errors in assumptions, judgements, methods and conclusions.

Consent

As with all assessment processes, informed consent prior to commencing the assessment piece is required. Having determined a person's communication needs and preferences, informed consent can be obtained via the communication method the individual has chosen. For many people, asynchronous communication (i.e., communicating something without expecting an immediate response, such as communicating by email or voice note) in relation to consent is preferable, as this allows the person time to process the information at their own pace and to determine whether they consent to it or not. For some, this may take the form of providing written material prior to the assessment process commencing. For others, for example, Dyslexic people or those with visual processing challenges, written information in relation to consent may be more challenging to access. Options in relation to providing this information via alternative methods should be considered and provided – for example, via pre-recorded video or audio explanation – while also ensuring that documents are accessible for text-to-speech software. Among other things, consent information needs to include information about what will happen during the assessment process, limits to confidentiality, how information is stored and whether it is shared, whether and how sessions will be recorded, etc.

Screening Questionnaires

While screening questionnaires can be useful, it is important to note that they should never be used in isolation to determine whether an autism assessment is warranted or not. Screening questionnaires alone should not be considered the gatekeepers to assessment, and further information is required in order to support a person in establishing whether proceeding with a full assessment would be helpful or not. At the time of writing, there are no screening questionnaires that we are aware of that are Neuro-Affirmative in their approach, and many of the screening questionnaires are significantly limited in the experiences they capture.

Within The Adult Autism Practice the only pre-assessment questionnaire used is the Camouflaging Autistic Traits Questionnaire (CAT-Q), which is a self-report measure of masking in adults. The CAT-Q measures masking in general as well as compensation (strategies used to actively compensate for challenges within social situations), masking (strategies used to hide Autistic characteristics or portray a non-autistic persona), and assimilation (strategies used to try to fit in with others in social situations). The CAT-Q is a helpful tool in exploring the masking experience of adults, but cannot be used in isolation. It must also be considered that there are many Autistic people who do not mask, and so they will not score within range on the CAT-Q.

Session Amount, Length and Content

The majority of people seeking to explore an Autistic assessment (whether they are seeking a private or public pathway) have questioned the possibility of being Autistic long before they attend for a consultation or assessment. They might have watched videos, learned about Autistic experiences, read books, discussed it with friends and/or family, etc. Essentially, they have tried themselves to make sense of whether they might be Autistic or not. In contrast, for those already attending services, if the service or professional they attend identifies that an assessment of Autistic identity might be needed, this may be the first time anyone has discussed the possibility of being Autistic with the person. It is important to remember again that regardless of whether a person is undertaking an assessment within a public or private system, the process should be collaborative, and so the sessions that are carried out as part of an assessment process should be conducted in an open and honest way.

Assessment sessions consist of a large amount of identity exploration, 'making sense' of experiences, establishing connections and determining explanations. They can be experienced by many people as very overwhelming and energy-consuming as they raise a lot of memories (both positive and challenging) and different emotions. It must also be remembered that for many people it might be the first time they are communicating about the possibility of being Autistic, despite the fact that many have had some level of input from mental health services in the past. It is vital to consider that each person approaches an assessment with different expectations. For example, previous personal experiences with mental health services can influence the beliefs and expectations a person might hold about the process of an assessment of Autistic identity. They might expect that the professional will 'interview' them and so they might not be expecting the collaborative aspect of the assessment. Providing information in advance of the process about what will happen during the process can be really helpful in this regard.

As a result of societal pressure to mask, many Autistic people are very aware of what is 'expected' of them within a neurotypical society. It is likely that without realizing it the person may replicate masking behaviours during the assessment process, therefore responding in ways that they believe are expected of them rather than how they might naturally engage. It is important to discuss and 'deconstruct' the idea of a formal assessment as well as the possibility of masking with a person, which leads to a much more collaborative and consistent process.

Reflection Point

Moving from a formal assessment procedure to a collaborative assessment framework for most services is a process in itself that takes time, reflection and learning. For most professionals, their training placed them in an 'expert' position, and moving away from this towards a collaborative piece of exploration is a new way of working for many. Within The Adult Autism Practice, developing a Neuro-Affirmative framework for assessment was central and intentional from the very beginning. Prior to offering a service to any person, significant consideration was given to what the process and experience of assessment would and should be like for all people, and the service was purposefully designed with this in mind. Working collaboratively with people to engage in an exploration of Autistic identity is a central component of the engagement, and is one that has continued to develop over time as those on the team and those joining the team have been open to working in this way and have developed their skills in this area. For the majority of people seeking an assessment, they have reflected that they enjoy this approach, feel empowered by it, feel safer within it, and that the outcome is more reliable and meaningful. Many are not expecting it and are pleasantly surprised by how much better it works for them in comparison to their previous experience of services. A small group of people have found the open collaborative nature more challenging, as they feel that they want a 'professional' to assess their experiences and to tell them what the best understanding of their experiences is. While the majority of people benefit from the shared collaboration of identity exploration, working collaboratively means listening to and respecting the needs of the person within the process.

Assessment processes vary between clinicians and people attending for assessment, and some will require a bespoke process depending on a person's circumstances and needs within communication. In our experience, most people complete the full assessment piece within three sessions, of 1 to 1.5 hours per session. This will, of course, vary according to the person's needs, and occasionally, a significant minority require a further session to explore different aspects of their experiences, for example trauma or mental health experiences. A vital component of the process is also in providing appropriate and adequate post-assessment support once the assessment process is complete. Our role as clinicians is to make the experience as straightforward, comfortable, safe and collaborative as possible for the person. As clinicians, we are there to assist a person in this process so that we can understand their rationale, learn about their life experiences, and bear witness to their strengths, passions, struggles and challenges in an effort to support them with making sense of their identity. Creating a comfortable and safe space for the exploration to take place where that person has agency allows them to be themselves as much as they feel safe to do so, and also allows for meaningful engagement with the process.

Pre-Assessment Consultation

Many people benefit from or even require a pre-assessment consultation session. This is particularly the case if they are unsure about whether a full assessment is the 'right track' for them or not, and they would like to further discuss this prior to proceeding. For many, having a pre-assessment consultation also means that they can meet with the clinician they will be working with so that they can safely and reliably evaluate whether the clinician is the 'right fit' for them to work with. This can be particularly important where a person has had a challenging experience previously with mental health services. A pre-assessment consultation can also be very helpful for some in determining what the next best step is for them. It is often very clear to a person that they are Autistic, and they may wish to explore the possible pros and cons of formal identification versus self-identification, which is a valid approach within the Autistic community.

Session One

The first session of an assessment process is an opportunity for the person attending the assessment to elaborate on their own understanding of why and how being Autistic makes sense to them. Listening to how the possibility that they might be Autistic arose for a person and what they have explored so far provides a clear context and foundation for the process. It is helpful to follow this by asking the person about their current work or studies, as this is usually a safer and easier topic for a person to start with. Asking about what a person enjoys or does not enjoy about their work or studies can be hugely informative in the exploration of Autistic identity. In our experience, for many people this is where their Autistic strengths come to the fore in terms of what they have been attracted to in terms of work or study and how they engage with it. Hearing about a person's passions, interests and hyperfocus, and listening to how they like to engage in their work in terms of attending to detail, problem-solving, approaching tasks analytically, etc. provides very helpful information to the process. It is also useful to explore the social aspects of work, that is, how a person relates to their colleagues, what challenges and benefits the person has faced within group or team dynamics at work, how these are managed, etc.

Within the first session, the process of gathering information about a person's experiences in relation to some of the areas within Autistic criteria begins – in relation to the person's strengths, preferences, needs, experiences and the challenges that have arisen in each area. In our experience, it is usually possible to explore in this first session the first half of the different areas within the criteria. This includes the areas of communicating and interacting with others, the person's experience of non-spoken communication, and their experience of friendships and relationships. It is important to consider that, as a clinician, you might be the first professional a person is meeting with in relation to the possibility that they may be Autistic. Many people will have had previous experiences with other services or professionals, but the possibility that they may be Autistic might not yet have been considered, explored or identified. Therefore, the first session is a collaborative process between the person and the clinician, where both are working to explore a person's inner experiences, and to consider together how they might relate or align to Autistic experiences.

Session Two

During the second session, the person's narrative will continue to be explored and there is a continuation of gathering information in relation to a person's internal experiences within the different areas of the criteria being used. In our experience, it is usually possible to explore the second half of the criteria within the second session. This includes the person's experience of hand or body movements or vocalizations that may be calming or energizing, their needs in relation to routines or managing change, their interests and passions and how they like to engage with them, and their sensory experiences. Our role as clinicians continues to be to support a person to understand their life experiences in the context of Autistic criteria in a respectful, ethical and empathetic way. Within the second session, it is also important to explore whether there is anything else within the person's history that might possibly offer a different explanation for their experiences, or whether there are co-occurring conditions. Due consideration should be given to their medical history, mental health history and experience of significant events in their life that may have been traumatic (i.e., the impact of trauma). On occasion, a further session may be required to allow space for continued exploration and information gathering before proceeding with the final session. This, again, highlights the collaborative nature of the assessment, with the person themselves setting the pace and not being held to the professional's time or agenda.

Final Assessment Session

The final session in the assessment process consists of a collaborative discussion about how the person's experiences align with Autistic experiences, and how they can be understood within the context of Autistic criteria. If an Autistic identity is confirmed, it is important to consider that this can be perceived and received differently for each person. Most often, within the context of a collaborative Neuro-Affirmative assessment framework, the assessment process is perceived as a very positive experience, bringing up different emotions, reactions and self-reflection. A Neuro-Affirmative conversation in this regard can assist the person in moving towards a more self-compassionate place of self-understanding and insight into their own experiences.

Within the final assessment session, consideration needs to be given to the next steps for the person following the assessment process and confirmation that they are Autistic (should this be the case). Reasonable accommodations a person may require in their workplace and/or education setting, and accommodations in relation to accessing healthcare require discussion. Letters, documentation and reports required relating to the identification that a person is Autistic are also explained to the person during this session. It is also a best practice recommendation to provide information about resources, services and initial information regarding linking with the Autistic community.

Multidisciplinary Approach to Assessment

Within an assessment process, it is an essential component to have input from the multidisciplinary team (MDT). There are almost always sensory processing differences, regulation needs and executive functioning differences that benefit from occupational therapy support. Communication differences and needs are also a core feature, and support from speech and language therapists is required in relation to supporting communication needs and self-advocacy. There are many Autistic people who experience co-occurring physical health needs, such as hypermobility, Ehlers-Danlos syndrome, etc., and who require physiotherapy support. Dietitians offer support in relation to managing the nutritional aspects of sensory needs – relating to eating and drinking – with interoception differences also requiring consideration. Access to support from psychotherapists, counsellors, psychologists and psychiatrists in relation to mental health support is essential for many.

Experienced clinicians across all disciplines play an important role within the assessment process in terms of both exploring Autistic identity, and also supporting a person's needs following the assessment process.

Post-Assessment Support

Within the final assessment session, it is essential that information is also provided about post-assessment support services and support options for the person. Every person requires access to post-assessment support as they adjust to their Autistic identity being confirmed, manage their sensory needs and mental health needs, consider disclosure, identify and access accommodations, etc. Post-assessment support should not be seen as 'an optional extra'; rather, it is an essential component within the process for all.

For further information in relation to the post-assessment support that is required and how to provide it, please see Chapter 13.

Reflection Point

In our experience of having engaged in both medical model assessments and Neuro-Affirmative exploration of Autistic identity, the contrast between the two approaches is stark, for the person attending for assessment and for a professional working in this area. Most importantly, feedback from people who attend for assessment indicates that they have a much more positive experience via the Neuro-Affirmative approach. Many people have been through medical model approaches prior to engaging in a Neuro-Affirmative assessment approach, or they have been involved with medical model assessments via their children or people they are close to, and speak very clearly about the experience as being 'othering', disempowering, invalidating, and at times, very confusing. In contrast, they speak about feeling empowered, validated, acknowledged and having a better self-understanding at the end of a Neuro-Affirmative process. While the experience of the person attending for assessment is the most important factor, there is also a difference experienced by professionals who have changed their practice from a medical model approach to a Neuro-Affirmative approach. In our own experience, a Neuro-Affirmative approach to assessment is empowering and validating, and supports a framework for a deeper sense of identity for a person, and this often brings about a life-changing moment for that person. Being involved in these pieces of work is highly meaningful and deeply rewarding as a clinician. There is a strong sense of being a part of making a meaningful difference in a person's life that changes how they know themselves and how they understand their needs. The meaning within the assessment piece and the life-changing aspect for the person is not just about the outcome and identifying whether a person is Autistic or not; it is within the witnessing of a person's experiences, sharing in their understanding, supporting them to develop an understanding of their needs, learning that who they are is valid, worthy and accepted, realizing that they are valued as a human being, beginning the process of re-framing their past experiences, and being a part of shaping their future experiences.

Gathering and Interpreting Information

During the course of an assessment of Autistic identity, it is vital to gather a wealth of detailed information. This needs to be carried out with due regard for the person's communication preferences and the level of stress or discomfort they may experience when engaging with an unfamiliar person. It is vitally important that there is a flexible approach to the assessment process that allows for different preferences in terms of how different people best communicate and engage, bearing in mind that preferences can change over time and within different circumstances (see Chapter 11).

Determine communication preferences and the most appropriate methods for information gathering

At the outset, a person's communication preferences need to be determined and adhered to. Autistic people are best placed to provide information about what works best for them (Gotham et al. 2015), and individuals require access to their preferred communication method by which to engage in the assessment process (e.g., face-to-face, video call, text-based methods, etc.) For many individuals, a mixed communication approach can work well, whereas for others they find exclusive written communication or exclusive spoken communication is preferable and/or necessary.

Within The Adult Autism Practice and Thriving Autistic, we have had experience of variable communication needs within the assessment process. In our experience, providing choice and options in relation to the communication method used results in a safer and more comfortable process for the person, which leads to more enriched information being gathered and a more detailed assessment being undertaken.

Some people have found text-based methods of information gathering (e.g., completing forms, writing information, emailing to communicate their information, etc.) work best for them, while others have found spoken methods (e.g., talking during sessions, monologuing, using voice notes, etc.) work better. Adjusting the process to align with the communication needs of the person is an essential requirement within every assessment process.

Reflection Point

Professionals need to consider what communication options are currently accessible within their service or practice. What options could be added?

Facilitating a person's needs in relation to communication is a vital component of the Neuro-Affirmative approach. It is respectful, will help to reduce a person's levels of stress, increases the likelihood of meaningful engagement, communicates a willingness to understand and accommodate a person's needs, and places a value on there being different methods of communicating.

Determine mental health needs and manage risk

Prior to engaging in an assessment process with a person, and particularly if working within a private setting that can be more isolating in terms of accessing other services and supports, it is important to determine whether a person is experiencing any mental health challenges requiring support, and whether they are experiencing any suicidal ideation or risk of harm. Although a Neuro-Affirmative assessment is largely a positive experience, contemplating the prospect of and then ultimately engaging in an assessment of Autistic identity as an adult can be quite a stressful process for many, as it involves exploring past experiences that might have been difficult.

> In our experience, many people experience the assessment process as overwhelming, although the degree of overwhelm can vary. Even for those who are very sure they are Autistic before beginning the process, the experience of this being formally confirmed can be overwhelming. For those who are unsure about whether they are Autistic or not, it can be significantly overwhelming to discover that they are.
>
> Many people speak about their difficult feelings in relation to what might have been different in their lives had they known they were Autistic sooner. Within our service, many people have described how it is helpful to have additional support with these feelings, and many will access additional therapeutic support before they begin the assessment. Some request pausing an assessment while they access additional support. Many people describe how they find it helpful for it to be acknowledged within the assessment process that it is typical for many others to feel overwhelmed, as this helps them to feel a sense of relatability and connection in what is happening for them. Working at the pace of the person is really helpful, with some finding that they need to move quickly through the process, while others need significant time between sessions in order to process their experiences.

Should there be any significant prior or current mental health needs, it is important to ensure that a person is supported prior to, during and after the assessment process, bearing in mind that this may involve them accessing therapeutic support and may require an assessment process to be paused. Even if a person's mental health needs are not at the level where further therapeutic support is required, it is important that their emotional wellbeing during the course of the process is supported (see Appendix 3, for a sample 'Looking After Myself Plan').

Gather information about previous diagnoses

Prior to undertaking an exploration of Autistic identity with a person, it is extremely important to gather information about whether they have received any previous diagnoses, and how they feel about these. Previous diagnoses might be in relation to other neurodivergencies, for example, ADHD, Dyslexia, Dyspraxia, etc., or in relation to a person's mental health experiences, such as mood, anxiety, PTSD, personality disorders, etc. Along with asking a person whether any previous diagnoses have been made, it is essential to also ask whether the person agrees or disagrees with them. Which ones, if any, make sense to the person in terms of how they understand themselves? Within The Adult Autism Practice, this information is gathered via the person's intake form, which is accessed by the person writing their information or speaking their information, with another person within the service transcribing their information. Overall, most people have significant clarity and insight into whether they identify with a particular diagnosis or not, or whether they are unsure whether it fits or not. Occasionally, possible diagnoses have been suggested by previous professionals, but neither confirmed nor ruled out. This can be particularly difficult for the person in terms of developing their sense of self and identity, with people reporting that they feel confused, misunderstood and frustrated, as though they have been 'left in limbo' by services when this has happened to them.

Having information about previous diagnoses and whether a person agrees with them or not provides a framework for a richer identity exploration where all parts of the self can be integrated and understood. Within this context, undertaking a Neuro-Affirmative approach to exploring an Autistic identity can then allow for the journey towards a holistic and rounded self-understanding to continue.

Gather information in relation to Autistic criteria – re-framing current classification systems

The current internationally recognized criteria for benchmarking Autistic assessments against are the DSM-5-TR or ICD-11 criteria. These outline the different areas within communication, interaction, relationships, interests, sensory experiences, routines, body movements, etc. that are related to Autistic experiences. While current best practice approaches to assessment indicate that a recognized classification system needs to be considered as part of the assessment process, there are significant issues relating to current classification systems. The two main issues to consider are:

- Current classification systems are significantly 'deficit'-focused in their language and descriptors of Autistic experiences. They typically mention 'abnormalities', 'disorder' and 'delay', and seek for the professional to make observations in relation to a person's 'deficiencies'. This approach is completely out of step with current understanding of Autistic experiences from a Neuro-Affirmative perspective as it holds neurotypical communication and engagement to be the default standard to be measured against rather than appreciating the natural variations between neurotypes as being equal.

- Current classification systems fail to recognize vital aspects of Autistic experiences, such as Autistic sensory perception, Autistic communication, creativity, masking, executive functioning, experiences of empathy, abilities relating to hyperfocus, having a strong sense of social justice, etc.

Reflection Point

When gathering information as part of the process of assessment, while the main areas outlined within the international criteria need to be considered, **how** we consider these areas needs to be interpreted differently. The areas themselves are broadly useful in thinking about Autistic experiences, but the language outlined in current classification systems implies that people who experience the world in a different way to the majority are 'impaired' in some way.

Instead of thinking about a person's 'deficits' or 'abnormalities' as compared to neurotypicals, it is important to think about what a person's experiences are in relation to the different areas. What are their preferences and needs in relation to each area, how do they best function in each area, how do they thrive or best engage in each area, what works best for them, what are their strengths in the different areas, etc.? It is also important to explore within each area what the challenges are that have arisen, what does not work well for the person, and how they prefer not to engage or do things, etc. When each of these aspects is explored, it must then be considered whether a person's experiences, strengths and the challenges that have arisen align with the experiences of Autistic people.

The following table offers a re-framing of many aspects of current criteria to a more Neuro-Affirmative approach.

Deficit-focused statements or aspects of current classification systems	Re-framed from a Neuro-Affirmative perspective
Persistent deficits	Consider how a person's experiences may change across their lifespan
Deficits in social communication and interaction, abnormal social interaction, failure to engage in normal interaction, etc.	Experience of social-emotional reciprocity, e.g., social approach, conversation styles, sharing of interests/emotions/affect, initiating and responding to social interactions Within this area, consider a person's communication and interaction preferences. What works best for them in terms of how they communicate with others? What do they like to communicate about? How do they experience neurotypical expectations for communicating and interacting, e.g., 'small talk', conversations, etc.? How do their experiences in these areas relate to 'masking'?
Deficits in non-verbal communication, poor use of communication, abnormalities in non-verbal communication, deficits in understanding non-verbal communication, a lack of non-verbal communication	Experience of non-spoken communication, e.g., eye contact, body language, gestures, facial expressions Within this area, consider a person's experience of non-spoken communication with others. How do they experience eye contact? Do they find it more comfortable or easier to communicate if eye contact is not expected (e.g., when driving in a car with someone or walking alongside them)? Is body language clear or confusing? How do their experiences in these areas relate to 'masking'? Would it be helpful for the person to learn more about others' experiences of masking?
Deficits in friendships and relationships, impairments in adapting to a situation, problems with sharing play and making friends, no interest in peers	Experience of friendships and relationships Within this area, it is important to explore a person's preferences in relation to friendships and relationships. How do they feel about having friendships or being in relationships? Is this something they would like, or are they more comfortable not being in friendships or relationships? If the person has friendships and/or relationships with others, how do they like to engage in these relationships? How often do they like to meet with others, and what form does the engagement take? How does the person relate to Autistic or neurodivergent people?
Restricted or repetitive behaviours	Calming, alerting, and/or balancing movements/activities, task engagement preferences, interests and sensory experiences
Repetitive or stereotyped movements, speech or play of objects. Atypical or unusual movements	Particular or repeated hand or body movements, use of objects or vocalizations/use of speech that a person may find balancing or self-regulating Within this area, ask about whether a person does anything with their hands or body that they find calming or energizing. Do they make any sounds or noises that they enjoy or find calming or alerting? Do they do anything with objects that they find balancing (either calming or energizing)? Did they do any of these things in the past?

cont.

Deficit-focused statements or aspects of current classification systems	Re-framed from a Neuro-Affirmative perspective
Persistence in wanting things to stay the same, inflexibility, ritualized behaviour, rigidity, lack of adaptability, excessive adherence to rules	Preference or need for routines and specific ways of doing things, response to change and transitions. Preference and/or need for familiarity Within this area, consider a person's experience of change, both planned and unexpected. Do they prefer familiar surroundings? How do they manage transitions? How do they experience new surroundings? Does the person thrive within structure or a routine? Do they have particular preferences for how they arrange their belongings? Or how their food is prepared? How do they experience it when other people do things differently to them? How do they experience uncertainty? Are they more comfortable if things are predictable? Do they have a strong sense of social justice? How do they feel about lying?
Interests that are restricted or fixed, abnormal focus	Particular interests or passions for particular topics or activities Within this area, it is important to explore what a person's interests are. What are they passionate about? Are there particular things they have been interested in all their lives, or do they 'cycle' through interests? How do they like to engage with their interests? Do they engage with interests via multiple modalities (e.g., reading about them, watching programmes, talking about them, listening to podcasts, etc.)? Do they experience hyperfocus? Does hyperfocus interfere with self-care tasks such as feeding themselves or remembering to move or use the bathroom? Are they able to sustain their attention on their interests for long periods?
Hyper- or hypo-response to excessive, persistent or unusual interest in sensory information	Hyper- and/or hypo-reactivity to sensory input or interest in sensory aspects of the environment, seeking out certain sensory pleasures Within this area, it is important to explore how a person experiences sensory aspects of their environment – what they find difficult to tolerate and what they seek out more of or enjoy. Ask about their experiences within all eight senses – visual (sight), gustatory (taste), tactile (touch), auditory (hearing), olfactory (smell), vestibular (balance), proprioception (movement) and interoception (internal communication between sense and emotional states), which refers to recognizing signals within the body such as hunger, thirst, pain, and needing to use the toilet. Does the person recognize body signals as signs of emotional states?
Social awareness, inappropriate social behaviour	Experience of masking Within this area, explore the person's experience of masking their Autistic experiences. Do they put effort into appearing to be like others? Do they engage in particular movements in private? Have they put a lot of effort into trying to make sense of the behaviour of others, e.g., by researching or role-playing? Do they prepare scripts in advance of interactions?

Understanding the emotional states and thoughts of others	Experience of emotion, empathy and compassion
	Within this area, consider a person's experiences of emotion. Are they able to identify and understand their own emotions? Do they experience alexithymia? What is the person's experience of others' emotions? Do they experience others' emotions intensely? How does the person understand others' behaviour within different contexts?
Ability to share interests with others	Experience of sharing experiences of the world with others
	Within this area, consider the person's preferences in relation to how they engage with others about their experiences of the world. Does the person seek to share experiences with others? Are they content to engage with experiences in their own way and/or without others' involvement? Explore with the person (or if they feel comfortable to ask a person who knew them when they were younger) how they liked to play when they were children. What toys or objects did they like to play with, and what did they like to do with them? Did they like to play by themselves or with another person or people? If they liked to play with others, what games did they enjoy?
Onset of symptoms occurs in the early developmental period	Within each of the areas above, explore with a person their experiences in each area when they were younger. If the person feels comfortable doing so, information can also be sought from family members or documentation relating to their experiences when younger
Autism symptoms give rise to impairment in various aspects of a person's life	Consider the support needs a person has. Explore with them the accommodations they require across different areas of their life

Reflection Point

In thinking about current classification systems for Autistic criteria, it is clear that these frameworks view Autistic experiences in a disrespectful and non-affirmative manner, and fall short of capturing Autistic experiences. In trying to adapt the current criteria into a Neuro-Affirmative paradigm, it is clear that the frameworks are unsuitable. Although it is possible to consider the criteria in their current state from a Neuro-Affirmative perspective (as demonstrated above), this is reflective of trying to 'fit a square peg into a round hole'. A new approach in terms of 'criteria' or a framework for understanding Autistic experiences is badly needed. This new framework must be Autistic-led in terms of what the experience of being Autistic is, rather than what the experience of not being a neurotypical is.

Gather information outside of the current diagnostic classifications

When exploring with a person whether their experiences align with Autistic experiences or not, while it is currently important to consider the areas within the formal diagnostic criteria from a Neuro-Affirmative perspective, it is also vital that Autistic experiences outside of the formal criteria are explored. Information needs to be gathered about these areas, and this information is extremely important to the overall process of identity exploration and to a person's sense of self and self-understanding. Often, these areas are the primary areas where a person might experience differences or challenge, and they can be the areas that impact the most on a person's functioning and wellbeing. Some of these areas (as informed by the Autistic community generally, our learning from the Thriving Autistic and The Adult Autism Practice and, of course, from both teams' shared clinical experiences) include:

1. **Autistic communication:** Instead of seeking to observe 'deficits' or 'deficiencies' in neurotypical communication, it is important to gather information about a person's experiences in relation to Autistic communication. Do they communicate in Autistic ways? Are the things that are important to them in communication aligned with Autistic communication? What are an individual's preferences for communication, and do these align with the preferences of Autistic people? Autistic people might use spoken communication, or they might be Non-Speaking. They might prefer to articulate their communication verbally, or they might prefer written communication. Some Autistic adults prefer communication that is visual. This might be in written format (using email, text, emojis, messenger services, etc.), or picture format. Some Autistic people prefer information to be presented in a format that allows them time to process and respond in their own time. Stimming (i.e., self-stimulatory behaviour that includes but is not limited to pacing, hand flapping, body rocking, etc.) is also a form of communication, and many Autistic people communicate about their emotional experiences, such as frustration and joy, and sensory needs via stimming.

   Not only are there differences in terms of the format within which Autistic people tend to prefer to communicate, but there are also differences in terms of the style of communication. Autistic people often place value on sharing detailed information about topics they are passionate about, they often value honesty in communication, and frequently prefer direct and straightforward communication. Some Autistic people prefer asynchronous communication (i.e., communicating something without expecting an immediate response such as communicating by email or voice note), to synchronous communication (i.e., communicating and expecting an immediate response, such as in a neurotypical back-and-forth spoken conversation). Synchronous communication between mixed neurotypes often has a high demand, which can cause considerable anxiety and exhaustion for Autistic people as they don't have enough time to process the information and plan their response. When thinking about the area of communication within an Autistic assessment, it is vital to consider Autistic communication and whether an individual's experiences align with this.

2. **Creativity:** Within 'deficit'-based approaches to Autistic experiences, there is an assumption that Autistic people engage in logical or analytical thinking and that they are therefore not as imaginative or creative as neurotypical people. Indeed, an apparent 'lack of social imagination' is often used as one of the ways of identifying autism in formal medical model assessments. While it is true that many Autistic people describe their thinking patterns as being 'black or white', it is grossly incorrect to assume that Autistic people are therefore not creative.

Best et al. (2015, p.4064) attempted to investigate the 'paradox of creativity in autism' and whether those with Autistic traits have cognitive styles conducive to creativity, or whether they are disadvantaged by the 'implied cognitive and behavioural rigidity of the autism phenotype'. They examined the relationship between divergent thinking (a cognitive component of creativity), perception of ambiguous figures and self-reported Autistic traits. The tests of creativity involved generating as many innovative uses for common objects or interpretations of vague figures as they could in one minute. The outcome of this study indicated that those with higher levels of Autistic traits made fewer suggestions than those with lower levels, but the suggestions from those with higher levels of Autistic traits had greater originality. The authors concluded that as generation of novel ideas is a prerequisite for creative problem-solving, this may be an adaptive advantage associated with Autistic traits, but needs to be considered cautiously as the research was carried out with people with Autistic traits and not with Autistic people per se. This finding is borne out in the anecdotal evidence of there being many creative Autistic individuals working in creative and artistic industries, such as acting, writing, graphic design, animation, teaching, art, music composition, etc. It is also common for Autistic people to find a sense of calm within creative activities, such as craftwork, art, music, etc., and to experience flow states. It is therefore vital when exploring Autistic experiences with a person that we explore individual experiences and avoid assumptions that lead us towards limited ways of viewing an experience.

3. **Masking:** When engaging in an exploration of Autistic identity with a person, it is essential to consider their experience of masking, while also being aware that this may not be a conscious experience for them. It is widely understood that masking has a negative impact on people, and it is a complex area to explore. When exploring this area with a person, ask about whether they have put in a lot of effort into learning to understand others, and why they act as they do. Have they put effort into acting a certain way in certain situations? Do they often 'mask' or 'camouflage' in certain situations? Some of the more common areas in which people mask relate to making the 'right amount' of eye contact that is expected by a neurotypical society when they find it uncomfortable, not talking about their interests as others can judge this negatively, or hiding from others any stimming behaviours that they find balancing. Others may mask though compensatory strategies, for example, people pleasing, or assimilation strategies, such as dressing like others, behaving as others do in order to 'fit in', etc.

4. **Executive functioning:** Executive functioning includes skills such as planning, organization, managing time, initiating tasks, perseverance, adapting to situations and working memory. These skills have significant implications for a person's ability to engage with education programmes, carry out daily functioning tasks, and maintain employment, etc., particularly where accommodations are not accessible. While many Autistic people have the ability to manage the demands of education and employment, they often struggle with the executive functioning skills that are necessary for daily tasks and self-care. Self-reported daily executive functioning has been shown to be a valuable predictor of academic progress within young Autistic adults (Dijkhuis et al. 2020), and it is reduced executive functioning, not cognitive aptitude, that leads to discontinuation of academic study.

   Executive functioning challenges can also impact on a person's progress within their careers and employment and can make daily living tasks challenging, but they are not universal and are not necessarily the experience of all Autistic people. In exploring this, it is important to ask about people's experiences of study, work, employment and managing home life. How have they experienced these things in the past? What was their experience of secondary school and university like? How did they find undertaking assignments and exams? If they are working, what are the aspects of their job that they enjoy? What aspects do they not enjoy? How do they experience tasks related to 'life admin', such as managing bills, grocery shopping, making and keeping medical or dental appointments, etc.?

5. **Experiences of empathy:** It has long been held that Autistic people

universally struggle with empathy and 'theory of mind' in that they lack the ability to identify and understand the thoughts and feelings of others. It was believed that this therefore leads Autistic people to have 'inappropriate' emotional responses to the feelings of others (Krahn and Fenton 2012). Related to this is the theory of 'extreme male brain' (Baron-Cohen 2002), which holds that Autistic people have an intense drive to systemize and a low drive to empathize. However, these views are now being challenged by the lived experience and further research in relation to Autistic experiences of empathy (see Chapter 4 for further information about Autistic empathy).

The landscape in relation to understanding Autistic experiences of empathy is shifting away from a focus on cognitive empathy (recognizing and understanding another's mental state) and more towards Autistic experiences of affective empathy (feeling the emotions of others). Affective empathy can be strong and overwhelming for Autistic people. There is research to suggest that Autistic children experience overwhelming affective empathy, which can therefore make it challenging to interact and engage with others (Markram and Markram 2010; Smith 2009). It has been suggested that the expression of emotion in Autistic individuals is different rather than non-existent, as there tends to be less facial expression and different body language, but the emotion is actually felt rather intensely (Smith 2009). This can then result in neurotypical individuals misreading or not understanding the emotional experience of Autistic individuals (Goodall 2013), which gives rise to mutual misreading and lack of empathy and understanding on both neurotypical and Autistic sides (the double empathy problem; see Milton 2012). Another aspect of empathy experience is the concept of alexithymia, which refers to an inability to recognize and label the emotion an individual might feel. Although alexithymia is prevalent among Autistic people (Griffin, Lombardo and Auyeung 2016; Poquérusse et al. 2018), it is not a universal experience, and individuals who experience alexithymia find it more challenging to express empathy, regardless of whether they are Autistic or not (Mul et al. 2018).

In considering all of the above and the evolving understanding of Autistic experiences of empathy, it is important to explore this area during assessment with individuals. Does the person find it easy to identify their feelings? How have they experienced previous counselling or therapeutic interactions where they have been asked to identify and explore their feelings? How do they experience the emotions of others?

6. **Abilities relating to 'hyperfocus':** There is a distinct lack of understanding of hyperfocus states within Autistic identity, with there being no studies to

date that specifically measure behaviour or cognitive performance during hyperfocus states within Autistic people (Ashinoff and Abu-Akel 2021). Ashinoff and Abu-Akel (2021) describe hyperfocus as having four main features: that it is induced by task engagement, that it is an intense state of sustained or selective attention, that during hyperfocus there is diminished perception of non-task-relevant stimuli, and that task performance improves.

Within the literature, the tendency for Autistic people to intensely focus on a particular behaviour or topic is often explicitly referred to as hyperfocus (see, for example, Mayes 2014; Fein 2015; Bombaci 2012) or monotropism (see Chapter 5). There is a clear relationship between hyperfocus and flow states, and Autistic people appear to more easily experience flow as compared to non-autistic people. While flow experiences are not always related to hyperfocus, hyperfocus can lead to an intense flow experience for Autistic people, but within the literature and within Autistic criteria, the ability to hyperfocus and to establish a flow state can be viewed as a deficit rather than a strength or ability. As is the case with any strength, if something is over-used it can cause a negative impact for the person, for example, being in flow or hyperfocusing can cause a person to neglect their self-care. However, this strength can also bring about deep and detailed knowledge, specialist expertise, intense pleasure and deep joy.

A person's experience of hyperfocus and flow states needs to be explored within an Autistic assessment process. What is a person passionate about? How do they like to engage with their interests? When engaging with their interests, do they experience a hyperfocus state? Do they experience flow states? Are they aware of external stimuli or interoception when engaging with their interests?

7. **Strong sense of social justice:** A particularly common trait among Autistic individuals is an innate sense of justice. Many Autistic individuals find injustice intolerable – both directed to them and to others – and are strong advocates for those experiencing injustice. Autistic people may be more likely to have traits such as care, loyalty, authority, sanctity and especially fairness (Kapp 2016), as well as values such as honesty, integrity and adhering to rules, which all converge to arrive at a sense of justice and fairness for all. Within the assessment context, it is important to explore a person's experience of these areas. Do they feel they have a strong sense of social justice? How do they feel about artifice or lying? Do they find it very difficult to understand unkindness, cruelty and injustice?

Gather information about strengths and whether they align to Autistic strengths

Despite the deficit-based approach of formal Autistic criteria, there is widespread recognition that there are many valuable, positive and advantageous attributes associated with being Autistic. However, it can be difficult for individuals to identify their skills and strengths, as it is more likely that they have experienced feedback from society on what their perceived 'deficiencies' are. It is essential that Autistic strengths are explored during the course of any assessment process as a person's profile of strengths may align with those of Autistic experiences, and can consequently support the exploration and cultivation of their identity. Having a sense of their Autistic strengths allows a person a greater sense of self and provides a greater depth to their self-understanding and self-compassion. It also allows a platform from which to build self-esteem and self-concept, where a person might have previously held a low view of themselves due to constant exposure within society to the idea that they are 'less than' others. Having a balanced perspective is essential for mental health and wellbeing.

When exploring Autistic strengths with a person, consider their observational skills and their ability to attend to detail. Are they thorough and accurate in their approach to tasks, and do they notice the detail? Do they have a strong ability to engage in detailed research and to source facts and information? Are they able to develop deep expertise in an area and to immerse themselves in the information they have gathered, recalling it when necessary? What are a person's attention and concentration skills like? Are they able to focus for long periods and to a deeper level? Does the person take a methodical approach to tasks and in solving problems? What are the person's core values? Do their values align with common Autistic values of honesty, loyalty, trust, transparency, being non-judgemental, etc.? Does the person demonstrate creative strengths in their thinking style, their passions and in problem-solving?

Gather information about previous or current mental health diagnoses

As discussed in Chapter 10, Autistic people experience higher rates of co-occurring mental health conditions and suicidality when compared to the general population. The intersectionality between being Autistic and mental health is well documented, yet there continues to be poor recognition of Autistic people within mental health populations. A recent systematic review by Tromans et al. (2018) focusing on unrecognized Autistic adults among psychiatric inpatients estimated a prevalence of between 2.4 per cent and 9.9 per cent, while Nyrenius et al. (2022) estimated prevalence in outpatient psychiatry clinics as at least 18.9 per cent, with another

5–10 per cent having 'subthreshold' symptoms. Geurts and Jansen (2012) found that most Autistic adults were known within mental health services prior to confirmation of being Autistic, with the time lapse between first contact with services and confirmation of Autistic identity ranging from 0–56 years, with a median of 12 years. In approaching an autism assessment, clinicians need to be aware of the intersectionality between being Autistic and mental health. This relates to mental health challenges being more prevalent among Autistic individuals, and also confirmation of Autistic identity often being missed as challenges are perceived as being related to mental health or misdiagnosed as mental health conditions.

When undertaking an autism assessment, it is vital to gather information about previous or current mental health diagnoses, including whether the person agrees with these diagnoses or not, and if not, why not. What are the aspects of a diagnosis that don't make sense to the person in terms of how they understand themselves? In exploring these areas, it can then be determined whether a person's experiences primarily relate to being Autistic, mental health, or a combination of both.

Gather information about medical history

Information about a person's medical history is essential in exploring whether they are Autistic or not. The importance and relevance of a person's medical history relates to two areas:

- Whether there may be any aspect of a person's medical history that might possibly account for aspects of their Autistic experiences.

- If a person is Autistic, and they also experience co-occurring medical conditions, they will require the barriers that exist for Autistic people in accessing healthcare to be removed.

In terms of determining whether there are factors within a person's medical history that need to be considered within an autism assessment, information in relation to the following is helpful (although please note that this list is not exhaustive):

- Genetic or chromosomal factors.

- History of head injury.

- History of illnesses involving the brain.

- Epilepsy.

- The presence of any chronic health conditions.

- Current medication.

Gather information about significant life events or potential trauma

In undertaking an autism assessment with an adult, information must be gathered regarding the person's exposure to and experience of trauma and significant events in their life. This is essential so that a person has a full and thorough understanding of their whole identity and sense of self. As stated previously (see Chapter 10), Autistic people are more likely to have experienced higher levels of trauma in their lives than neurotypical people, and so it is possible that being Autistic and experiencing trauma are co-occurring. Autistic people are more likely to have been exposed to traumatic events in their life, such as bullying, abuse or assault, and also due to the trauma of masking, camouflaging and living within a society that actively excludes other neurotypes. On the other hand, it must also be considered whether a person's trauma experience might offer a better explanation for their overall sense of identity than an Autistic framework.

While many people will have experienced significant events in their lives, whether or not it gives rise to the experience of trauma is subjective and depends on a number of objective and subjective factors (Weinberg and Gil 2016). When considering the impact of significant events during the course of an exploration of Autistic identity, information is required in relation to the following:

- Whether a person has experienced what they deem to be significant events in their life.

- How the person has responded to the events.

- Whether the person considers themselves to have experienced trauma as a result of the events they have experienced.

- Whether the person feels they have had an opportunity to access support in relation to the trauma they have experienced.

- What the impact of trauma has been.

- Whether the person feels they have processed their traumatic experiences, or whether they still need support and an opportunity to do this.

- How does the person themselves feel they understand the role of trauma in their life alongside their Autistic experiences? Does it make sense to them in how they understand themselves that trauma and being Autistic co-occur in their experiences, or do they have a question about the possibility of one being a more fitting framework than the other?

The final point is extremely important in a collaborative assessment process, and increases the likelihood of a reliable and valid outcome that is a helpful framework in moving forward positively for the person. In considering the occurrence of identity exploration within an Autistic assessment process, it is essential that time and consideration is devoted to exploring and supporting a person in making sense of their own experiences from both trauma and Autistic perspectives (for a full discussion in relation to trauma in the context of Autistic experiences, see Chapter 10).

There is a significant risk of diagnostic overshadowing in relation to the co-occurrence of trauma or PTSD and being Autistic, with the presence of trauma often overshadowing an Autistic identity. There have been countless occasions of Autistic people being misunderstood and misdiagnosed due to the presence of trauma in their lives. There is often a failure to recognize a person's Autistic identity due to clinicians misattributing some Autistic experiences to trauma symptoms, for example an Autistic person who experiences shutdowns or meltdowns due to sensory overwhelm being viewed through a trauma lens of flashbacks and significant emotional distress. Diagnostic overshadowing in relation to trauma and Autistic experiences not only denies the person from having a full understanding of their sense of self and identity; it also denies the person the opportunity to access appropriate support with their trauma experiences through an Autistic lens therapeutically.

When gathering information in relation to significant life events and possible trauma, it is important to consider a person's experience of having to communicate about difficult experiences. Some people will feel comfortable expressing their experiences, and some won't. This may depend on a number of factors, including whether a person has had an opportunity yet to process their experience of trauma, or whether the impact continues to be active. The pacing of this piece requires consideration, as does the role of the clinician and the possibility or not of them being in a position to offer continued support to the person should it transpire that they require additional support due to active trauma, or whether the experience of recounting their trauma experiences triggers distress. If a clinician is not in a position to offer longer term support, then safeguarding in relation to managing distress needs to be considered prior to communicating about trauma, particularly in situations where it is known that there is likely to be a presence of trauma in a person's experiences.

Of significant importance when communicating about trauma during the course of an autism assessment is that a person is given a choice in relation to how they communicate about their experiences, that is, do they wish to communicate through spoken communication or would they feel more comfortable writing about their experiences? Some people prefer a combination of communication methods.

Due to the fact that there is a high co-occurrence of being Autistic and exposure to traumatic experiences, it can sometimes feel challenging for non-autistic clinicians to feel confident in their ability to determine the presence of an Autistic identity where there is a high level of trauma experience. In considering this piece, it is important for clinicians to keep in mind the following:

- The assessment process is a collaborative exploration of identity with a person. Determining whether an Autistic identity co-occurs with trauma experiences is the outcome of a joint and shared process with a clinician and client in partnership with each other. It is of primary importance that a framework is proposed that makes sense to a client in terms of how they know and understand themselves. Some people are very clear and sure about how they understand their Autistic identity alongside their experience of trauma. Others will require the support of a clinician who can facilitate an open and safe space within which to explore this.

- In determining whether an Autistic identity and trauma co-occur, it can be more difficult to determine this if only the challenges a person experiences are considered. Many challenges Autistic people experience can often also be considered as related to a trauma experience (e.g., feeling uncomfortable around other people, different sleep patterns, meltdowns/shutdowns). Focusing on Autistic strengths and whether a person experiences these will assist in exploring whether an Autistic identity co-occurs with an individual's experiences of trauma. The presence of Autistic strengths such as attention to detail, deep focus, methodical/novel approaches, creativity, expertise, ability to retain facts, etc., can all indicate that a person's experiences relate to Autistic experiences, and that being Autistic co-occurs alongside trauma.

Issues in relation to gathering evidence from childhood

Within the current diagnostic classification systems, reference is made within Autistic criteria to evidence of Autistic traits being required within early childhood. Both the ICD-11 criteria (WHO 2019) and the DSM-5 and DSM-5-TR criteria (APA 2013, 2022) state that Autistic traits should be evident during the developmental period, but both also specify that characteristics may not manifest until later in life, when social expectations move beyond what a person is deemed capable of responding to or engaging with.

There are a number of challenges and considerations when approaching the reference to evidence in early life when undertaking an autism assessment with adults. First, and of prime importance, the autonomy and respect for the person who is exploring their identity needs to be kept at the core of the process. It is our experience that many people have found it immensely disrespectful that their own account of their experiences, including their early years experiences, are not simply accepted as truth and as valid information. Within a Neuro-Affirmative assessment framework, it cannot be a requirement that an outside source must be provided in order to confirm or provide information if a person does not wish to include this.

Further consideration needs to be given to the challenges of gathering information about a person's early developmental period when that time period might have been a long time ago. Adults attend for assessment at all ages and stages of their lives. It is not unusual for people in their 60s and 70s to seek assessment. The older a person is, the more amount of time has passed since their early childhood, and with the passage of time it is less likely that reliable information can be gathered from memory. For those who do wish to include family members in the assessment process, older people may have less opportunity to ask parents or family members about their childhood experiences if family members have now died or are infirm, and memories of observations from siblings or others can often be limited and possibly inaccurate due to the passage of time and the likelihood that the reporter was also a child themselves at the time of observation.

This can also raise challenging emotions for the person, in relation to a sense of loss in not having the chance to explore with their parent(s) or relative(s) their experiences through an Autistic lens. Furthermore, with the landscape of understanding in relation to Autistic experiences changing so rapidly in recent years, it is often the case that Autistic experiences were poorly understood when many adults attending for assessment were children, and therefore their experiences were understood through a different lens, which can also influence reported observations from others.

When considering different methods for gathering information about childhood experiences, the following might be helpful:

- Experiences recalled by the person themselves.

- Information from parents.

- Information from siblings.

- Information from extended family members (e.g., aunts, uncles, cousins, etc.).

- Information from childhood friends.

- Childhood photographs.

- Childhood videos.

- School reports.

- Formal assessment reports from childhood.

- Records of health or developmental checks.

- Medical records.

When gathering information about a person's experiences in childhood, it is helpful to explore the following:

- What they were like as a baby and toddler?

- What were their speech and language skills like?

- What were their social and emotional experiences as a child?

- Did they ever meet with any professionals as a child, and why?

- How did they experience change as a child?

- What did they love doing as a child?

- What did they hate as a child?

- What helped to calm them as a child?

- How were their activity levels as a child?

- Did they make any hand, body or vocal sounds as a child that were repeated?

- How did they experience school?

- What activities did they choose to do?

- How was their sleep as a child?

- What were their friendships like?

- How did they manage daily tasks such as brushing teeth, dressing, feeding themselves, etc.?

- How did they experience sensory aspects of their environment?

Reflection Point

In our experience, the process of gathering information from childhood during an adult assessment is variable. Some people recall huge amounts of detail in relation to their childhood experiences, and others don't. Some are comfortable to involve family members, and for some that isn't possible for a variety of reasons. It is vital to always check with the person whether they wish to include other people in their assessment process or not. If they do choose to include information from others, it is essential to check with the person whether they agree with the accuracy of the information or not. In our practice, it has frequently occurred that information provided by a family member is completely at odds with a person's own recollection of their experiences. Or a person's internal experience differed hugely from what was outwardly observed by others. It is respectful and more accurate to seek feedback from the person themselves about other people's information about them.

Reflection Point

In many assessment processes, there is no information about an individual's childhood experiences. Either the person finds it difficult to recall specific experiences, and/or there is no information from any other sources. Lack of information about childhood experiences is not a barrier to completing the assessment piece, and a conclusion can be drawn on the information that is available. This may change should new information come to light, but based on the information available, a conclusion to the piece should be arrived at.

There has been an exponential increase in the number of people being identified as Autistic for the first time in adulthood. One UK population-based study examined time trends in Autistic identification, and found a 787 per cent increase in confirmation of Autistic identity among the general population over the time period from 1998 to 2018, with the greatest increase in identification among adults when compared with children and adolescents (Russell et al. 2021). For many individuals, there is clear evidence of Autistic experiences within their childhood. This evidence either comes from the person's own memory of their early preferences and experiences, or it may come from the observations of others who knew them when they were younger, if a person wishes to include information from others in their assessment process. For others, despite detailed information gathering, there is little to no evidence of Autistic traits in childhood, even though the person's experiences clearly align with Autistic experiences as an adult, and nothing else has occurred that might explain why that is (Russell et al. 2021).

Rødgaard et al. (2021) investigated whether Autistic identification in adulthood might be explained by misdiagnosis in childhood or diagnostic overshadowing. They found that while most childhood diagnoses (e.g., ADHD, anxiety, stress, clinical low mood, etc.) were highly prevalent in adults, 69 per cent of males and 61 per cent of females did not have any other psychiatric or neurological diagnoses in childhood, and for those who did, they mostly received these after the age of 12. This suggests that for this cohort, late identification cannot be explained by misdiagnosis or overshadowing. The authors concluded that there could be several explanations for delayed confirmation of Autistic identity for these people, including masking and Autistic developmental trajectories. Research in the area of evidence of Autistic experiences within childhood for Autistic adults is in its very early stages. Further research is required to investigate how Autistic experiences may have manifested in childhood for the adult-identified population.

Involving Family Members and/or Others in the Assessment Process

The involvement of a parent or other person in an assessment process requires careful consideration and consultation with a client within a Neuro-Affirmative assessment approach. The decision to involve others should be determined in consultation with a person, with the person having the final say. Many people are comfortable with involving others in the assessment process. For some, this might be a parent or a sibling, or someone who can provide information about an individual's experiences and preferences in childhood. A spouse or partner, a friend or a co-worker might provide information about current strengths and challenges they have noticed a person to experience. Information might be provided by a family member or friend joining a session with the person also present, or it could be gathered via written formats, for example a questionnaire. The person should always have the opportunity to hear or read the information that is provided by others about them as part of the process if they wish to review it. This also facilitates the person to give feedback on how others' views of them make sense to their sense of self, and it allows for any differences between internal experiences and outward projections to be considered and made sense of. This can give rise to a richer understanding of a person and a more rounded sense of identity.

Although it can be helpful to the information-gathering process in order to understand a person from different perspectives and across their lifespan, there can be many reasons why gathering information from others is not possible, or is not appropriate. Some Autistic adults who demonstrated Autistic characteristics as children have grown up in environments where their Autistic needs were not recognized or understood. Some have been exposed to deep invalidation of their identity and their needs through the mal-intention of others, and some were exposed to invalidation from well-intended but misinformed family members or others. Many are acutely aware of this and are deeply traumatized and uncertain of their identity as a result.

Many would likely experience a re-traumatization as a result of being invalidated again via the involvement of another in their assessment process. Some have fractured relationships with family members following a childhood of being misunderstood, or other factors such as parental mental health challenges, abuse or neglect. For these reasons, it is important that the decision to involve others in the assessment process is collaborative and meaningful for the person. In our practice, the decision on whether to involve anyone else is made solely by the person themselves, without pressure or judgement, as receiving information about others' reflections on one's behaviour can bring up a range of different emotions, from amusement to upset. It is important that the person leads the decision on whether to involve a family member as it can have benefits or repercussions that extend beyond the assessment process.

Reports, Letters and Documents

Within The Adult Autism Practice, when it has been collaboratively confirmed that a person is Autistic, they are issued a 'suite of letters' that are tailored to their specific needs. These letters cover a range of different needs a person has, including (but not limited to) confirmation of Autistic identity, accommodations required, support with applications for welfare payments, letters informing other services of a person's Autistic identity, etc. For the vast majority of people, a full 'clinical report' is not required, and brief documentation that gives access to what is needed is what is most helpful, with letters outlining accommodations required being reported as the most helpful. Very occasionally, a person seeks or requires a full clinical report.

Typically, this may be to support their processing of their identity, or it may be that they are seeking to access other services, such as mental health services, and a more detailed report is helpful.

As the neurodiversity movement progresses and the landscape of understanding Autistic experiences changes, it is hoped that formal documentation in relation to confirming an Autistic identity will eventually no longer be required in order for adults to access supports. It is hoped that there will come a time when there is widespread acceptance of self-identification of being Autistic, if a person wishes to do so, and that everyone can choose and access the accommodations and supports they need with or without having supporting documentation to do so. Indeed, the introduction of universal accommodations along with greater understanding, kindness towards and acceptance of each other within society would eventually mean that any accommodations that currently have to be 'implemented' are just automatically part of our societal experience. Some people may still require support to identify what would be helpful to them, but most already have an intuitive sense of what they need and what they would like, and they rightfully find it frustrating that many systems insist on formal documentation as evidence of this, which is often expensive, time-consuming and difficult to obtain. Insisting on formal and often unnecessarily exposing documentation for an adult person to have any access to supports invalidates their expertise about themselves, and is unobtainable and prohibitive for many.

Although it is hoped that society will continue to move towards universal accommodations with free access for all, the situation in most, if not all, countries is that this is not currently the case. Despite self-identification being considered valid within the Autistic community, formal identification with associated documentation is generally required if a person requires access to services, supports and accommodations. As a result, there is currently a continuing need for formal documentation at the conclusion of an assessment process, and this is likely to remain the case for the immediate future. It is also the case that many people find written reports and documentation helpful in terms of understanding themselves and how their experiences fit with Autistic experiences.

When concluding an assessment process with a person, the documentation that outlines the outcome of the process and the next steps of support provision is important and needs careful consideration. What will be required will depend on each person's situation, the context of their work and education environments, and whether they are already or will need to be linked with any other services.

> All documentation that is issued must be affirmative, validating, reflective of the person and their own experiences, and must include information about the person's Autistic strengths (if being Autistic is confirmed) and the challenges they experience.

Following a Neuro-Affirmative assessment process, it is important to be aware that there is often a need to explain an Autistic identity from a Neuro-Affirmative perspective to other professionals and to mental health services within documentation that is issued (see Chapter 4 for further discussion on what being Autistic is). Helpful things to outline in letters include:

- Being Autistic is not a 'condition' or an illness.

- Explain Autistic experience as a neurotype and a valid way to be in the world.

- Discuss the need for accommodations within neurotypical environments.

- Give recommendations for reading or for obtaining further information if the recipient would like to enhance their knowledge.

Other professionals and services may already embody a Neuro-Affirmative understanding of being Autistic, and in this circumstance, outlining it in documentation will only serve to confirm what the Autistic person already knows. However, if they are not aware, then it is extremely important that we educate and advocate, not only for our own clients but also for those who may already be within services or who will be referred in the future.

A bespoke approach for each person is the most helpful when considering the documentation to be issued following an assessment process. Each person varies in terms of what they require and what is relative to their needs. The following are the central and core aspects of the functions that documentation needs to fulfil:

- A statement of whether a person is Autistic or not.

- Which classification of Autistic criteria the person met.

- Information on how the person meets the criteria.

- Information on what the person requires in terms of accommodations and supports.

The following types of letters and documents should be considered following an assessment process. Not all will be required by each person, and it should be discussed with the person as to what they feel is required for their particular situation and circumstances:

1. Document outlining experiences mapped onto areas within the criteria: Everyone who seeks a full assessment piece will require written information about how their experiences align with Autistic experiences or fit with Autistic criteria. This is an extremely important document as it supports a person's understanding of their sense of identity, and how their experiences align with the different areas of an Autistic identity. This document can be developed collaboratively with a person as part of the assessment process (see Appendix 5 for a sample of mapping documents using the DSM-5-TR criteria and ICD-11 criteria).

2. Brief letter confirming assessment outcome: A brief letter consisting of two to three sentences confirming that the person is Autistic in line with whichever classification system was used as part of the assessment process is very helpful. There are many circumstances where a person is required to show evidence or 'proof' that they are Autistic, for example, if they are accessing assistance within an airport, but further information or details in relation to how they meet Autistic criteria is not required, or the person does not feel comfortable sharing it. Having a brief letter confirming the outcome of the assessment is very helpful in this regard.

3. Documentation relating to reasonable accommodations: Reasonable accommodations can be requested in a variety of situations. Most typically, they can be considered for a workplace; a learning environment, such as university, college, etc.; and accessing healthcare, for example, attending GP appointments, hospital appointments, etc. Formal documentation outlining the accommodations a person requires in each of these settings is still often required. Most people are unsure about what accommodations are possible, and it is helpful to provide them with a list of options that they can review and consider before recommendations are developed and documented (see Appendix 4 for exercises to support development of workplace accommodations and Appendix 6 for a blank healthcare passport).

Examples of Possible Reasonable Accommodations in College and/or in the Workplace:

Note: Accommodations should be tailored to the needs of the person within their specific environment. The following list is not exhaustive.

- College staff, tutors and colleagues should familiarize themselves with Autistic experiences by researching information provided by Autistic people themselves.

- Be aware of possible auditory processing difficulties when speaking to the Autistic person, in particular in busy environments where multiple people are present.

- Clear and direct communication is required, and agreed actions should be communicated in written and spoken formats.

- Targets should be mutually agreed and realistic.

- Clear and simple guidance should be provided when giving instructions, which should come from one person only.

- Communicate decisions, changes and exceptions explicitly, to avoid ambiguity and assumption.

- Allow additional time for the Autistic person to process, respond and follow through on instructions.

- Non-complex tasks should be available to switch to when other tasks are overloading.

- There may be a need for movement if the person has difficulties sitting still for long periods of time. Fidgeting and moving around should be accepted as necessary for the Autistic person to pay attention and concentrate.

- Non-spoken communication, such as eye contact, should not be an automatic expectation in communication, as for Autistic people eye contact is not necessary for communication, and not making eye contact is not a sign that the person is not paying attention or engaging in the conversation.

- A quiet location is useful for taking exams or carrying out work.

- Provide a quiet location for break times.

- Give access to regular break times to support regulation.

- Provide the option for the person to wear headphones, ear defenders, ear plugs, sunglasses, etc. to support sensory regulation.

- Give the person access to a workplace or college mentor.

- Be flexible in the workplace culture around food, such as if the person wants to eat on their own.

- If applicable, offer working from home or a part-time option, where possible.

- Allow adjustments to uniform or dress code.

4. A full Neuro-Affirmative assessment report: Whether or not a full assessment report is required needs consideration and discussion with the person. For most adults who are not linked in with specific services and who are not going to be linked in with services, a full formal report is not necessarily required. However, a full report may be helpful to some in terms of processing the outcome and beginning the process of understanding their Autistic identity. Where a person is being referred to a specific team or service, a full report may be required in order to access the service, as information is needed in relation to how a person meets the criteria, whether other potential explanations were considered, and what the person requires in terms of supports. As is the case with all other outcome documentation, a full report should be Neuro-Affirmative.

Should a full Neuro-Affirmative assessment report be required, it should consist of:

- Information about a person's background.

- Detailed information about the person's preferences, needs, strengths, challenges and experiences within the different areas of the criteria.

- Information about potential other understandings of a person's experiences and how these are understood in the context of other things, such as their medical history, mental health history and experience of trauma.

- Information about the collaborative conclusion that was reached.

- Recommendations in relation to the accommodations and supports required.

Applying for Welfare Payments (e.g., Disability Allowance, Personal Independence Payment)

Depending on individual circumstances, some people may wish to apply for a specific welfare payment to support their financial needs. In Ireland, this payment is called Disability Allowance, in the UK it is the Personal Independence Payment, and there are equivalents in other jurisdictions. At the current time, it is very challenging to create documentation that is Neuro-Affirmative and that also satisfies the requirements of state welfare systems. Such systems are most likely to be medicalized in their approach and expect there to be reference to 'severe-to-profound impairments', 'inability', 'deficiencies', etc. within the documentation in order for the welfare support to be granted. This, and the overall application process, can be very challenging for people to navigate when they have been through a Neuro-Affirmative assessment process that validates their identity and bears witness to their challenges from a non-impaired perspective.

Should a person wish to apply for these welfare payments, they will likely require a separate letter outlining their needs from the perspective of the impact on their ability to work. If a Neuro-Affirmative assessment has been conducted, clients will need to be aware that they need to inform their diagnosing clinician that they intend to apply for a welfare payment, and additional documentation using particular language will need to be issued separately to a Neuro-Affirmative report. This document needs to be deficit-focused and outline all of the ways that being Autistic negatively impacts on a person's ability to work and to engage in daily living tasks. People attending for assessment will need to be advised that the language and phrasing used within a document for the purpose of welfare payment applications is not Neuro-Affirmative and is not reflective of the person as a whole, but has to be used to satisfy the requirements of the welfare system.

While acknowledging with a person that the documentation in support of their application for welfare support is not Neuro-Affirmative, and subsequently issuing such documentation, it is also important that we acknowledge our role in advocating for system change. The current systems within Ireland, the UK and elsewhere are typically extremely challenging for people to navigate. The application forms are extensive, information about deficits is required, supporting documentation is required (often from multiple sources) and sign-off is required from the person's GP or primary healthcare professional. Meeting all of these requirements is hugely challenging for most while they are also managing higher levels of internal stress, adjusting to learning about a change in their identity and possible financial concerns, etc. For those who do undertake the process, the application is often denied.

While it is acknowledged that there must be certainty that welfare support is only being given to those who need it, consideration needs to be given to defining better methods of assessing need, providing evidence in support of applications and recognizing that there can be a Neuro-Affirmative approach to understanding and conveying a person's experience of being Autistic while also finding engaging in work overwhelming.

Considering Previous Diagnoses

A comprehensive autism assessment includes screening and/or further assessment in relation to mental health and personality factors, with further follow-up where indicated. However, it is often the case that many people who seek and attend for an autism assessment have already previously been identified as other neurodivergencies, as well as having mental health challenges, or as having 'personality disorders' (see Chapter 10). Through the course of a comprehensive Autistic assessment, it can often become very clear that the previous diagnoses that were either suggested or confirmed are not the best understanding of a person's experiences, particularly when an Autistic lens is applied to their experiences. Although best practice guidelines indicate that there should be a holistic review, the issue remains in clinical practice that there often tends to be no review of previous confirmed diagnostic labels, and quite often people may have been discharged from a service that made a previous diagnosis. There have also been many occasions where services have suggested the possibility of a diagnosis, for example, 'borderline personality disorder', but have neither confirmed nor ruled this out, which leaves the person with no clarity on how best to understand themselves and their experiences. This has also meant that many Autistic people have been treated as if they do have a diagnosis of 'borderline personality disorder', which leads to further trauma, and sometimes fatal outcomes.

Within the scope of a comprehensive Autistic assessment, it is important to explore with a person what aspects within their previous diagnoses make sense to them in how they understand themselves, and what does not. Where it is clear that a previous diagnosis is relevant or not to a person's experiences, this should be confirmed either way as part of a full assessment process. It is a fundamental care piece to explore this with a person (within the bounds of your professional competencies or within the scope of your team), particularly when it is clear that a previous diagnosis is not applicable, or if a previous diagnosis has been suggested but neither confirmed nor denied. It is often the case that with 'personality disorder' there has been no formal or detailed assessment carried out, and yet the label is very 'sticky' in that once it is mentioned, it becomes attached. It is very difficult for a person to tolerate having diagnoses attached to them that don't make sense to them, and if clarity can be offered, then it is ethically appropriate that it is. With a formal previous diagnosis, and where a person is still actively involved with the service or professional who has made the previous diagnosis, then a collaborative approach is advised so that all involved can reach a consensus on the most appropriate understanding of a person's experiences, which allows for an integrated framework moving forward.

Where a person has many previous diagnoses, some of which might not make sense to them in terms of how they understand themselves, it is typically not helpful to add another diagnosis while also leaving the others there. An adult Autistic assessment is a process of identity exploration with a person in order to support them to arrive at the best understanding of how they know themselves and understand their experiences. If a person has multiple diagnoses, it is important to support them to explore how they understand each of those diagnoses, and how they might interact with each other. There needs to be a broad overview on what the conclusions are based on the information to hand at the current time of assessment. What makes the most sense in a person's self-understanding? There may be five previous diagnoses that make sense to a person, but it could be the case that actually three of those don't make sense and there are two left that fully explain things. Undertaking this broad review of diagnostic exploration encompassing previous diagnoses alongside current ones being considered is part of a Neuro-Affirmative assessment process.

Listening to Autistic people talking about their experiences of exploring and acquiring diagnoses is profound. Where a diagnosis is made in a non-collaborative way that doesn't make sense to the person, the consequences can be devastating. People frequently experience PTSD/complex PTSD, lower self-esteem, lower self-confidence, depression and anxiety, and their trust in services and professionals and belief that there is help and support can be profoundly impacted. Conversely, diagnoses that make sense to a person in how they know themselves can be extremely helpful in moving forward positively and in cultivating identity. There are diagnoses that people are born with (e.g., being Autistic, ADHD, Dyslexic, epilepsy, etc.) and there are ones that people acquire (e.g., PTSD/complex PTSD, etc.). Having a clear understanding of these gives a framework for moving forward positively with a strong sense of self and an awareness of strengths and challenges.

Support When Being Autistic Is Not Identified

For most people seeking a private autism assessment, they have carefully considered and carried out their own research into Autistic experiences, and have developed very good insight into whether they feel their own experiences align with Autistic experiences. This is also very often the case for those accessing a public assessment pathway. For some, however, it is challenging to determine whether their experiences are fully explained by an Autistic identity, or whether there is possibly a better explanation elsewhere. Some who attend feel that their experiences do align with Autistic experiences, but haven't considered a likely better alternative, and the assessment process allows them the opportunity to explore this. Some attend for assessment believing that the outcome will indicate that they are Autistic, but ultimately come to the understanding that their experiences can be better explained by other factors.

Engaging in a collaborative process with a person is key in supporting them with an assessment outcome that indicates they are not Autistic. If a collaborative process has been undertaken, then the steps to arriving at the conclusion are taken jointly, and both parties are discovering the outcome of the process together at the same time. If the outcome is not what the person was expecting, then discovering this gradually and jointly is more helpful to the person than hearing it suddenly, as they will have worked through the steps (in a supportive way) to understand why that is the outcome, and what an alternative explanation might be.

Reflection Point

Within a Neuro-Affirmative Autistic assessment process, it is important to prepare a person attending for assessment for what they may experience within other services they engage with post assessment that are not Neuro-Affirmative in their approach. Within a Neuro-Affirmative assessment process, the person will have been respected, supported and empowered throughout, and their autonomy will have been held throughout. It is often reported that returning to or being referred into other services that are not Neuro-Affirmative in their approach can be challenging for many people, and can be a sharply contrasting experience. It is important to prepare people for the distinct possibility that other professionals they meet may not be aware of and/or use a Neuro-Affirmative framework in their approach.

Reflections for Clinicians within the Process

Conducting a Neuro-Affirmative exploration of Autistic identity with a person is typically a highly rewarding piece of work as a clinician, whether you are an Autistic or non-autistic clinician. In our practice, we have found huge fulfilment in the therapeutic pieces we have engaged in with people, and it has been a privilege to walk this part of a person's Autistic journey with them, as they trust us with their deepest thoughts and most personal experiences. It is usually the case that for most people the prospect of undertaking an assessment has been carefully considered, and the process of making sense of their experiences, re-framing past experiences, further developing their sense of identity and understanding their strengths and needs is a hugely positive experience. Having said that, for some, the experience can be extremely overwhelming as they contemplate how their lives might have been different had they known they were Autistic at a younger age, and as they come to terms with learning about their Autistic identity.

There are many layers to consider in conducting the process, and if you are not an Autistic clinician, there is an additional layer of deepening and developing your knowledge about Autistic experiences. It is extremely important for all clinicians to access Neuro-Affirmative supervision during the process or to engage in Neuro-Affirmative peer supervision with colleagues. Be aware of tone, body language and facial expressions during assessment sessions, as many Autistic people report being confused by these not matching what a clinician might be saying. Ensure that you are clear, concise and consistent in all interactions with a person. Seek feedback from the person, and revise your approach in line with their feedback. Offer alternative ways of working and information gathering, and collaboratively construct, deconstruct and reconstruct assessment practices that meet the person's unique needs, offering support where needed. Be open to changing the pace of the process, and be mindful of the demands a person might be managing outside of the assessment process.

13

Post-Assessment Support and Recommendations

Introduction

All support following an autism assessment should focus on the person's specific, individual needs. As stated numerous times previously in this book, each human being is unique, and given that the Autistic neurotype is simply a **different** neurotype to the typical, there is clearly no inherent recommendation for treatment of a specific neurotype (i.e., autism in this case). **Individual** differences, however, are vitally important to consider when recommending future support to the newly diagnosed Autistic person.

In post-assessment support our initial enquiry is **why** the person sought an assessment in the first instance. This alone usually gives us an abundance of rich data to develop a working hypothesis of the support that may be required.

In our experience as a team, adults come to us for an autism assessment for a range of reasons, although certain themes do emerge. Adults today who grew up in the 1960s, 1970s, 1980s and even the 1990s were more likely than not to have been missed as children, particularly if they were multiply marginalized or high-camouflaging (see Chapter 10). Even more recently still, young people and adults who fall outside the stereotypical conceptualization of an Autistic white, cisgender male are more likely to be missed. Autistic adults who may have come into contact with mental health services prior to seeking assessment have been diagnosed with depression, 'borderline personality disorder', anxiety disorder, or any number of other conditions. At times, adults seek assessment because none of these diagnoses fully resonated with them. Other salient reasons include that their child has been assessed as Autistic and they have seen themselves reflected in descriptions of Autistic experience as explored in relation to their children. Often, parents will have assumed these ways of being were simply family traits. Others may have come into contact with some Autistic adults and discovered a number of shared experiences.

When working with late-identified Autistic adults, it is important to note that the vast majority have generally spent the best part of their lifetime feeling like a failed version of 'typical'. Living as a neuro-minority within a system not designed for you is a harsh environment in which to grow and develop. Add to this the experience of late-identified adults who are aware of their differences but unaware as to the reason they find aspects of life so difficult, and it is common for an additional level of chronic stress and potentially traumatic events to be present in someone's history (Dodds 2021). Given that there is a large overlap between neuro-minorities and other marginalized identities, those occupying multiple marginalized identities will have intensified experiences and are **more** likely to have experienced traumatic events.

How Best to Signpost and Support People Post Assessment

Here are some of the ways that you, as the assessing professional (or post-assessment support professional), can best signpost and support people post assessment:

1. Discuss and explore the person's experience of the assessment process

There is no recommended guide to the length of time or number of sessions an individual person will need to explore their experience of the assessment process, as each person's journey is unique. At Thriving Autistic, we offer single support sessions, group workshops and blocks of sessions to support people's exploration of the assessment and their emotions. We find that many people who come to a single support session will want to continue working with their practitioner for as long as needed to explore the impact the assessment has had on them.

2. Review pivotal moments of the person's life through the new lens of Autistic experience

Validation of the person's experience throughout post-assessment support is vitally important, and assisting them to review potent past events through the lens of their neurotype is exceptionally helpful. Much of this self-reflection work will likely happen outside of the support space, triggered by thoughts, memories and even dreams, so normalizing and preparing people for this can be useful and reassuring for them to know. It is also important to appreciate that there is an unprecedented opportunity in this 'psychological restructuring' for the person's attitude towards themselves to shift towards that of self-acceptance, self-appreciation and self-advocacy.

3. Help the person realign their life to fit their neurology

A priority for therapists in Thriving Autistic is to support late-identified adults in realigning their lives to fit better with their neurology. Late-identified Autistic adults have spent a lifetime as outsiders, with the vast majority of them attempting to live a life as a neurology that isn't their own. The consequences of having done this are far-reaching, and so the person will need a complete overhaul if they are to have a chance to thrive as the wonderful, authentic beings they already are. Autistic adults are not failed versions of normal, yet that's the message they typically have spent their lives internalizing.

Broadly, then, there are several areas that need attending to so that late-identified adults can live authentically as themselves. Crucial to this exploration of realigning life to fit better with the person's neurology is understanding their sensory experience. For example, working from the outside inward, be curious about the following: how does the person experience the world through their senses? Which senses are more highly tuned in, and which less so? In what contexts?

Many newly diagnosed adults will be able to relay difficulties with sensory processing in some contexts whereas they have no difficulties in others. This is an important point to make note of. For many, background stress, lack of sleep and sickness can be a contributory factor to acute sensory processing distress. We need to be curious and open-minded when enquiring about these internal experiences, as many of our late-diagnosed clients will have pushed through or been very hard on themselves about these intermittent difficulties, not recognizing them as legitimate disabling factors.

Answers to these questions will give us a glimpse into the specific future support recommendations that our clients may benefit from.

4. Support people to foster a positive Autistic identity

Overall, a successful conclusion to post-assessment support could be viewed as supporting an Autistic adult in their personal journey to foster a positive Autistic self-identity. Some points to keep in mind when co-creating support goals could be:

- Recognize and increase personal strengths.

- Value and cultivate opportunities for flow states.

- Value own internal drives, such as the need for stimming.

- Value own communication preferences.

- Value own learning or work preferences.

- Promote autonomy.

- Promote self-advocacy.

- Promote self-acceptance.

- Connect with Autistic and neurodivergent peers and wider community.

- Understand and appreciate the social model of disability and the impact disabling factors within society have had on the person's life to date.

- Unpack own internalized ableism.

- Develop a personal perspective on the components of a good life.

5. Discuss camouflaging and masking and support people to begin the process of becoming more authentically themselves while remaining safe

One important point to note about the experience of unmasking is that it takes conscious effort for an Autistic person to be **authentically** themselves, on a moment-by-moment basis, and resist the urge to mask. Masking for many has developed as a psychological safety device. It will very likely be excruciatingly difficult for late-diagnosed adults to resist the overwhelming social pressure to comply in any given situation.

Please be aware that within the support space, the person will likely need constant encouragement and reassurance that they can be their authentic selves with you, and that they don't need to mask. It's not enough to expect them to tell you if they feel uncomfortable; you need to constantly reach out of your own comfort zone of social norms within the therapeutic environment and re-connect with their needs.

One element of masking is the often-experienced shame and difficulty many late-identified Autistic adults experience in their relationship with stimming. All humans stim. Stimming is important and has an important function. Some late-identified adults may not even realize that they stim because it has been suppressed out of them as children. There can be a strong sense of shame in adults who have been forced to suppress their natural way of stimming to self-regulate or expressing joy by prejudicial attitudes in their family or wider society. Normalize the act of stimming, and you will support your client to experiment and explore what feels best to them.

Reflection Point

It's important to note if you work in support services that some Autistic people may have extremely negative and hostile views of their mask. They may experience emotions such as anger towards their mask, or describe it as something that has controlled large periods of their life and put them in many vulnerable and traumatizing situations. They may be highly frustrated or enraged at their mask. They may describe feeling powerless against it and at a loss as to how to stop masking. Practitioners need to realize that for some Autistic clients this could be the first time they have had a safe space to talk about masking, thus an important part of the journey towards becoming their authentic selves is to provide a safe space to vent and express their anger about the control masking has had over their lives, while always remaining respectful of the diverse experiences people have of masking.

6. Promote self-advocacy

In contrast to masking, self-advocacy is building on what the person needs to change in the environment so that they can access it on an equitable footing. Becoming comfortable with advocating for themselves is a doorway into unmasking and being more authentically their self. A constant question we are asked in post-assessment support services is, 'How do I unmask?' The response must therefore be that unmasking is an active, continual process, and understanding your needs, then advocating for them, is the first step to living as your authentic self across all life domains.

7. Connect people with the Autistic community

Possibly one of the most valuable interventions you can provide for your clients is to simply connect the newly diagnosed Autistic person in with the wider Autistic community. A sense of belonging is **crucial** to overall wellbeing, and for the vast majority of Autistic people, finding they are accepted and welcomed into a community as diverse as the Autistic community brings a sense of relief and acceptance like nothing before.

The Autistic community has blossomed since the development of social media. One of the more positive stories of the evolution of social media and the internet and global village is that Autistic and otherwise neurodivergent people have found community online. They have found ways to connect around shared experience. Indeed, many Autistic people have sought official diagnosis only after already finding the community online and hearing their inner experiences described in others' accounts of their own neurotype.

Communities have formed online on every social media channel, spreading across what seems every nuance and co-occurring experience that Autistic people share. There are subcommunities for different professions (e.g., #AutisticsInAcademia on Twitter and Facebook, Autistic Doctors International, Autistic Therapists, Autistic Lawyers), gender and sexuality (Rainbow Autistics, Trans Autistics, Autistic Women and Girls), race (#BlackAutistics on Twitter, BIPOC Autistic groups on Facebook and TikTok) and health (e.g., Autistic EDS and hypermobility groups, Autistic epileptic groups, Autistic and mental health groups).

8. Signpost people to peer support

The community peer support model for mental health recovery is an interesting one when applied to recently diagnosed or self-identified Autistic adults. Clearly, the fact of being Autistic is not in itself a mental health issue, although it's important to be aware that Autistic people are more vulnerable to experiencing negative mental health due to the mismatch between societal norms and the Autistic way of being and experiencing the world (see Chapters 4 and 5).

In peer support, a person who has a shared experience and can relate to where someone is on a specific point of their life journey is trained to provide a listening ear and offer signposting and resources to support another's wellbeing. We have found facilitating peer support meetings a wonderful opportunity for recently identified Autistic adults to connect with others and to discuss shared experiences. The feedback from many has been that the experience of being in a room of others experiencing similar adjustments following diagnosis is profoundly helpful.

Within the Autistic community itself, peers naturally offer support to each other inside the individual groups and subgroups. At Thriving Autistic, we are piloting a peer support model of support alongside our multidisciplinary team of neurodivergent professionals, and so far, feedback has been astoundingly positive.

9. Discuss with the person the benefits and risks of disclosure

One of the most important decisions each person has to make is about disclosing their diagnosis. This decision is, of course, intensely personal, and one with multiple dimensions that need consideration. Factors include weighing up the pros and cons of disclosing within the different settings and people the person interacts with. For example, at the time of writing, workplace disclosure may be an asset or a liability depending on the culture towards neurodiversity within the environment. Employers are legally required to provide accommodations, and these may be exceptionally helpful to the person, and go a long way towards supporting the person's wellbeing in the workplace. On the other hand, a workplace culture with a highly stigmatic attitude towards difference may become an even more toxic environment for the Autistic person if the letter of the law is followed, but the underlying culture is isolating and stigmatizing.

Late-diagnosed adults often relate one of the greatest difficulties with disclosure to family and friends being that of meeting ignorance among those they disclose to. Common disclosure experiences include being invalidated, dismissed and told they 'don't look Autistic' to assumptions they 'must be high functioning' or 'mildly Autistic'. These responses are difficult for the newly identified adult to navigate, both emotionally and practically. They are still themselves coming to terms with this new information about themselves. During this time of psychological 'restructuring', until they feel themselves to be on solid ground in their own understanding of their neurology and life narrative, meeting this level of misunderstanding can often result in the person questioning themselves more, perhaps even to the point of questioning their diagnosis and thus delaying the process of adapting to and benefiting from the positive aspects of finally gaining a deeper understanding of who they are and how they experience the world.

10. Discuss burnout and energy accounting

When you listen closely to Autistic adults' descriptions of their lives, you'll start to notice that many will have experienced periods of time where they had no choice but to walk away from all workplace or educational commitments due to physical and emotional exhaustion. These periods of what is known as Autistic burnout may have been mistaken for depression, as the symptoms can seem to mirror each other. When drilling down into the causes, however, it becomes clear that the person will have exhausted all their internal resources and need a complete break from everyday demands for a stretch of time. This stretch may last from days to years, depending on how much energy the person has depleted. Research is sparse at the time of writing, and anecdotal evidence suggests a complete absence of demands is the greatest need.

Learning Through Practice

For example, 'G' is a parent of young children. G finds the school run each day very stressful. By the time G has left the house each morning G is emotionally and physically drained from getting the children up, washed, fed and dressed. G finds small talk excruciating and they have to steel themselves every morning to face the other school parents and muddle through the social interactions. Once the children are safely inside the school doors, G makes excuses to avoid joining the other parents for their morning activities (coffee, exercise, etc.) and rushes home. Once inside the door G collapses and sobs from the strain of it all. G lies on the couch for hours.

To recuperate, the person needs to simply **be** for a time. It's very much worth exploring people's experiences of burnout as, along with offering illuminating self-insight, it will give clues as to what led to the burnout(s) in the first instance, so that you can support them to put plans in place to prevent it.

Maja Toudal, an Autistic educator and writer, developed the concept and tool 'energy accounting'. To use the example of a bank account, Autistic people learn to audit their daily lives within the context of how much energy they are depositing versus spending in an effort to manage stress levels and therefore reduce the prospect of burnout. It can be considered a self-care tool, and one that we find exceptionally effective within our post-assessment support service.

11. Discuss and support sensory differences or sensitivities

One of the areas where differences in sensory experience can cause difficulty for a person is when there are competing needs within a family. Stepping back to look at the larger picture, we all experience the world through our senses. The neurotypical way of experiencing the world is a qualitatively different experience than that of neurodivergent people such as Autistic people. If you remember back to your childhood, perhaps you can think of a time that you were told to wear a coat outside because your parent thought you would be too cold, or to take off a jacket because they determined it was too hot? This example is of an adult determining what your sensory experience is likely to be. Consider that a parent may respond to the child based on their own sensory experience and perception of temperature. If it is objectively an extreme temperature, then for the neurotypical child, the parent is likely to have been correct, and at a certain point you recognized they were correct and were grateful for their sage advice. For a neurodivergent child with a difference in sensory perception and experience to the parent, the experience is more likely to have been both excruciating, and a lesson in learning to mask their true feelings and way of being in order to comply with their parent's wishes and gain their approval. The child may comply and gain approval, or resist and be in conflict with the parent.

A third alternative, which we are only recently learning more about with regards to sensory perception differences, is that the child may have a reduced or heightened interoceptive sense. Interoception is our internal sense of signals – the communicator between all of our senses and what is coming from our bodies (Mahler 2016). Those with low interoception awareness may not be aware of their body's signals until they are screaming at them. This has implications for pain awareness, awareness of heat and cold, awareness of hunger, thirst, tiredness and other signals such as the need to urinate or defecate. Those with heightened interoceptive awareness may have a heightened awareness of body sense; this has implications for hunger (they may feel starving at only the slightest pang of hunger) or they may go to the bathroom a lot (as even a slightly full bladder feels like too much). Body signals may be too small (they go unnoticed), too big (they are too strong, overpowering or too much at once to make sense of) or distorted (body signals are noticeable but not clear enough to work out where the specific location or type of feeling is).

In the earlier outlined scenario, the child with low interoceptive awareness may find the parent was correct that they needed to take off or put on the coat. Over time this repeated exposure to experiences of being unable to trust their own sensory experience can build up to a reduced sense of self-efficacy and over-reliance on others' opinions. Mahler (2021) describes how a caregiver's best attempts to soothe and provide feel-good sensations are based on their **own** interoceptive experiences in the world. What a neurotypical parent finds soothing may not be what an Autistic child finds soothing, as their neurology requires a unique set of feel-good sensations that may be completely unknown to the loving parent. For example, a parent may find deep pressure soothing based on their own interoceptive needs, and may therefore hug their child to console and soothe them. However, if their child finds deep touch aversive, they may experience a lack of attunement and invalidation, meaning that they become more distressed **despite the best intentions of the caregiver** (Mahler 2021). Over time, we can see how this may impact on the parent–child relationship and on the child's learning about their own body signals, emotions and regulation strategies.

Individual differences in how children respond to their sensory differences being invalidated do, of course, apply. Our practice, and the experiences as related by Autistic adults more generally, show that the outcome typically is that late-diagnosed adults often don't know what their individual sensory profile or needs actually are. They may have spent a lifetime putting their needs aside, pushing them away while attempting to fit the neurotypical expectation of what they 'should' be experiencing if they possessed the typical brain type. This process of self-discovery is a revelation and truly imperative if we are to support late-identified adults to become more wholly free to be themselves.

Learning Through Practice

For example, Client A related experiencing extreme pain and fatigue when in a busy coffee shop, trying to focus on the conversation between themselves and a potential manager, during an informal interview. The pain was related to the background sounds of people chatting and coffee machines grinding, steaming and till registers pinging. Client A felt a pain in their ears and a difficulty in focusing on the words coming out of the manager's mouth. All the sounds blended together, and it was difficult to separate them out, process a response, and then verbalize the response, all while surrounded by the noisy, hot, crowded environment. A fatigue set over them from the cognitive and sensory cost of being in such an inhospitable environment for their sensory system. Even though the meeting had apparently gone well, Client A got the job, and to anyone looking on from the outside, nothing would have appeared amiss. Client A related that the entire journey home they couldn't speak, they went straight to their room and went to bed for 48 hours, too exhausted to re-join the family, as all their internal resources had been used up.

In this example, Client A's auditory processing capacity was overwhelmed, and the knock-on effect was dysregulation of their nervous system and the loss of two days. Recommendations were clear-cut that they complete a full sensory audit with a trained sensory specialist to ascertain which accommodations they could put in place to help make the environment more suitable for their sensory system. Simple solutions such as meeting in quiet places, wearing noise-cancelling headphones and limiting time spent trying to focus on a single sound source when several are present proved liberating for them. They had spent their entire life thus far 'pushing through' and berating themselves when they found themselves inevitably exhausted after these types of scenarios. The fact that alongside these difficulties with sound, they also happen to thoroughly enjoy loud music of their own choosing, meant they discounted their difficulties in some contexts as valid (and had contributed to their being missed in autism screenings previously).

12. Discuss and support possible competing family needs

One of the areas that needs exploring is that of competing needs within the family. These are when one person has a need that is the exact opposite to another person's (e.g., the need for peace and quiet within the home versus the need for lots of loud noise – often experienced by the sensory-avoidant and sensory-seeker preferences for sound).

From our practice-based observation, and of the shared experiences online by Autistic adults, many Autistic people live within a 'neurodivergent bubble', that is, they will often have become attracted to, and partnered with, other neurodivergent people. This makes a lot of sense considering the research by Crompton, Milton and others into the double empathy problem and Autistic communication. Added to this the emerging appreciation that the Autistic neurotype is handed down through generations, it's clear that the rule rather than the exception is that many families are comprised of neurodivergent people. As each person has their own unique sensory profile and preferences (needs), it's perhaps becoming clearer why oftentimes a major source of distress or disharmony within a household is managing competing needs.

For a recently identified Autistic adult, this concept can be a complete revelation to them. It may be the first time in their lives they have an explanation for why they find home (or work) life so difficult to manage. This can be at the heart of many difficulties in relationships and environments, and understanding, unpacking and exploring sensory preferences and needs, along with fluid ways to fulfil and honour those needs for each person within the person's sphere, can go a long way towards increasing their wellbeing exponentially.

Learning Through Practice

For example, Client M cannot focus if there is any background noise in their environment. They are acutely sensitive to sound. They feel pain when sitting under fluorescent lights, as the sound from the electricity feels like their brain being stabbed. They are working in a busy office environment a as a solicitor. They spend hours each day in this painful environment reading and writing legal documents. When they come home in the evening their two children are bouncing around the house, shouting, singing and screaming. Their children are both also diagnosed

Autistic and ADHD. The children have a need for lots of sensory input. They have been sitting still all day in mainstream school attempting to focus their attention on their schoolwork and trying to listen to their teachers' instructions. They have been feeling confined and restrained, unable to move as their bodies need. As soon as they come home they are bursting with energy, at exactly the moment Client M arrives home needing quiet and respite from the chaos and pain of the workplace.

Once the concept has been explained, it can often be a simple enough matter to explore what the main competing needs in a person's life are and to find workarounds. As a best practice, however, we recommend supporting the person to more fully explore their sensory preferences and profile. Occupational therapists with specialist sensory training are those most likely to be able to support a client with this exploration.

13. Celebrate and support passions and interests

When viewed through the Neuro-Affirmative lens, the DSM-5's deficit-framed proposition of Autistic people experiencing limited and bound interests that are marked in vigour can actually be one of the Autistic person's greatest strengths. The theory of monotropism (see Chapter 5) introduces us to the Autistic person's tendency to focus, at depth, on what captures their interest. This tendency towards narrow, deep focus for extended periods of time is a core feature shared by experts across different fields, and is most commonly known as 'hyperfocus'. These interests or passions, if allowed to thrive during childhood, can often become the focus of the person's career, or a deeply satisfying hobby.

A giant in the field of positive psychology, Mihaly Csikszentmihalyi, contributed to our understanding of what makes a fulfilled life by introducing us to the construct of 'flow' with his book *Flow: The Psychology of Optimal Experience* (1990). Flow is experienced both in peak performance, by those at the pinnacle in their respective domains of excellence, and in everyday life, by those with the ability to 'lose themselves' in the moment. Flow is a state of complete absorption and concentration of attention in the activity at hand, where temporal concerns (hunger, time, ego, etc.) don't exist. It brings a sense of wellbeing where a person feels they are 'in the zone', acting from an intrinsic motivation.

The parallels between the common experience described as hyperfocus, and Csikszentmihalyi's flow are evident. Autistic people commonly describe hyperfocus as being an all-encompassing, immersive experience. Time can 'stand still', and when deeply engaged, the person feels at one with the activity, often not noticing the need to eat or drink for hours at a time. This also appears to align with the monotropism theory of attention discussed in Chapter 5.

Interruption of flow is frequently described by Autistic people as physically painful. Autistic artist and advocate Erin Human created a comic strip illustration describing the experience, which has been shared countless times across social media, and is commonly cited as resonating perfectly with many Autistic people's experience. The comic strip proposes 'tendril theory', and explores the experience of hyperfocus from the first person's perspective. In the comic, Human shows us how the hyperfocuser's brain sends out millions of tiny tendrils as they move deeper into the experience. We visualize the process through the drawing when just as suddenly the tendrils are ripped out during an interruption. This disruption of flow is an explanation for how sharp transitions can be so painful for Autistic people, and how they can have such a negative impact on their wellbeing.

Now that we have set the scene and explored the experience of flow/hyperfocus and interruption/transitions, it's time to turn our focus to Autistic people's passions and interests. Within this context, we can see how important it is to people's wellbeing to have the opportunity to let their brains focus in the most natural way for them, via the passions and interests they are naturally drawn to.

The Autistic child who is lining up cars, dolls or other items is experiencing flow and hyperfocus. Their brain is naturally drawn to develop in its own trajectory. Given time and space, that child's interest will deepen as they grow into an adult. They will experience a sense of mastery as their interests and play are respectfully accepted as an authentic representation of who they are at their core. They may grow to be an engineer, a scientist, an artist, a therapist, an athlete – their interest will determine their trajectory if left unhindered and allowed to flourish.

Of course, as we know from the science of psychological strengths, any strength that is over-used can become a liability depending on the context. One of the areas to check in on with your client is if they frequently find that their ability to hyperfocus comes with a downside. Often, the experience is so absorbing the person is not aware of bodily signals to eat, hydrate or move. They may be so absorbed they regularly lose track of time completely, and then an area for support is to look at strategies that they could put in place to alleviate those challenges. These could include, for example:

- Setting timers to eat, drink or move, or setting aside time to eat, drink or use the bathroom before beginning the activity.

- Providing quiet hours in the workplace when they won't be disturbed.

- Turning off all notifications on their devices so they can work uninterrupted.

- Providing uninterrupted time in the workplace daily to hyperfocus.

- Setting aside specific times to check external communications (e.g., email messages) rather than a continual interruption of flow.

14. Support access to disability services, if appropriate

If appropriate for the person, discuss and support their access to whatever disability services may be available to them. It can be helpful to have a list of resources readily available that you can share with them. Be available to write letters of support for their access to services. If they have the financial means, and disability services are not accessible for them, discuss what supports they could perhaps privately fund. Either through public or private means, being able to get supports could make a real difference to their quality of life. The supports will look different for each person, as each person's needs are unique. They may range from occupational health, work with a sensory-trained occupational therapist, a personal assistant to support them with paperwork, someone to help with housekeeping, cooking and laundry, attending appointments with them or psychological supports. Please see Appendix 7 and Appendix 8 for further valuable resources for Autistic adults to use when accessing healthcare.

15. If needed, support people to find a Neuro-Affirmative therapist, or provide Neuro-Affirmative therapy yourself

Not all people are going to need, or want, in-depth therapeutic support post assessment, although it is likely to be helpful for the vast majority, if conducted in a Neuro-Affirmative manner. Also, not all professionals, teams or practices are going to have the facilities to provide this post-assessment therapeutic support. If therapy is to be provided, it is vital that it is Neuro-Affirmative therapy. Thriving Autistic provides training for professionals looking for more in-depth training in this area.

Research shows the primary predictor in confidence among clinicians in supporting Autistic people is not years of practice, but specific training. The top three questions people have reported about accessing supports (National Autistic Society and Mind 2021) are:

1. Does the practitioner understand autism?

2. What will therapy be like?

3. What is the process to access therapy?

The law requires reasonable accommodations and adaptations for all disabled people. Many of the adaptations most useful for Autistic people will benefit all your clients, so the principle of universal design is a worthwhile construct to keep in mind as you audit your service and make adaptations (see Chapter 4).

Recommendations for Adapting the Journey

Let's consider adapting the journey each person makes thorough your service, from first contact, through to co-creating therapy goals and finally measuring outcomes.

First, ensure each member of your team (or yourself, if a solo practitioner) has a thorough understanding of autism. As mentioned above, the primary predictor of confidence among therapists in working with Autistic people is training. Seek out training led by Autistic professionals. Listen and learn from the Autistic community. Learn about minority stress and intersectionality. Understand the social model of disability. Gain cultural competence and take a person-centred approach to your work while gaining an appreciation of common co-occurring conditions that Autistic people may have.

While some Autistic adults are comfortable educating professionals about their experience, others find it exhausting, so don't expect to gain your education from your clients!

Recommendations for First Contact

Whatever the point of first contact with your practice or service, ensure that it is Autistic-friendly by considering the following:

- Written materials (website, adverts, handouts and resource materials) should offer clear, concise and specific information about your service, therapy delivery and your communication options.

- Offer multiple methods for people to make appointments with you. Telephone calls are generally inaccessible for the vast majority of Autistic people, so offering online booking systems or email contact to set appointments is a must.

- Consider making a short video introduction to yourself and your service. It will help put people at ease as they can get a sense of you before you meet. If the sessions are in-person, consider making a walkthrough video of the journey from the street to your office, so people can visualize the journey and allay anxieties. Give concise, clear location directions for in-office visits.

- Conduct a sensory audit on the environment you intend to welcome your clients into. Ideally hire a local Autistic professional to consult on this, as they will be more likely to identify elements that would be potentially overwhelming for Autistic people. Look at the physical environment from the point of view of the senses: consider if the lighting needs adapting (e.g., avoid fluorescent lighting), download a decibel reader app and check for underlying sounds that may cause distress, avoid strong scents and chemical smells, de-clutter rooms and keep visual input clean (note that Autistic people vary in their sensory preferences, so the environment that perfectly suits one person may not suit another – these are general guidelines). Keep a basket of fidget toys in the room that can be freely used. If possible, allow space for the person to move around if they so wish. Have fresh water available nearby.

- If possible, share power with your client by inviting them to choose where each of you will sit in the therapy room.

- Consider the possibility of outdoor sessions. Many Autistic people think better when moving. Is there a calm, quiet place in nature that you could move and conduct a session? There are obviously many considerations to think about when deciding on what therapeutic delivery options you can offer. Consider matters of privacy and safety when weighing up the possibility of outdoor sessions.

- Offer asynchronous support options if possible. Many Autistic people need time to process and consider responses, and conversation can flow better when barriers to communication are removed. We find many people can express themselves extremely eloquently and thrive in therapeutic settings that allow for their preferred communication styles. Of course, clear boundaries with regard to time allocated to sessions need to be considered when offering asynchronous therapeutic support. Other considerations are the risk profile of the person and a back-up plan for if an urgent disclosure is made.

- Telehealth, or online support options, can be extremely beneficial to many Autistic people. Benefits are that they are in their own environment where they may be most at ease, and they avoid the unnecessary stress with all the potential sensory overwhelm that travelling to a therapy centre can bring. They can remain in their most comfortable clothing, have their camera switched off if they prefer, and can use a text box to write their answers rather than using their voice, if they prefer.

- Duration of sessions – consider building time flexibility into your sessions. Some people need longer than the traditional hour session to allow themselves time to process the conversation and take a slower pace, whereas others find sessions overwhelming and shorter sessions much more manageable. Many people report needing several sessions to build trust and stability with their practitioner before being in a place to move forward with possible therapeutic interventions.

- Explicitly offer the option of the person bringing a close friend or support person with them to sessions. They can be a source of comfort to your client and help build trust.

- Share a written summary with your client following the session. This provides a clear overview of what was discussed and the content of the session, and also offers an opportunity for your client to process the session in their own time and reflect back to you any differences in your shared understanding of the therapy session.

Recommendations for Co-Creating Therapeutic Goals

At this point you will already appreciate that the fact of being Autistic is not in itself a target for therapy. There is no therapy that can change a person's neurotype, and nor should there be. Our world needs the richness, diversity and perspectives of all neurotypes, and each neurotype is entitled to the human right to thrive as their authentic selves.

The most important piece in determining therapeutic goals is to co-create them with the person themselves. Explain the different therapeutic options and see which they resonate best with. Become competent in distinguishing normative and curative goals from goals that support the person to embrace their neurology, to self-advocate for their needs, to gain self-acceptance of the negative impact of living in a world that is not designed for them, and how to uncover and utilize their strengths. Work on unpacking your own internalized ableism and be alert to your client's too, as we have all been born into a society that was built on the delusion of there being one 'gold standard' way of being. Regardless of neurotype, each of us will, of course, have an Achilles' heel and areas we wish to improve in our lives and our thought or emotional processing and relationships. Build on the foundation of autonomy, self-acceptance and validation, and work from there.

Recommendations for Measuring Outcomes

At each point in the process, explicitly request and be open to feedback. Anonymous surveys, voice and text feedback and wider consultation with the community you serve are all important to ensure you're aligned with best practice for Neuro-Affirmative care. Consider setting up or joining a Neuro-Affirmative practitioners network locally, so that you have a safe space to reflect and honestly discuss and unpack issues as they arise. Keep up to date with research in the neurodiversity field, and continually reflect on your practice as research and community preferences evolve.

When using assessment tools, adapt them as necessary. At the time of writing, all our standardized tools for assessing mental wellbeing and risk have been developed for the neurotypical population. They will need to be adapted for the person you are working with. First, ensure you explain the purpose of the assessment in a clear, direct manner. Next, consider the person's preferred communication style. Would they prefer an asynchronous assessment where they have time to consider their response to each question? Would written or verbal information work better for them? Do they have difficulty labelling emotions and feelings, and does the language in the assessment need to be made clearer and less abstract? Give examples where appropriate to clarify abstract questions. Don't assume the person shares the same meaning of colours attached to emotions (red may equal peaceful, green may equal agitated). Many Autistic people experience synaesthesia where senses overlap and so they may have unique ways of experiencing colour, sound or words.

The Neuro-Affirmative Language Guide

The Adult Autism Practice (www.adultautism.ie),
Thriving Autistic (www.thrivingautistic.org)

Use each Autistic individual's personal preference first. Otherwise, here is a list of general phrases or terms to use or not to use.

Do use	Don't use
Identity-first language: Autistic person/child/adult, Autistic experience, Autistic neurology	Person-first language: person with autism, person on the spectrum, your autism
Disabled person/is disabled	Person with a disability/has a disability
Difference, differences	Disorder, disease, illness
Talk about the individual's strengths and needs that account for different internal and external factors such as time, context, energy, mood, environment, etc.	High functioning, low functioning
Talk about the individual's strengths and needs that account for different internal and external factors such as time, context, energy, mood, environment, etc.	Mild, severe
Non-Speaking, Non-Speaking (at times)	Non-verbal, limited speech
Speech and language differences	Speech and language difficulties
Co-occurring conditions	Co-morbidities, co-morbid conditions/disorders
...is Autistic	Suffers from/has autism
Characteristics	Symptoms, impairments
Communication differences	Social impairments, lacks social skills
Communication, communicating distress	Challenging, problematic, disruptive behaviour
Double empathy, different communication style	Lacks theory of mind
Stimming, self-expression body language	Self-stimulatory behaviour, repetitive movements
Support, adaptions, accommodations	Treat, treatment
Needs, challenges accompanying autism	Difficulties attributed to being Autistic

cont.

Do use	Don't use
Description of the autism spectrum as non-linear and non-binary with a multitude of ways of being Autistic. Each Autistic person is different and has their own unique context and time-dependant neutralities, strengths and needs that are constantly changing and never fixed. Their ability to adapt to this world changes from situation to situation depending on many internal and external factors	Description of the autism spectrum as linear and binary
Attention to detail	Lacking central coherence
Thrives with predictability and structure	Deficit, lacks cognitive flexibility, rigidity of thought
Hyperfocused	Deficits in task switching
Energetic	Restless, hyperactive
Value Autistic ways of being	Odd, unusual, peculiar, aloof
Talkative	Talks too much
Use full words: autism, executive functioning, disability allowance	Abbreviations: AS, ASD, ED, DA, DCF
For full title use autism	Autism spectrum disorder or condition
Embrace autism, accept autism, be Neuro-Affirmative. Focus on the quality of life and internal wellbeing	Cure autism, fix autism, treat autism
Discourage masking, passing for non-autistic and social skills training. Be aware of the harmful psychological effects of masking to authentic development	Encouraging masking and social skills training
You either are or are not Autistic, but there are many ways of being Autistic	Everyone is a little bit Autistic
Different, Autistic pattern, neurotypical pattern, common pattern	(Ab)normal pattern
Passions, areas of expertise/strengths	Special interests, restrictive interests/obsessions
Autism	ASD, ASC, AS, Aspergers
Autistic sensory perception, sensory processing differences, sensory differences, perceptual differences	Sensory processing disorder, sensory atypicalities, sensory abnormalities
Autistic developmental trajectory	Developmental delay, developmental difficulties, problematic development
Autism is a neurotype and a neurodivergency. All humans are neurodiverse	Autism is a neurodiversity. Neurotypical people are not neurodivergent
Identity-first language should be used unless the person has expressed a desire for person-first language	Assuming you know what the Autistic person's language preferences will be

Appendix 2

Making Zoom More Comfortable for You

The Adult Autism Practice (www.adultautism.ie)

This is information that we, in The Adult Autism Practice, give to our clients before they come to us for an assessment.

We are aware of how difficult video calls and sustained eye contact can be for lots of people. Below are some potential issues and solutions to get the most from your sessions.

Tips to Reduce Anxiety Before Your Session

- Prepare a way to take notes if you want, and write down any question you might want to ask (these can be emailed in advance of the meeting as well).

- Stay hydrated – have water nearby.

- Use the bathroom before the meeting, but know you can take a bathroom break during the call at any time.

- Decide on a comfortable position to sit, with any seating supports you might need.

- We are happy for pets to join our video calls – feel free to have them with you!

- Get ready any sensory aids you may want to use during the call (e.g., deep pressure, weighted aids, fidget toys, stress ball, sunglasses).

Setting Up Zoom to Work Best for You

- Test your microphone and speaker settings in Zoom and adjust to a level you are comfortable with.

- Adjust the brightness of your screen or change to night filter to reduce visual input.

Sensory Environment

- Video interactions can require additional sensory processing.

- In offline meetings, there is only one environment to process. On video calls, you are managing the sensory inputs in both your own physical environment and in others'.

- We will do our part to ensure our environments are sensory calm by reducing background distractions, using low lighting and reducing background sounds. If you notice something distracting, please let us know, and we will try to address this.

- You can make your own environment more calming by using dim lighting to reduce visual stimuli and having a comfortable place to sit or stand in an area that limits background distractions.

During Your Session

- Research has shown that movement helps to improve cognitive functioning. During in-person conversations or on the phone, we tend to move around while interacting. Online video calls can feel restrictive. Often the camera is in a set place, meaning that we have to stay in the same spot. In an age where everyone is adjusting to online communication, much emphasis has been put on looking good on screen, which often involves holding unnatural posses that limit movement for long periods.

- Need more personal space? You don't always have to sit in front of the screen. Take a step back. You can increase your personal space by using Bluetooth headphones that allow you to be away from the screen but still be heard. Feel free to move around. Stimming can be a great way to reduce uncertainty.

- Visuals too overwhelming? We recommend taking breaks where you switch your camera off and just talk. Or you can change your position to look away from the screen.

- Too much talking? Feel free to communicate through the Chat function instead.

- Seeing our own face stare back at us during video meetings can be tiring as it can increase the feeling that we are being watched and need to perform. In offline interactions, we don't constantly observe ourselves interacting the way we do on video calls. Studies have shown that this constant view of ourselves can be a source of stress.

- We highly recommend reducing this stress by choosing to hide self-view in the Zoom video settings. Once you are happy with how you look in the camera, right-click on your image and select 'hide self-view'.

Tips for After Your Session

- After the session do some relaxing activity to relax and ground yourself. For example, give your eyes time to rest and recover by doing an activity that does not involve a screen.

- Go for a walk outside and get some fresh air.

- If you are feeling tense, give yourself a hug or squeeze your limbs. Lean against a wall and push yourself back up to get some deep pressure, which can help reduce nervous energy, anxiety and focus by helping your nervous system decrease your state of arousal.

- To get a whole-body sense of calm, tighten your muscles and hold for the count of 5 and then release, starting with your toes and working your way up through the different muscles in your body to help reduce tiredness.

- If you're feeling overwhelmed, you could try some breathing techniques, such as taking a deep breath in while you trace a square shape with your fingers. Start at the top left side of the square as you trace each side, breathe in for a count of 4 and then on the next side breathe out for the count of 4, then the next and the last side hold for the count of 4. Repeat this 4 times. This technique helps slow your breathing and tells your brain you are safe and can relax.

- We do ask for at least one Zoom video call. We are also happy to conduct shorter sessions if you would prefer to supplement them with sending us written information or responses to questions by email. We can also conduct some sessions over the phone if you would prefer.

Appendix 3

Looking After Myself Plan

The Adult Autism Practice (www.adultautism.ie)

Date: _____

I know I need to look after myself when I notice:

```



```

Some safe people I can contact are:

1.

2.

3.

4.

Some good ways to distract myself are:

1.

2.

3.

4.

Things that help when I feel this way are:

```



```

Other:

```



```

Ways to keep myself and my space safe:

1.

2.

3.

4.

Workplace Accommodations Self-Reflection Exercise

Written by Síofra Heraty for Thriving Autistic (www.thrivingautistic.org)

Identify aspects of your working environment that interfere with your wellbeing/ functionality considerably. There are a couple of ways to do this. Some useful questions to ask yourself could be:

- What times of day or tasks evoke negative feelings in me? Why?

- Were there any one-off incidents at work that had a negative effect on me? What about these incidents caused this distress?

- What types of invisible labour am I required to perform as part of my job? (Invisible labour in this case means engaging in activities which are normative for your workplace and its culture, but which require a disproportionate amount of energy for you, e.g., being required to attend phone meetings despite having difficulties with auditory processing, or being required to work in an open-plan office conducive to sensory overload.)

- What are my limits (or spoons, if you prefer this terminology) for each type of labour I am being asked to perform?

Mind map what possible changes could be put in place to mitigate the effect of each experience so that it doesn't affect you so negatively. Remember to consider all aspects of the work day/environment, for example:

- Sensory (How can I address issues with noise, light, texture, smells?)

- Routine (Do I work best with a fixed routine, a partially fixed routine with some flexibility, or a relatively open-plan day?)

- Social (How much social interaction can I manage in a day? How can I achieve this?)

- Cognitive load (How do I like to give, and receive, information? How much information can I process in one day? Is this different depending on the type of information?)

- Recovery time (Consider situations where there is high load of invisible labour required. Would it be helpful to schedule in some recovery time?)

Compile a list of the people/processes that will be affected in some way by your accommodations, so that your supervisor can understand the impact of what you are requesting and what they need to do to make it happen.

- Remember that you may not need to actually tell each of these people personally. You may just need to tell your supervisor and then they will do the rest.

- Can the objectives of your role still be met with the chosen accommodations in place?

- Will your accommodations require other people to change their behaviours?

- If you need a designated workspace, is this currently a space regularly used by others?

Consider how you would like your accommodation needs to be communicated. Points to consider here:

- If your accommodation affects colleagues, how would you like them to be notified?

- How would you like to tell these people, and what makes the most sense for the nature of the accommodation? (Go via HR, chat with supervisor, written, verbal, etc.)

- Boundaries: how to maintain accommodations, especially nebulous or less visible accommodations. (This can sometimes be a little confusing for colleagues. It can help others to get used to this by explaining the things they are still okay to do, for example, 'While I need to have tasks sent to me via email now so that I can keep track of them, please feel free to keep stopping by my desk to pick me up for lunch.')

Appendix 5

Neuro-Affirmative Autistic Criteria Mapping Document

Option 1

Please note: This document was prepared as part of a broader comprehensive assessment process in relation to the possibility of autism for XX. It details areas in which XX met these criteria.

Section 1

Area number	Area description	Information gathered
1	Experience of social-emotional reciprocity, e.g., communication preferences, interaction preferences, 'small talk', conversation style, sharing of interests/emotions/affect, initiating and responding to social interactions	Communication preferences:
2	Experience of non-spoken communication, e.g., eye contact, body language, gestures, facial expressions	
3	Experience of developing, maintaining and understanding friendships and relationships	

Section 2

Area number	Area description	Information gathered
1	Preference or need for particular or repeated motor movements, use of objects or vocalizations that might be balancing or regulating	
2	Preference or need for routines, particular ways of doing things, managing change and transitions, thinking patterns, specific greetings, taking the same route or eating the same food every day	
3	Particular interests or passions for particular topics or activities	
4	Sensory experiences	

Option 2

Please note: This document was prepared as part of a broader comprehensive assessment process in relation to the possibility of autism for XX. It details areas in which XX met these criteria.

Section 1: Experiences Of Communication and Engagement with Others. Consider How Experiences Might Change Across a Person's Lifespan, and Whether They Communicate Via Spoken and/or Non-Spoken Methods.

Consider the following areas:

Area number	Area description	Information gathered
1	Experience of social communication with others, e.g., experience of spoken and non-spoken communication with others, and understanding of behaviour in different contexts	Communication preferences:

2	Experience of non-spoken communication, e.g., eye contact, facial expression, body language and gestures, and how the person experiences non-spoken communication in conjunction with spoken communication	
3	Experience of using spoken communication with others	
4	Experience of masking	
5	Experience of developing, maintaining and understanding friendships and relationships	
6	Experience of emotion, empathy and compassion	
7	Experience of sharing experiences of the world with others	

Section 2: Calming and/or Energizing and Balancing Movements/Activities, Task Engagement Preferences, Interests and Sensory Experiences. These May Include:

Area number	Area description	Information gathered
1	Preference and/or need for familiarity	
2	Preference and/or need for routines and specific routes	
3	Preference and/or need for specific ways of doing things	
4	Preference and/or need for rules to be followed	
5	Particular or repeated hand or body movements that a person may find balancing or self- regulating	
6	Interests and passions. Preferred objects	
7	Sensory experiences	

Filled-In Option 1

Please note: This document was prepared as part of a broader comprehensive assessment process in relation to the possibility of autism for XX. It details areas in which XX met these criteria.

Section 1

Area number	Area description	Information gathered
1	Experience of social-emotional reciprocity, e.g., communication preferences, 'small talk' or conversation style, sharing of interests or emotions or affect, initiating and responding to social interactions	X stated that written communication is her preferred method as she has time to think about what what she will write and it is less distracting when compared to face-to-face or phone calls.
		Small groups of people (2–3) is described by X as the ideal social situation.
		X described how she finds it challenging to be part of group conversations when there are more than 2–3 people present as X has recently noticed that it feels she is always trying to 'catch up' the conversation and finds it very hard to articulate her ideas and express them in the presence of more people. She feels more anxious when there are more people around her. She makes herself pay attention to other people's body language and keeps checking if hers is appropriated to that particular situation. Her understanding of language can be very literal, and jokes can be difficult for her to understand.
		She reports finding 'small talk' difficult and feels anxious and under pressure when it happens. Situations such as taking and collecting her children to and from school, tea breaks in her work, etc., generate a lot of anxiety for her, and leave her feeling very overwhelmed.
		X describes experiencing the same when she was in primary and secondary school, especially during break times.
		X talks about and remembers engaging in masking from a very early age, and describes relying on her friend, who was very sociable, during break times.
		At the same time, X describes that she loves talking about some topics that she is passionate about, and in those situations finds it very easy to relate to people she might not know very well.
		X reported that she loved travelling on her own and how she found it very entertaining.
		X reports that she finds it difficult to verbalize emotions but is very good at writing about them.
		X finds it difficult to relate to others in a more emotional way because she feels that she is always trying to meet the other person's expectations when interacting with them.
		As a result, she finds herself exhausted after social interactions.

2	Experience of non-spoken communication, e.g., eye contact, body language, gestures and facial expressions	As a child X describes liking watching films and observing how the different characters interacted with each other.
		X also describes always observing other people's behaviours and reading books about body language.
		X feels she is constantly checking her own body language and facial expressions when around others.
		Eye contact is something that X can experience as very intrusive and uncomfortable.
		But X also experiences it as distracting, as X explains that she can pay better attention to the conversation she is having with the other person when she is not looking at them.
3	Experience of developing, maintaining and understanding friendships and relationships	X explains that throughout her childhood and adulthood she tended to have one best friend who she deeply connected with, but somehow friendships ended without her fully understanding the reason why.
		X also recalls that during school years she liked and preferred talking and helping her teachers instead of playing with other children.
		X describes her mother as a very sociable person and she (mother) always invited the children of her friends to play with X and her siblings, and she recalls playing with them and retreating to her room after a while, as she loved reading and playing with her dolls.
		She finds it difficult to invite friends of her children over as she describes finding it difficult to socialize with their mothers.
		Transitioning from primary to secondary school was socially difficult as she remembers being part of different groups but feeling she didn't belong to any in particular.
		When she started university she describes 'finding her gang' and loving being part of debating groups.
		She is still very friendly with one person she met at university and they communicate a lot via message or email.

Section 2

Area number	Area description	Information gathered
1	Preference for particular or repeated motor movements, use of objects or vocalizations that might be balancing or regulating	X describes loving rocking and pacing when she is at home.
		She taps her fingers in a particular order and gets distressed if the order is changed.
		X describes fidgeting a lot as a child, but as she started noticing that people commented on it a lot, she started chewing her tongue.
		She loves counting numbers in her own head, and finds it relaxing.

cont.

Area number	Area description	Information gathered
2	Preference for routines, particular ways of doing things, managing change and transitions, thinking patterns, specific greetings, taking the same route or eating the same food every day	This is one point that X has noticed since she was a child – she liked to know her routine in advance and once it was explained to her that there was a change in plans, she was okay with it. But if her mother didn't point it out beforehand, she would get quite upset and frustrated.
		As a child she liked having her books ordered by colour and in alphabetic order.
		As a teenager she preferred to eat the same food.
		Also as a teenager she describes herself as a very 'radical thinker' as her opinions about different subjects tended to be quite radical – she describes it as a 'black and white' thinking.
		She loves routine and 'drives' when she follows them.
		She also likes to set the dishes in a particular way in the dishwasher and loves to organize her clothes in her wardrobe.
3	Particular interests or passions for particular topics or activities	X describes a passion of numbers since she was very small and learned to add before she started reading.
		She loves photography, particularly how visually the images and colours are set in a photo.
		She also loves languages and has recently learned Portuguese.
		She loves knitting and has mastered it in no time!
		She has also identified that she gets very invested in some topics and that can result in the exclusion of other things. It is like she can't focus on anything else.
4	Sensory experiences	X describes feeling extremely well when she is in nature – she loves the sounds of the trees, the wind and the feeing it generates in her body.
		Noise is something that it is very difficult for her: loud noises, too many people talking at the same time and some noises that other people seem not to be bothered by (e.g, sound from electricity).
		As a child X used to have difficulties with certain clothes and that is something that she still experiences as an adult.
		She also recalls preferring certain foods (due to taste and/or smell).
		She has recently noticed that she needs to avoid the freezer area when she is in a supermarket, as the change in temperature can frustrate her.
		X loves to drink very hot tea and have very hot showers.
		She has also mentioned that when she was a child, she broke her arm and only noticed it the next day.

Appendix 6

Healthcare Passport for Autistic Adults

© Tara O'Donnell-Killen, Thriving Autistic CLG, 2020–2022

To staff:

Please consult this passport and make reasonable adjustments **before** you undertake any assessment, examination, treatment or care.

This document was designed in 2021 by Thriving Autistic, an Autistic-led support service, and is based on the HSE Health Passport for People with Intellectual Difficulties[1] and the National Autistic Society (UK) 'My health passport'.[2]

My Personal Details

Please take special note of my preferred name and my pronouns

My legal name is: _____

Please call me: _____

My pronouns are: _____

Date of birth: _____

Phone number: _____

Address: _____

My emergency contact person(s) are:

Name: _____ Relationship: _____ Phone number: _____

Name: _____ Relationship: _____ Phone number: _____

1   https://healthservice.hse.ie/filelibrary/onmsd/hse-health-passport-for-people-with-intellectual-disability.pdf
2   www.autism.org.uk/advice-and-guidance/topics/physical-health/my-health-passport

A Vital Thing to Know about Me Is:

My Current Medications

Please don't make changes without first consulting:

Name: _____

Role in my care: _____

Phone number: _____

Allergies or known side effects from:

A Vital Thing to Know about My Medical History Is:

How I communicate best:

For example, in writing/communication aids/mouth speaking

How you can communicate with me:

For example, use open versus closed questions, give me time to process and respond, use clear, specific language

How to help if I'm having difficulty communicating:

For example, reduce extra noise sources, give me physical space, provide me with a quiet area

A Vital Thing to Know about My Communication Is:

How I experience pain:

For example, some Autistic people are hyper- or hypo-sensitive

How I communicate pain:

For example, do you make sounds when something hurts, or rub the area?

How you can ask me about pain:

For example, do you make sounds when something hurts, or rub the area?

A Vital Thing to Know about My Pain Is:

My sensory needs:

For example, I may need to wear sunglasses or headphones

My passions:

I really enjoy talking about:

Other things you can do to make my experience tolerable:

A Vital Thing to Know about Me Is:

Autism COVID-19 Individual Health Action Plan, Universal Format

Autism COVID-19 Individual Health Action Plan, created by J. K. Doyle, Ireland 2020. Free to disseminate and amend, Original Irish format and universal format templates created by J. K. Doyle. For academic reference please cite. Contact: doylej30@tcd.ie

Section One

Do I Have any Symptoms of Covid-19?

You can mark your symptoms below or/and write your own.

Fever	Do I have a temperature above 38C?[1]	☐
Shortness of breath	This can feel like it's harder to breathe in and/or breathe out.	☐
Cough	This can be any kind of cough, usually dry, but not always.	☐

Other symptoms that I have are:

---

[1] If you don't have a thermometer: some signs of a fever include feeling unusually hot or cold, feeling clammy or sweating.

My Notes

Here I can write down and/or draw my notes.

> For example: What I want to tell my doctor, what my doctor tells me and/or any other, what I want to tell the people I love with or any information I want to record.

If you have any of the symptoms described or any other flu-like symptoms DO NOT go to the GP (doctor's) surgery, pharmacy or hospital. Stay at home, don't go outside, and if you live with other people, tell them your symptoms. Make contact with any health professional you need to see by phone or message first.

Section Two

How Can I Contact My GP (Doctor)?

Mark your choice or write your own:

What communication can I use?

I can send an email	☐
I can use the telephone	☐
I can send a message	☐

> I can:

What communication can my doctor use?

    My doctor has email   ☐

    My doctor has a telephone   ☐

    My doctor has a message device   ☐

> My doctor has:

Do I need help from another person to communicate with my doctor?

    I can contact my doctor on my own   ☐

    I need help to contact my doctor   ☐

Who Can I Contact and How Can I Contact Them if I Need Help?

You can write contact information and mark the type of communication you can use to contact that person below.

Contact details of someone I can contact if I need help

    Name: _____

    Phone number: _____

    Email: _____

    I can send an email   ☐

    I can use the telephone   ☐

    I can send a message   ☐

> I can:

Contact details of someone I can contact if I need help

Name: _____

Phone number: _____

Email: _____

I can send an email　　　　　☐

I can use the telephone　　　☐

I can send a message　　　　☐

I can:

Contact details of someone I can contact if I need help

Name:_____

Phone number:_____

Email:_____

I can send an email　　　　　☐

I can use the telephone　　　☐

I can send a message　　　　☐

I can:

Section Three

Your important information

My personal details

My full name is:[2] _____

My date of birth is: _____

My gender is: _____

My address is:_____

_____

My postcode is: _____

I have a diagnosis of:[3]_____

_____

My blood type is:[4] _____

My GP's (doctor's) information

List your GP (doctor's) information below.

My GP's (doctor's) name is _____

My GP's (doctor's) phone number is: _____

My GP's (doctor's) address is: _____

_____

My emergency contact's information

List your emergency contact's information below. This is also called 'Next of kin' and is someone the GP can contact for you if you are in an emergency.

My emergency contact's name is: _____

My emergency contact's phone number is: _____

My emergency contact's address is:_____

_____

---

2 Put down first and last name.
3 You can list previous diagnoses you have received from professionals.
4 Only write this down if you definitely know it; most people don't and that's okay.

Medication I take

List your prescribed and over-the-counter medication, such as vitamins and inhalers that you take.

(Some people don't take any medication, so it's not unusual to leave this blank.)

Name of the drug	Dosage	Frequency taken

Medications I am allergic to

List any medications you have had an allergic reaction to in the past.

(Lots of people are not allergic to any medication, so it's not unusual to leave this blank.)

Name of the drug	Reaction you had

Section Four

How I communicate

Below are a number of statements you can read and space to fill in your answers to let others know how you communicate. There is also a space to add your own, with some suggestions for each statement if you need help.

Statements	Fill in your answer	Suggestions
My strongest style of communication is:		People have different styles of communication, e.g., some people are better at writing things down, others are stronger using sign language, some people use devices, others prefer to talk by spoken word
The communication aids I use are:		Some people use aids to communicate, e.g., AAC devices, text-to-speech devices, visual aids, another person's help to communicate, writing things down
I can have difficulty communicating when:		For example, when some people are stressed or overloaded, they can find it hard to communicate the way they normally do
I find communication hard when:		For example, when some people are in loud or busy settings, they find it harder to communicate. Others find it hard when someone asks them lots of questions at one time
You can help me communicate by:		For example, not asking too many questions at one time, giving me time to process, supporting me to use my aids, providing me with clear, concrete information

Section Five

Emergency bag checklist in case i need to go to hospital

What I need in my emergency bag

Below are different categories of items you might want to put in your emergency bag. Everyone's emergency bag is different. Items listed are only suggestions; there are blank spaces where you can add your own. Tick off each item when it has gone into your bag.

Information items

This booklet when filled in	☐
Identification	☐

Sensory items

Headphones	☐
Fidget toy/chew stick	☐
Colouring book and pencils	☐
Teddy	☐
Sunglasses/eye mask	☐
Ear plugs/defenders	☐
Pen and paper	☐

Self-care items

Pyjamas ☐

Bottle of water ☐

Change of clothes + underwear/socks ☐

Toothbrush and toothpaste ☐

Non-perishable snack ☐

Technology items

Phone ☐

Communication aids ☐

Phone charger ☐

Charged power bank ☐

References

AAIDD (American Association on Intellectual Developmental Disabilities) (2010) Intellectual disability: Definition, classification, and systems of supports. www.aaidd.org/intellectual-disability/definition

Addiction Policy Forum (2020) DSM-5 Criteria for Addiction Simplified. https://www.addictionpolicy.org/post/dsm-5-facts-and-figures

APA (American Psychiatric Association) (ed.) (1980) *Diagnostic and Statistical Manual of Mental Disorders* (Third edn). APA.

APA (ed.) (2013) *Diagnostic and Statistical Manual of Mental Disorders* (Fifth edn). APA.

APA (ed.) (2022) *Diagnostic and Statistical Manual of Mental Disorders* (Fifth edition, Text Revision). APA.

Arkowitz, H. and Lilienfeld, S. O. (2017) *Facts and Fictions in Mental Health*. Chichester: John Wiley & Sons Inc.

Arwert, T. G. and Sizoo, B. B. (2020) Self-reported suicidality in male and female adults with autism spectrum disorders: Rumination and self-esteem. *Journal of Autism and Developmental Disorders* 50(10), 3598–3605. https://doi.org/10.1007/s10803-020-04372-z

ASAN (Autistic Self Advocacy Network) (2022) Open letter to the Lancet Commission on the future of care and clinical research in autism. 14 February. https://autisticadvocacy.org/2022/02/open-letter-to-the-lancet-commission-on-the-future-of-care-and-clinical-research-in-autism

Asherson, P. and Agnew-Blais, J. (2019) Annual research review: Does late-onset attention-deficit/hyperactivity disorder exist? *Journal of Child Psychology and Psychiatry* 60(4), 333–352. https://doi.org/10.1111/jcpp.13020

Ashinoff, B. K. and Abu-Akel, A. (2021) Hyperfocus: The forgotten frontier of attention. *Psychological Research* 85(1), 1–19. https://doi.org/10.1007/s00426-019-01245-8

Attanasio, M., Masedu, F., Quattrini, F., Pino, M. C., *et al.* (2021) Are autism spectrum disorder and asexuality connected? *Archives of Sexual Behavior*. https://doi.org/10.1007/s10508-021-02177-4

Attwood, T., Bolick, T., Faherty, C., Garnett, M., *et al.* (2019). *Autism and Girls*. Arlington, TX: Future Horizons Incorporated.

Autistamatic (2022) Monotropism: One step at a time (autism). YouTube, 4 March. https://youtu.be/wOe1fliDsoI

Au-Yeung, S. K., Bradley, L., Robertson, A. E., Shaw, R., Baron-Cohen, S. and Cassidy, S. (2019) Experience of mental health diagnosis and perceived misdiagnosis in autistic, possibly autistic and non-autistic adults. *Autism* 23(6), 1508–1518. https://doi.org/10.1177/1362361318818167

Ayres, A. J. (1972) *Sensory Integration and Learning Disorders*. Torrance, CA: Western Psychological Services.

Bailin, A. (2019) Clearing up some misconceptions about neurodiversity. *Scientific American*, 6 June. https://blogs.scientificamerican.com/observations/clearing-up-some-misconceptions-about-neurodiversity

Bargiela, S., Steward, R. and Mandy, W. (2016) The experiences of late-diagnosed women with autism spectrum conditions: An investigation of the female autism phenotype. *Journal of Autism and Developmental Disorders* 46(10), 3281–3294. https://doi.org/10.1007/s10803-016-2872-8

Barlow, C. and Walklate, S. (2022) *Coercive Control*. Abingdon: Routledge.

Barlow, C. and Whittle, M. (2019) *Policing Coercive Control Project Report*. London and Lancaster: The British Academy and Lancaster University Law School. https://eprints.lancs.ac.uk/id/eprint/135955/1/Policing_Coercive_Control_Project_Report_final.pdf

Barnett, J. P. and Maticka-Tyndale, E. (2015) Qualitative exploration of sexual experiences among adults on the autism spectrum: Implications for sex education. *Perspectives on Sexual and Reproductive Health* 47(4), 171–179. https://doi.org/10.1363/47e5715

Baron-Cohen, S. (2002) The extreme male brain theory of autism. *Trends in Cognitive Sciences* 6(6), 248–254. https://doi.org/10.1016/S1364-6613(02)01904-6

Baron-Cohen, S. and Wheelwright, S. (2004) The Empathy Quotient: An investigation of adults with Asperger Syndrome or high functioning autism, and normal sex differences. *Journal of Autism and Developmental Disorders* 34(2), 163–175. https://doi.org/10.1023/B:JADD.0000022607.19833.00

Barton, B. B., Segger, F., Fischer, K., Obermeier, M. and Musil, R. (2020) Update on weight-gain caused by antipsychotics: A systematic review and meta-analysis. *Expert Opinion on Drug Safety* 19(3), 295–314. doi:10.1080/14740338.2020.1713091.

Bascom, J. and Perry, D. M. (2022) Dividing up the autism spectrum will not end the way you think. *The Nation*, 31 January. www.thenation.com/article/society/autism-division

BDA (n.d.) Dyscalculia. https://www.bdadyslexia.org.uk/dyscalculia

Beat (n.d.) What are Eating Disorders? https://www.beateatingdisorders.org.uk/get-information-and-support/about-eating-disorders/types

Begeer, S., Mandell, D., Wijnker-Holmes, B., Venderbosch, S., *et al.* (2013) Sex differences in the timing of identification among children and adults with autism spectrum disorders. *Journal of Autism and Developmental Disorders* 43(5), 1151–1156. https://doi.org/10.1007/s10803-012-1656-z

Berg, K. L., Shiu, C.-S., Acharya, K., Stolbach, B. C. and Msall, M. E. (2016) Disparities in adversity among children with autism spectrum disorder: A population-based study. *Developmental Medicine & Child Neurology* 58(11), 1124–1131. https://doi.org/10.1111/dmcn.13161

Berger, B. (2014) *Power, Selfhood, and Identity: A Feminist Critique of Borderline Personality Disorder (The Advocates' Fourm)*. Chicago, IL: The University of Chicago.

Berney, T. (2020) *The Psychiatric Management of Autism in Adults*. CR228, College Report, July. London: Royal College of Psychiatrists. www.rcpsych.ac.uk/docs/default-source/improving-care/better-mh-policy/college-reports/college-report-cr228.pdf?sfvrsn=c64e10e3_2

Berthoz, S. and Hill, E. L. (2005) The validity of using self-reports to assess emotion regulation abilities in adults with autism spectrum disorder. *European Psychiatry* 20(3), 291–298. https://doi.org/10.1016/j.eurpsy.2004.06.013

Bertilsdotter Rosqvist, H. (2014) Becoming an 'autistic couple': Narratives of sexuality and couplehood within the Swedish autistic self-advocacy movement. *Sexuality and Disability* 32(3), 351–363. https://doi.org/10.1007/s11195-013-9336-2

Best, A. J. (2020) Is motor impairment in autism spectrum disorder distinct from developmental coordination disorder? A report from the SPARK Study. *Physical Therapy* 100(4), 633–644. doi:10.1093/ptj/pzz190.

Best, C., Arora, S., Porter, F. and Doherty, M. (2015) The relationship between subthreshold autistic traits, ambiguous figure perception and divergent thinking. *Journal of Autism and Developmental Disorders* 45(12), 4064–4073. https://doi.org/10.1007/s10803-015-2518-2

Bettin, J. (2022) Education about Autistic culture, the ND paradigm, and the ND movement – for medical professionals, by Autistic people. Autistic Collaboration, 1 June. https://autcollab.org

Bhat, A. N. (2020) Is Motor Impairment in Autism Spectrum Disorder Distinct From Developmental Coordination Disorder? A Report From the SPARK Study. *Physical Therapy* 100(4), 633–644. https://doi.org/10.1093/ptj/pzz190

Bird, G., Silani, G., Brindley, R., White, S., Frith, U. and Singer, T. (2010) Empathic brain responses in insula are modulated by levels of alexithymia but not autism. *Brain* 133(5), 1515–1525. https://doi.org/10.1093/brain/awq060

Bíró, S. and Russell, J. (2001) The execution of arbitrary procedures by children with autism. *Development and Psychopathology* 13(1), 97–110. https://doi.org/10.1017/S0954579401001079

Bishop-Fitzpatrick, L. and Rubenstein, E. (2019) The physical and mental health of middle aged and older adults on the autism spectrum and the impact of intellectual disability. *Research in Autism Spectrum Disorders* 63, 34–41. https://doi.org/10.1016/j.rasd.2019.01.001

Bloch, C., Burghof, L., Lehnhardt, F.-G., Vogeley, K. and Falter-Wagner, C. (2021) Alexithymia traits outweigh autism traits in the explanation of depression in adults with autism. *Scientific Reports* 11(1), 2258. https://doi.org/10.1038/s41598-021-81696-5

Bloom, P. (2017) *Against Empathy: The Case for Rational Compassion*. London: Vintage.

Blume, H. (1997) *Neurodiversity*. New York: The Atlantic Monthly Group, 3 September.

Bogdashina, O. (2016) *Sensory Perceptual Issues in Autism and Asperger Syndrome: Different Sensory Experiences – Different Perceptual Worlds* (Second edn). London: Jessica Kingsley Publishers.

Bombaci, N. (2012) Performing mindblindness: Gertrude Stein's autistic ethos of modernism. *Journal of Gender Studies* 21(2), 133–150. https://doi.org/10.1080/09589236.2012.661567

Bordes Edgar, V., Meneses, V., Shaw, D., Romero, R. A., Salinas, C. M. and Kissel, A. (2021) Clinical utility of the ECLECTIC framework in providing culturally-informed autism spectrum disorder evaluations: A pediatric case-based approach. *The Clinical Neuropsychologist*, 1–24. https://doi.org/10.1080/13854046.2021.1936187

Boren, R. (2021) Autigender and neuroqueer: Two words on the relationship between autism and gender that fit me. Ryan Boren, 14 April. https://boren.

blog/2021/04/14/autigender-and-neuroqueer-two-words-on-the-relationship-between-autism-and-gender-that-fit-me

Bottema-Beutel, K., Kapp, S. K., Lester, J. N., Sasson, N. J. and Hand, B. N. (2021) Avoiding ableist language: Suggestions for autism researchers. *Autism in Adulthood* 3(1), 18–29. https://doi.org/10.1089/aut.2020.0014

Braden, B. B., Smith, C. J., Thompson, A., Glaspy, T. K., *et al.* (2017) Executive function and functional and structural brain differences in middle-age adults with autism spectrum disorder. *Autism Research* 10(12), 1945–1959. https://doi.org/10.1002/aur.1842

Branford, D., Gerrard, D., Saleem, N., Shaw, C. and Webster, A. (2019) Stopping over-medication of people with an intellectual disability, autism or both (STOMP) in England, Part 2 – The story so far. *Advances in Mental Health and Intellectual Disabilities* 13, 1, 41–51. https://doi.org/10.1108/AMHID-02-2018-0005

Brimo, K., Dinkler, L., Gillberg, C., Lichtenstein, P., Lundström, S. and Åsberg Johnels, J. (2021) The co-occurrence of neurodevelopmental problems in dyslexia. *Dyslexia* 27(2), 1–17. doi:10.1002/dys.1681.

Brown, A., Tse, T. and Fortune, T. (2019) Defining sensory modulation: A review of the concept and a contemporary definition for application by occupational therapists. *Scandinavian Journal of Occupational Therapy* 26(7), 515–523. https://doi.org/10.1080/11038128.2018.1509370

Brown, C., Tollefson, N., Dunn, W., Cromwell, R. and Filion, D. (2001) The adult sensory profile: Measuring patterns of sensory processing. *American Journal of Occupational Therapy* 55(1), 75–82. https://doi.org/10.5014/ajot.55.1.75

Brown, K. R., Peña, E. V. and Rankin, S. (2017) Unwanted sexual contact: Students with autism and other disabilities at greater risk. *Journal of College Student Development* 58(5), 771–776. https://doi.org/10.1353/csd.2017.0059

Brown, T. (2020) Autism and Addiction. In D. Milton (ed.) *The Neurodiversity Reader: Exploring Concepts, Lived Experience and Implications for Practice.* Shoreham-by-Sea: Pavilion Publishing and Media.

Brown-Lavoie, S. M., Viecili, M. A. and Weiss, J. A. (2014) Sexual knowledge and victimization in adults with autism spectrum disorders. *Journal of Autism and Developmental Disorders* 44 (9), 2185–96.1899–1911. https://doi.org/10.1007/s10803-014-2093-y

Buckle, K. L., Leadbitter, K., Poliakoff, E. and Gowen, E. (2021) 'No way out except from external intervention': First-hand accounts of autistic inertia. *Frontiers in Psychology* 12, 631596. https://doi.org/10.3389/fpsyg.2021.631596

Butwicka, A., Långström, N., Larsson, H., Lundström, S., *et al.* (2017) Increased risk for substance use-related problems in autism spectrum disorders: A population-based cohort study. *Journal of Autism and Developmental Disorders* 47(1), 80–89. https://doi.org/10.1007/s10803-016-2914-2

Cage, E. and Troxell-Whitman, Z. (2019) Understanding the reasons, contexts and costs of camouflaging for autistic adults. *Journal of Autism and Developmental Disorders* 49(5), 1899–1911. https://doi.org/10.1007/s10803-018-03878-x

Cambridge Academic (no date) Morality. https://dictionary.cambridge.org/dictionary/english/morality

Camden, C., Hérault, E., Fallon, F. and Couture, M. (2022) Children with autism and potential developmental coordination disorder: Results from a literature review to inform the diagnosis process. *Current Developmental Disorders Reports* 9(1), 1–8. https://doi.org/10.1007/s40474-021-00242-0

Camm-Crosbie, L., Bradley, L., Shaw, R., Baron-Cohen, S. and Cassidy, S. (2019) 'People like me don't get support': Autistic adults' experiences of support and treatment for mental health difficulties, self-injury and suicidality. *Autism* 23(6), 1431–1441. https://doi.org/10.1177/1362361318816053

Cardoso, D., Pascoal, P. M. and Maiochi, F. H. (2021) Defining polyamory: A thematic analysis of lay people's definitions. *Archives of Sexual Behavior* 50(4), 1239–1252. https://doi.org/10.1007/s10508-021-02002-y

Carpenter, B., Happé, F. and Egerton, J. (eds) (2019) *Girls and Autism: Educational, Family and Personal Perspectives.* London: Routledge.

Casanova, E. L., Baeza-Velasco, C., Buchanan, C. B. and Casanova, M. F. (2020) The relationship between autism and Ehlers-Danlos syndromes/hypermobility spectrum disorders. *Journal of Personalized Medicine* 10(4), 260. https://doi.org/10.3390/jpm10040260

Casanova, E. L., Sharp, J., Edelson, S., Kelly, D. and Casanova, M. (2018) A cohort study comparing women with autism spectrum disorder with and without generalized joint hypermobility. *Behavioral Sciences* 8(3), 35. https://doi.org/10.3390/bs8030035

Casanova, M. F., van Kooten, I. A. J., Switala, A. E., van Engeland, H., *et al.* (2006). Minicolumnar abnormalities in autism. *Acta Neuropathologica* 112(3), 287–303. https://doi.org/10.1007/s00401-006-0085-5

Cashin, A., Buckley, T., Trollor, J. N. and Lennox, N. (2018) A scoping review of what is known of the physical health of adults with autism spectrum disorder. *Journal of Intellectual Disabilities* 22(1), 96–108. https://doi.org/10.1177/1744629516665242

Cassidy, S., Bradley, L., Shaw, R. and Baron-Cohen, S. (2018) Risk markers for suicidality in autistic adults. *Molecular Autism* 9(1), 42. https://doi.org/10.1186/s13229-018-0226-4

Cassidy, S., Goodwin, J., Robertson, A. and Rodgers, R. (2021) INSAR Policy Brief: Autism community priorities for suicide prevention. International Society for Autism Research. https://cdn.ymaws.com/www.autism-insar.org/resource/resmgr/files/policybriefs/2021-insar_policy_brief.pdf

Cassidy, S., Bradley, P., Robinson, J., Allison, C., McHugh, M. and Baron-Cohen, S. (2014) Suicidal ideation and suicide plans or attempts in adults with Asperger's syndrome attending a specialist diagnostic clinic: A clinical cohort study. *The Lancet Psychiatry 1*(2), 142–147. https://doi.org/10.1016/S2215-0366(14)70248-2

Cassidy, S., Au-Yeung, S., Robertson, A., Cogger-Ward, H., *et al.* (2022) Autism and autistic traits in those who died by suicide in England. *The British Journal of Psychiatry*, 1–9. https://doi.org/10.1192/bjp.2022.21

Cederlöf, M., Larsson, H., Lichtenstein, P., Almqvist, C., Serlachius, E. and Ludvigsson, J. F. (2016) Nationwide population-based cohort study of psychiatric disorders in individuals with Ehlers–Danlos syndrome or hypermobility syndrome and their siblings. *BMC Psychiatry 16*(1), 207. https://doi.org/10.1186/s12888-016-0922-6

Chance, P. and Løvaas, I. (1974) 'After you hit a child, you just can't get up and leave him; you are hooked to that kid.' Converstaion with Ivar Løvaas. *Psychology Today*, January, 76–84.

Chaplin, E., Spain, D. and McCarthy, J. M. (eds) (2020) Substance Use Disorders. In *A Clinician's Guide to Mental Health Conditions in Adults with Autism Spectrum Disorders: Assessment and Interventions (pp.373–388)*. London: Jessica Kingsley Publishers.

Chiang, S.-Y., Fleming, T., Lucassen, M., Fenaughty, J., Clark, T. and Denny, S. (2017) Mental health status of double minority adolescents: Findings from national cross-sectional health surveys. *Journal of Immigrant and Minority Health 19*(3), 499–510. https://doi.org/10.1007/s10903-016-0530-z

Chown, N. (2017) *Understanding and Evaluating Autism Theory*. London: Jessica Kingsley Publishers.

Cooper, K., Smith, L. G. E. and Russell, A. J. (2018) Gender identity in autism: Sex differences in social affiliation with gender groups. *Journal of Autism and Developmental Disorders 48*(12), 3995–4006. https://doi.org/10.1007/s10803-018-3590-1

Corbett, B. A., Constantine, L. J., Hendren, R., Rocke, D. and Ozonoff, S. (2009) Examining executive functioning in children with autism spectrum disorder, attention deficit hyperactivity disorder and typical development. *Psychiatry Research 166*(2–3), 210–222. https://doi.org/10.1016/j.psychres.2008.02.005

Cory, J. M. (2021) White privilege in neuropsychology: An 'invisible knapsack' in need of unpacking? *The Clinical Neuropsychologist 35*(2), 206–218. https://doi.org/10.1080/13854046.2020.1801845

Costa, A. P., Loor, C. and Steffgen, G. (2020) Suicidality in adults with autism spectrum disorder: The role of depressive symptomatology, alexithymia, and antidepressants. *Journal of Autism and Developmental Disorders 50*(10), 3585–3597. https://doi.org/10.1007/s10803-020-04433-3

Crane, L., Lui, L. M., Davies, J. and Pellicano, E. (2021) Short report: Autistic parents' views and experiences of talking about autism with their autistic children. *Autism*. https://doi.org/10.1177/1362361320981317

Croen, L. A., Zerbo, O., Qian, Y., Massolo, M. L., *et al.* (2015) The health status of adults on the autism spectrum. *Autism 19*(7), 814–823. https://doi.org/10.1177/1362361315577517

Crompton, C. J., Hallett, S., Ropar, D., Flynn, E. and Fletcher-Watson, S. (2020a) 'I never realised everybody felt as happy as I do when I am around autistic people': A thematic analysis of autistic adults' relationships with autistic and neurotypical friends and family. *Autism 24*(6), 1438–1448. https://doi.org/10.1177/1362361320908976

Crompton, C. J., Ropar, D., Evans-Williams, C. V., Flynn, E. G. and Fletcher-Watson, S. (2020b) Autistic peer-to-peer information transfer is highly effective. *Autism 24*(7), 1704–1712. https://doi.org/10.1177/1362361320919286

Crompton, C. J., Michael, C., Dawson, M. and Fletcher-Watson, S. (2020c) Residential care for older autistic adults: Insights from three multiexpert summits. *Autism in Adulthood 2*(2), 121–127. https://doi.org/10.1089/aut.2019.0080

Csikszentmihalyi, M. (1990) *Flow: The Psychology of Optimal Experience*. New York: Harper & Row.

Davis, R. and Crompton, C. J. (2021) What do new findings about social interaction in Autistic adults mean for neurodevelopmental research? *Perspectives on Psychological Science 16*(3), 649–653. https://doi.org/10.1177/1745691620958010

de Graaf, G., Buckley, F. and Skotko, B. G. (2020) Estimation of the number of people with Down syndrome in Europe. *European Journal of Human Genetics 29*, 402–410. doi:10.1038/s41431-020-00748-y.

De Hert, M., Correll, C. U., Bobes, J., Cetkovich-Bakmas, M., *et al.* (2011) Physical illness in patients with severe mental disorders. I. Prevalence, impact of medications and disparities in health care. *World Psychiatry 10*(1), 52–77. doi:10.1002/j.2051-5545.2011.tb00014.x.

de Vignemont, F. and Singer, T. (2006) The empathic brain: How, when and why? *Trends in Cognitive Sciences 10*(10), 435–441. https://doi.org/10.1016/j.tics.2006.08.008

de Waal, F. (2010) *The Age of Empathy: Nature's Lessons for a Kinder Society*. New York: Broadway Books.

Decety, J. and Cowell, J. M. (2014) Friends or foes: Is empathy necessary for moral behavior? *Perspectives on Psychological Science 9*(5), 525–537. https://doi.org/10.1177/1745691614545130

Demetriou, E. A., Lampit, A., Quintana, D. S., Naismith, S. L., *et al.* (2018) Autism spectrum disorders: A meta-analysis of executive function. *Molecular Psychiatry* 23(5), 1198–1204. https://doi.org/10.1038/mp.2017.75

Dewinter, J., De Graaf, H. and Begeer, S. (2017) Sexual orientation, gender identity, and romantic relationships in adolescents and adults with autism spectrum disorder. *Journal of Autism and Developmental Disorders* 47(9), 2927–2934. https://doi.org/10.1007/s10803-017-3199-9

Dhejne, C., van Vlerken, R., Heylens, G. and Arcelus, J. (2016) Mental health and gender dysphoria: A review of the literature. *International Review of Psychiatry* 28(1), 44–57. https://doi.org/10.3109/09540261.2015.1115753

Dijkhuis, R., de Sonneville, L., Ziermans, T., Staal, W. and Swaab, H. (2020) Autism symptoms, executive functioning and academic orogress in higher education students. *Journal of Autism and Developmental Disorders* 50(4), 1353–1363. https://doi.org/10.1007/s10803-019-04267-8

Dike, J. E., DeLucia, E. A., Semones, O., Andrzejewski, T. and McDonnell, C. G. (2022) A systematic review of sexual violence among autistic individuals. *Review Journal of Autism and Developmental Disorders*. https://doi.org/10.1007/s40489-022-00310-0

Dodds, R. L. (2021) An exploratory review of the associations between adverse experiences and autism. *Journal of Aggression, Maltreatment & Trauma* 30, 8, 1093–1112. doi:10.1080/10926771.2020.1783736.

Dodson, W. (2022) ADHD brain: Unraveling secrets of your ADD nervous system. *Additude*, 10 January. www.additudemag.com/secrets-of-the-adhd-brain

Doherty, M., Neilson, S., O'Sullivan, J., Carravallah, L., *et al.* (2022) Barriers to healthcare and self-reported adverse outcomes for autistic adults: A cross-sectional study. *BMJ Open* 12(2), e056904. https://doi.org/10.1136/bmjopen-2021-056904

Donaldson, A. L., corbin, endever* and McCoy, J. (2021) 'Everyone deserves AAC': Preliminary study of the experiences of speaking autistic adults who use augmentative and alternative communication. *Perspectives of the ASHA Special Interest Groups* 6(2), 315–326. https://doi.org/10.1044/2021_PERSP-20-00220

Downing, J. M. and Przedworski, J. M. (2018) Health of transgender adults in the US, 2014–2016. *American Journal of Preventive Medicine* 55(3), 336–344. https://doi.org/10.1016/j.amepre.2018.04.045

Doyle, J. K. and Wilson, C. (2020) Exploring the Links between Perception, Cognition and Anxiety in Autistic Adults through the Lens of Hierarchical Predictive Coding. Undergraduate Thesis. Trinity College Dublin.

Dunn, W. (2001) The sensations of everyday life: Empirical, theoretical, and pragmatic considerations. *American Journal of Occupational Therapy* 55(6), 608–620. https://doi.org/10.5014/ajot.55.6.608

Dyspraxia Foundation (2016) *Teaching for Neurodiversity: A Guide to Specific Learning Difficulties.* www.dyspraxiafoundation.org.uk/wp-content/uploads/2016/09/P16-A_Guide_to_SpLD_copy_2.pdf

Eagleman, D. (2014) What is synesthesia? World Science Festival. YouTube, 27 August. https://youtu.be/FDLKWDSx4g0

Espadas, C., Ballester, P., Londoño, A. C., Almenara, S. *et al.* (2020) Multimorbidity and psychotropic polypharmacy among participants with autism spectrum disorder with intellectual disability. *Psychiatry Research* 292, 113321.

Faraone, S. V., Asherson, P., Banaschewski, T., Biederman, J., *et al.* (2015) Attention-deficit/hyperactivity disorder. *Nature Reviews Disease Primers* 1(1), 15020. https://doi.org/10.1038/nrdp.2015.20

Fein, E. (2015) Making meaningful worlds: Role-playing subcultures and the autism spectrum. *Culture, Medicine, and Psychiatry* 39(2), 299–321. https://doi.org/10.1007/s11013-015-9443-x

Fietz, J., Valencia, N. and Silani, G. (2018) Alexithymia and autistic traits as possible predictors for traits related to depression, anxiety, and stress: A multivariate statistical approach. *Journal of Evaluation in Clinical Practice* 24(4), 901–908. https://doi.org/10.1111/jep.12961

Fitzgerald, M. (2020) The myth of borderline personality disorder. *Autism Study*. https://doi.org/10.13140/RG.2.2.13443.53283

Fletcher-Watson, S. and Bird, G. (2020) Autism and empathy: What are the real links? *Autism* 24(1), 3–6. https://doi.org/10.1177/1362361319883506

Fletcher-Watson, S. and Happé, F. (2019) *Autism: A New Introduction to Psychological Theory and Current Debate*. Abingdon: Routledge.

Flygare Wallén, E., Ljunggren, G., Carlsson, A. C., Pettersson, D. and Wändell, P. (2018) High prevalence of diabetes mellitus, hypertension and obesity among persons with a recorded diagnosis of intellectual disability or autism spectrum disorder. *Journal of Intellectual Disability Research* 62(4), 269–280. https://doi.org/10.1111/jir.12462

Fombonne, E. (2003) Epidemiological surveys of autism and other pervasive developmental disorders: An update. *Journal of Autism and Developmental Disorders* 33, 365–382. https://doi.org/10.1023/A:1025054610557

Friston, K. (2010) The free-energy principle: A unified brain theory? *Nature Reviews Neuroscience* 11(2), 127–138. https://doi.org/10.1038/nrn2787

Friston, K. (2018) Does predictive coding have a future? *Nature Neuroscience 21*(8), 1019–1021. https://doi.org/10.1038/s41593-018-0200-7

Friston, K. and Kiebel, S. (2009) Predictive coding under the free-energy principle. *Philosophical Transactions of the Royal Society B: Biological Sciences 364*(1521), 1211–1221. https://doi.org/10.1098/rstb.2008.0300

Friston, K., FitzGerald, T., Rigoli, F., Schwartenbeck, P. and Pezzulo, G. (2017) Active inference: A process theory. *Neural Computation 29*(1), 1–49. https://doi.org/10.1162/NECO_a_00912

Fujii, D. E. M. (2018) Developing a cultural context for conducting a neuropsychological evaluation with a culturally diverse client: The ECLECTIC framework. *The Clinical Neuropsychologist 32*(8), 1356–1392. https://doi.org/10.1080/13854046.2018.1435826

Fuld, S. (2018) Autism spectrum disorder: The impact of stressful and traumatic life events and implications for clinical practice. *Clinical Social Work Journal 46*(3), 210–219. https://doi.org/10.1007/s10615-018-0649-6

Gaigg, S. B., Cornell, A. S. and Bird, G. (2018) The psychophysiological mechanisms of alexithymia in autism spectrum disorder. *Autism 22*(2), 227–231. https://doi.org/10.1177/1362361316667062

George, R. and Stokes, M. A. (2018a) Sexual orientation in autism spectrum disorder: Sexual orientation in ASD. *Autism Research 11*(1), 133–141. https://doi.org/10.1002/aur.1892

George, R. and Stokes, M. A. (2018b) Gender identity and sexual orientation in autism spectrum disorder. *Autism 22*(8), 970–982. https://doi.org/10.1177/1362361317714587

Geurts, H. M. and Jansen, M. D. (2012) A retrospective chart study: The pathway to a diagnosis for adults referred for ASD assessment. *Autism 16*(3), 299–305. https://doi.org/10.1177/1362361311421775

Gibbs, V., Hudson, J., Hwang, Y. I., Arnold, S., Trollor, J. and Pellicano, E. (2021) Experiences of physical and sexual violence as reported by autistic adults without intellectual disability: Rate, gender patterns and clinical correlates. *Research in Autism Spectrum Disorders 89*, 101866. https://doi.org/10.1016/j.rasd.2021.101866

Gillespie-Lynch, K. and Botha, M. (2021) Come as you are: Examining autistic identity development and the neurodiversity movement through an intersectional lens. https://doi.org/10.13140/RG.2.2.33966.02881

Giwa Onaiwu, M. (2020) 'They don't know, don't show, or don't care': Autism's white privilege problem. *Autism in Adulthood 2*(4), 270–272. https://doi.org/10.1089/aut.2020.0077

Glover, G., Bernard, S., Branford, D., Holland, A. and Strydom, A. (2014) Use of medication for challenging behaviour in people with intellectual disability. *The British Journal of Psychiatry 205*(1), 6–7.

Goddu, A. P., O'Conor, K. J., Lanzkron, S., Saheed, M. O., *et al.* (2018) Do words matter? Stigmatizing language and the transmission of bias in the medical record. *Journal of General Internal Medicine 33*(5), 685–691. https://doi.org/10.1007/s11606-017-4289-2

Golson, M. E., Ficklin, E., Haverkamp, C. R., McClain, M. B. and Harris, B. (2022) Cultural differences in social communication and interaction: A gap in autism research. *Autism Research 15*(2), 208–214. https://doi.org/10.1002/aur.2657

Goodall, E. (2013) *Understanding and Facilitating the Achievement of Autistic Potential.* CreateSpace Independent Publishing Platform.

Gotham, K., Marvin, A. R., Taylor, J. L., Warren, Z., *et al.* (2015) Characterizing the daily life, needs, and priorities of adults with autism spectrum disorder from Interactive Autism Network data. *Autism 19*(7), 794–804. https://doi.org/10.1177/1362361315583818

Gray, S., Kirby, A. V. and Graham Holmes, L. (2021) Autistic narratives of sensory features, sexuality, and relationships. *Autism in Adulthood 3*(3), 238–246. https://doi.org/10.1089/aut.2020.0049

Griffin, C., Lombardo, M. V. and Auyeung, B. (2016) Alexithymia in children with and without autism spectrum disorders: Alexithymia in childhood. *Autism Research 9*(7), 773–780. https://doi.org/10.1002/aur.1569

Groenman, A. P., Torenvliet, C., Radhoe, T. A., Agelink van Rentergem, J. A. and Geurts, H. M. (2021) Menstruation and menopause in autistic adults: Periods of importance? *Autism.* https://doi.org/10.1177/13623613211059721

Gros, D. F., Morland, L. A., Greene, C. J., Acierno, R., *et al.* (2013) Delivery of evidence-based psychotherapy via video telehealth. *Journal of Psychopathology and Behavioral Assessment 35*(4), 506–521. https://doi.org/10.1007/s10862-013-9363-4

Gross, R. D. (2015) Psychology as a Science. In N. Holt, A. Bremner, E. Sutherland, M. Vliek, M. Passer and R. Smith (eds) *Psychology: The Science of Mind and Behaviour* (Chapter 3). New York: McGraw Hill Education. http://public.eblib.com/choice/publicfullrecord.aspx?p=2066675

Gupta, S. and Kiran, S. (2019) Obsessive–compulsive disorder and child safeguarding. *BJPsych Advances 25*(3), 185–186. https://doi.org/10.1192/bja.2018.60

Haberstroh, S. and Schulte-Körne, G. (2019) The diagnosis and treatment of dyscalculia. *Deutsches Ärzteblatt International 116*, 107–114. https://doi.org/10.3238/arztebl.2019.0107

Haddock, J. N. and Hagopian, L. P. (2020) Suicidality and Self-Harm in Autism Spectrum Conditions. In S. W. White, B. B. Maddox and C. A. Mazefsky (eds) *The Oxford Handbook of Autism and Co-Occurring*

Psychiatric Conditions (pp.348–368). Oxford: Oxford University Press. https://doi.org/10.1093/oxfordhb/9780190910761.013.18

Haker, H., Schneebeli, M. and Stephan, K. E. (2016) Can Bayesian theories of autism spectrum disorder help improve clinical practice? *Frontiers in Psychiatry 7*. https://doi.org/10.3389/fpsyt.2016.00107

Hall, J. P., Batza, K., Streed, C. G., Boyd, B. A. and Kurth, N. K. (2020) Health disparities among sexual and gender minorities with autism spectrum disorder. *Journal of Autism and Developmental Disorders 50*(8), 3071–3077. https://doi.org/10.1007/s10803-020-04399-2

Hansson Halleröd, S. L., Anckarsäter, H., Råstam, M. and Hansson Scherman, M. (2015) Experienced consequences of being diagnosed with ADHD as an adult – A qualitative study. *BMC Psychiatry 15*(1), 31. https://doi.org/10.1186/s12888-015-0410-4

Happé, F. G. E. (1996) Studying weak central coherence at low levels: Children with autism do not succumb to visual illusions. A research note. *The Journal of Child Psychology and Psychiatry 37*(7), 873–877. https://doi.org/10.1111/j.1469-7610.1996.tb01483.x

Happé, F. G. E. and Frith, U. (1996) Theory of mind and social impairment in children with conduct disorder. *British Journal of Developmental Psychology 14*(4), 385–398. https://doi.org/10.1111/j.2044-835X.1996.tb00713.x

Harvey, K. (2012) *Trauma-Informed Behavioral Interventions: What Works and What Doesn't.* Silver Spring, MD: American Association on Intellectual and Developmental Disabilities (AAIDD). www.aaidd.org/publications/bookstore-home/product-listing/trauma-informed-behavioral-interventions-what-works-and-what-doesnot

Higgins, A., Doyle, L., Downes, C., Murphy, R., *et al.* (2016) *The LGBT Ireland Report: National Study of the Mental Health and Wellbeing of Lesbian, Gay, Bisexual, Transgender and Intersex People in Ireland.* Dublin: GLEN and BeLong To.

Hillier, A., Gallop, N., Mendes, E., Tellez, D., *et al.* (2020) LGBTQ + and autism spectrum disorder: Experiences and challenges. *International Journal of Transgender Health 21*(1), 98–110. https://doi.org/10.1080/15532739.2019.1594484

Hines, M., Balandin, S. and Togher, L. (2011) Communication and AAC in the lives of adults with autism: The stories of their older parents. *Augmentative and Alternative Communication 27*(4), 256–266. https://doi.org/10.3109/07434618.2011.587830

Hisle-Gorman, E., Landis, C. A., Susi, A., Schvey, N. A., *et al.* (2019) Gender dysphoria in children with autism spectrum disorder. *LGBT Health 6*(3), 95–100. https://doi.org/10.1089/lgbt.2018.0252

Hoffman, M. L. (2010) *Empathy and Moral Development: Implications for Caring and Justice.* New York: Cambridge University Press.

Hollocks, M. J., Lerh, J. W., Magiati, I., Meiser-Stedman, R. and Brugha, T. S. (2019) Anxiety and depression in adults with autism spectrum disorder: A systematic review and meta-analysis. *Psychological Medicine 49*(4), 559–572. https://doi.org/10.1017/S0033291718002283

Hood, B. M. (1995) Gravity rules for 2- to 4-year olds? *Cognitive Development 10*(4), 577–598. https://doi.org/10.1016/0885-2014(95)90027-6

Hoofs, V., Princen, M. M., Poljac, E., Stolk, A. and Poljac, E. (2018) Task switching in autism: An EEG study on intentions and actions. *Neuropsychologia 117*, 398–407. https://doi.org/10.1016/j.neuropsychologia.2018.07.008

Houghton, R., Liu, C. and Bolognani, F. (2018) Psychiatric comorbidities and psychotropic medication use in autism: A matched cohort study with ADHD and general population comparator groups in the United Kingdom. *Autism Research 11*(12), 1690–1700. https://doi.org/10.1002/aur.2040

Huang, J.-S., Yang, F.-C., Chien, W.-C., Yeh, T.-C., *et al.* (2021) Risk of substance use disorder and its associations with comorbidities and psychotropic agents in patients with autism. *JAMA Pediatrics 175*(2), e205371. https://doi.org/10.1001/jamapediatrics.2020.5371

Huang, M., Liang, C., Li, S., Zhang, J., *et al.* (2020) Two autism/dyslexia linked variations of DOCK4 disrupt the gene function on Rac1/Rap1 activation, neurite outgrowth, and synapse development. *Frontiers in Cellular Neuroscience 13*, 577. https://doi.org/10.3389/fncel.2019.00577

Hughes, E. (2015) Does the different presentation of Asperger syndrome in girls affect their problem areas and chances of diagnosis and support? *Autonomy, the Critical Journal of Interdisciplinary Autism Studies 1*(4). www.larry-arnold.net/Autonomy/index.php/autonomy/article/view/AR17

Hull, L., Mandy, W., Lai, M.-C., Baron-Cohen, S., *et al.* (2019) Development and validation of the Camouflaging Autistic Traits Questionnaire (CAT-Q). *Journal of Autism and Developmental Disorders 49*(3), 819–833. https://doi.org/10.1007/s10803-018-3792-6

Hull, L., Petrides, K. V., Allison, C., Smith, P., *et al.* (2017) 'Putting on my best normal': Social camouflaging in adults with autism spectrum conditions. *Journal of Autism and Developmental Disorders 47*(8), 2519–2534. https://doi.org/10.1007/s10803-017-3166-5

Human Rights Council (2018) *Mental Health and Human Rights, Report of the United Nations High Commissioner for Human Rights*. Thirty-Ninth Session, 10–28 September. www.ohchr.org/Documents/Issues/MentalHealth/A_HRC_39_36_EN.pdf

Hwang, A. and Francesco, A. M. (2010) The influence of individualism – Collectivism and power distance on use of feedback channels and consequences for learning. *Academy of Management Learning & Education* 9(2), 243–257.

Intriago, K. E. C., Rodríguez, L. M. A. and Cevallos, L. A. T. (2021) Specific learning difficulty: Autism, dyscalculia, dyslexia and dysgraphia. *International Research Journal of Engineering, IT & Scientific Research* 7(3), 97–106.

Janssen, A., Huang, H. and Duncan, C. (2016) Gender variance among youth with autism spectrum disorders: A retrospective chart review. *Transgender Health* 1(1), 63–68. https://doi.org/10.1089/trgh.2015.0007

Jones, D. R., Nicolaidis, C., Ellwood, L. J., Garcia, A., *et al.* (2020) An expert discussion on structural racism in autism research and practice. *Autism in Adulthood* 2(4), 273–281. https://doi.org/10.1089/aut.2020.29015.drj

Kaihlanen, A.-M., Hietapakka, L. and Heponiemi, T. (2019) Increasing cultural awareness: Qualitative study of nurses' perceptions about cultural competence training. *BMC Nursing* 18(1), 38. https://doi.org/10.1186/s12912-019-0363-x

Kaltiala-Heino, R., Sumia, M., Työläjärvi, M. and Lindberg, N. (2015) Two years of gender identity service for minors: Overrepresentation of natal girls with severe problems in adolescent development. *Child and Adolescent Psychiatry and Mental Health* 9(1), 9. https://doi.org/10.1186/s13034-015-0042-y

Kandeh, M. S., Kandeh, M. K., Martin, N. and Krupa, J. (2020) Autism in black, Asian and minority ethnic communities: A report on the first Autism Voice UK Symposium. *Advances in Autism* 6(2), 165–175. https://doi.org/10.1108/AIA-12-2018-0051

Kanner, L. (1943) Autistic disturbances of affective contact. *Nervous Child* 2, 217–250.

Kapp, S. (2016) Social Justice and Autism: Links to Personality and Advocacy. PhD Dissertation, UCLA. https://escholarship.org/uc/item/6fm925m3

Kelly, C., Sharma, S., Jieman, A.-T. and Ramon, S. (2022) Sense-making narratives of autistic women diagnosed in adulthood: A systematic review of the qualitative research. *Disability & Society*, 1–33. doi:10.1080/09687599.2022.2076582.

Kenny, L., Hattersley, C., Molins, B., Buckley, C., Povey, C. and Pellicano, E. (2016) Which terms should be used to describe autism? Perspectives from the UK autism community. *Autism* 20, 442–462. doi:10.1177/1362361315588200.

Kerns, C. M., Rast, J. E. and Shattuck, P. T. (2020) Prevalence and correlates of caregiver-reported mental health conditions in youth with autism spectrum disorder in the United States. *The Journal of Clinical Psychiatry* 82(1). https://doi.org/10.4088/JCP.20m13242

Kerns, C. M., Lankenau, S., Shattuck, P. T., Robins, D. L., Newschaffer, C. J. and Berkowitz, S. J. (2022) Exploring potential sources of childhood trauma: A qualitative study with autistic adults and caregivers. *Autism*. doi:10.1177/13623613211070637.

Kerr-Gaffney, J., Halls, D., Harrison, A. and Tchanturia, K. (2020) Exploring relationships between autism spectrum disorder symptoms and eating disorder symptoms in adults with anorexia nervosa: A network approach. *Frontiers in Psychiatry* 11, 401. https://doi.org/10.3389/fpsyt.2020.00401

Kervin, R., Berger, C., Moon, S. J., Hill, H., Park, D. and Kim, J. W. (2021) Behavioral addiction and autism spectrum disorder: A systematic review. *Research in Developmental Disabilities* 117, 104033. https://doi.org/10.1016/j.ridd.2021.104033

Kindgren, E., Quiñones Perez, A. and Knez, R. (2021) Prevalence of ADHD and autism spectrum disorder in children with hypermobility spectrum disorders or hypermobile Ehlers-Danlos syndrome: A retrospective study. *Neuropsychiatric Disease and Treatment* 17, 379–388. https://doi.org/10.2147/NDT.S290494

Kink Guidelines (2019) *Clinical Practice Guidelines for Working with People with Kink Interests*. www.kinkguidelines.com/the-guidelines

Kinnaird, E., Stewart, C. and Tchanturia, K. (2020) Investigating alexithymia in autism: A systematic review and meta-analysis. *European Psychiatry* 55, 80–89. https://doi.org/10.1016/j.eurpsy.2018.09.004

Kinnaird, E., Norton, C., Stewart, C. and Tchanturia, K. (2019) Same behaviours, different reasons: What do patients with co-occurring anorexia and autism want from treatment? *International Review of Psychiatry* 31(4), 308–317. https://doi.org/10.1080/09540261.2018.1531831

Kõlves, K., Fitzgerald, C., Nordentoft, M., Wood, S. J. and Erlangsen, A. (2021) Assessment of suicidal behaviors among individuals with autism spectrum disorder in Denmark. *JAMA Network Open* 4(1), e2033565. https://doi.org/10.1001/jamanetworkopen.2020.33565

Kourti, M. (ed.) (2021) *Working with Autistic Transgender and Non-Binary People*. London: Jessica Kingsley Publishers.

Kourti, M. and MacLeod, A. (2019) 'I don't feel like a gender, I feel like myself': Autistic individuals raised as girls exploring gender identity. *Autism in Adulthood 1*(1), 52–59. https://doi.org/10.1089/aut.2018.0001

Krahn, T. M. and Fenton, A. (2012) The extreme male brain theory of autism and the potential adverse effects for boys and girls with autism. *Journal of Bioethical Inquiry 9*(1), 93–103. https://doi.org/10.1007/s11673-011-9350-y

Kudryashov, L. (2021) Participatory Design of Augmentative and Alternative Communication (AAC) Technology with Autistic Adults. Master's Thesis. https://doi.org/10.7302/1729

Lachambre, C., Proteau-Lemieux, M., Lepage, J.-F., Bussières, E.-L., *et al.* (2021) Attentional and executive functions in children and adolescents with developmental coordination disorder and the influence of comorbid disorders: A systematic review of the literature. *PLoS ONE 16*(6), E0252043. https://doi.org/10.1371/journal.pone.0252043

Lai, M.-C., Kassee, C., Besney, R., Bonato, S., *et al.* (2019) Prevalence of co-occurring mental health diagnoses in the autism population: A systematic review and meta-analysis. *The Lancet Psychiatry 6*(10), 819–829. https://doi.org/10.1016/S2215-0366(19)30289-5

Lai, M.-C., Lombardo, M. V. and Baron-Cohen, S. (2014) Autism. *The Lancet 383*(9920), 896–910. https://doi.org/10.1016/S0140-6736(13)61539-1

Lai, M.-C., Lombardo, M. V., Ruigrok, A. N., Chakrabarti, B., *et al.* (2017) Quantifying and exploring camouflaging in men and women with autism. *Autism 21*(6), 690–702. https://doi.org/10.1177/1362361316671012

Lawson, R. P., Rees, G. and Friston, K. J. (2014) An aberrant precision account of autism. *Frontiers in Human Neuroscience 8*. https://doi.org/10.3389/fnhum.2014.00302

Leadbitter, K., Buckle, K. L., Ellis, C. and Dekker, M. (2021) Autistic self-advocacy and the neurodiversity movement: Implications for autism early intervention research and practice. *Frontiers in Psychology 12*, 635690. https://doi.org/10.3389/fpsyg.2021.635690

Lehmann, K. and Leavey, G. (2017) Individuals with gender dysphoria and autism: Barriers to good clinical practice. *Journal of Psychiatric and Mental Health Nursing 24*(2–3), 171–177. https://doi.org/10.1111/jpm.12351

Lever, A. G. and Geurts, H. M. (2016) Psychiatric co-occurring symptoms and disorders in young, middle-aged, and older adults with autism spectrum disorder. *Journal of Autism and Developmental Disorders 46*(6), 1916–1930. https://doi.org/10.1007/s10803-016-2722-8

Leweke, F., Leichsenring, F., Kruse, J. and Hermes, S. (2012) Is alexithymia associated with specific mental disorders? *Psychopathology 45*(1), 22–28. https://doi.org/10.1159/000325170

Lewis, L. F. (2017) A mixed methods study of barriers to formal diagnosis of autism spectrum disorder in adults. *Journal of Autism and Developmental Disorders 47*(8), 2410–2424. https://doi.org/10.1007/s10803-017-3168-3

Liu, X., Sun, X., Sun, C., Zou, M., *et al.* (2021) Prevalence of epilepsy in autism spectrum disorders: A systematic review and meta-analysis. *Autism.* https://doi.org/10.1177/13623613211045029

Lorincz, A. (2018) Colors of autism spectrum: A single paradigm explains the heterogeneity in autism spectrum disorder. *Behavioral Sciences.* https://doi.org/10.20944/preprints201804.0302.v1

Luterman, S. (2020) The biggest autism advocacy group is still failing too many autistic people. The *Washington Post*, 14 February. www.washingtonpost.com/outlook/2020/02/14/biggest-autism-advocacy-group-is-still-failing-too-many-autistic-people

Lynch, C. L. (2019) 7 cool aspects of autistic culture. NeuroClastic, 5 April. https://neuroclastic.com/7-cool-aspects-of-autistic-culture

Made by Dyslexia and EY (2019) *The Value of Dyslexia: Dyslexic Capability and Organisations of the Future*. https://assets.ey.com/content/dam/ey-sites/ey-com/en_uk/topics/diversity/ey-the-value-of-dyslexia-dyslexic-capability-and-organisations-of-the-future.pdf

Made by Dyslexia (2021) What is Dyslexia? *Join the Dots Workplace Guide*. https://www.madebydyslexia.org/wp-content/uploads/2021/08/Join-The-Dots-Workplace-Guide-1.pdf

Maenner, M. J., Shaw, K. A., Bakian, A. V., Bilder, D. A., *et al.* (2021) Prevalence and characteristics of autism spectrum disorder among children aged 8 years – Autism and Developmental Disabilities Monitoring Network, 11 sites, United States, 2018. *Morbidity and Mortality Weekly Report. Surveillance Summaries 70*(11), 1–16. https://doi.org/10.15585/mmwr.ss7011a1

Mahler, K. (2016) *Interoception: The Eighth Sensory System*. Shawnee, KS: AAPC Publishing.

Mahler, K. (2021) An interoception-based approach for supporting traumatized learners. 22 September. www.kelly-mahler.com/live-online-courses/an-interoception-based-approach-for-supporting-traumatized-learners

Mahler, K. and Vermeulen, P. (2021) Theory of own mind: Helping neurodivergents become the manager of their own emotions. Webinar, 21 April.

Mailhot Amborski, A., Bussières, E.-L., Vaillancourt-Morel, M.-P. and Joyal, C. C. (2021) Sexual violence against persons with disabilities: A meta-analysis. *Trauma, Violence, & Abuse*. https://doi.org/10.1177/1524838021995975

Mallipeddi, N. V. and VanDaalen, R. A. (2021) Intersectionality Within Critical Autism Studies: A Narrative Review. *Autism in Adulthood*. https://doi.org/10.1089/aut.2021.0014

Mandell, D. S., Ittenbach, R. F., Levy, S. E. and Pinto-Martin, J. A. (2007) Disparities in diagnoses received prior to a diagnosis of autism spectrum disorder. *Journal of Autism and Developmental Disorders* 37(9), 1795–1802. https://doi.org/10.1007/s10803-006-0314-8

Markram, K. and Markram, H. (2010) The intense world theory – A unifying theory of the neurobiology of autism. *Frontiers in Human Neuroscience* 4. https://doi.org/10.3389/fnhum.2010.00224

Mason, D., Ingham, B., Urbanowicz, A., Michael, C., *et al.* (2019b) A systematic review of what barriers and facilitators prevent and enable physical healthcare services access for autistic adults. *Journal of Autism and Developmental Disorders* 49(8), 3387–3400. https://doi.org/10.1007/s10803-019-04049-2

Mason, D., Mackintosh, J., McConachie, H., Rodgers, J., Finch, T. and Parr, J. R. (2019a) Quality of life for older autistic people: The impact of mental health difficulties. *Research in Autism Spectrum Disorders* 63, 13–22. https://doi.org/10.1016/j.rasd.2019.02.007

Maurer, D., Gibson, L. C. and Spector, F. (2013) Synesthesia in Infants and Very Young Children. In J. Simner and E. Hubbard (eds) *The Oxford Handbook of Synesthesia* (pp.46–63). Oxford: Oxford University Press.

Mayes, S. (2014) Diagnosing Autism with Checklist for Autism Spectrum Disorder (CASD). In V. B. Patel, V. R. Preedy and C. R. Martin (eds) *Comprehensive Guide to Autism* (pp.285–298). New York: Springer New York. https://doi.org/10.1007/978-1-4614-4788-7_11

McAlonan, G. M. (2004) Mapping the brain in autism. A voxel-based MRI study of volumetric differences and intercorrelations in autism. *Brain* 128(2), 268–276. https://doi.org/10.1093/brain/awh332

McConnell, E. A., Janulis, P., Phillips, G., Truong, R. and Birkett, M. (2018) Multiple minority stress and LGBT community resilience among sexual minority men. *Psychology of Sexual Orientation and Gender Diversity* 5(1), 1–12. https://doi.org/10.1037/sgd0000265

McLemore, K. A. (2018) A minority stress perspective on transgender individuals' experiences with misgendering. *Stigma and Health* 3(1), 53–64. https://doi.org/10.1037/sah0000070

Memmott, A. (2019) Autistic children – Are we helping them after trauma? PTSD. cPTSD. Ann's Autism Blog, 19 April. http://annsautism.blogspot.com/2019/04/autistic-children-are-we-helping-them.html

Merriam-Webster (no date) Morality. www.merriam-webster.com/dictionary/morality

Metcalfe, D., McKenzie, K., McCarty, K. and Murray, G. (2020) Screening tools for autism spectrum disorder, used with people with an intellectual disability: A systematic review. *Research in Autism Spectrum Disorders* 74, 101549. https://doi.org/10.1016/j.rasd.2020.101549

Meyer, I. H. (2015) Resilience in the study of minority stress and health of sexual and gender minorities. *Psychology of Sexual Orientation and Gender Diversity* 2(3), 209–213. https://doi.org/10.1037/sgd0000132

Miller, H. L., Sherrod, G. M., Mauk, J. E., Fears, N. E., *et al.* (2021) Shared features or co-occurrence? Evaluating symptoms of developmental coordination disorder in children and adolescents with autism spectrum disorder. *Journal of Autism and Developmental Disorders* 51, 3443–3455. doi:10.1007/s10803-020-04766-z.

Miller, R. A., Nachman, B. R. and Wynn, R. D. (2020) 'I feel like they are all interconnected': Understanding the identity management narratives of autistic LGBTQ college students. *College Student Affairs Journal* 38(1), 1–15. https://files.eric.ed.gov/fulltext/EJ1255491.pdf

Milot, T., Éthier, L. S., St-Laurent, D. and Provost, M. A. (2010) The role of trauma symptoms in the development of behavioral problems in maltreated preschoolers. *Child Abuse & Neglect* 34(4), 225–234. https://doi.org/10.1016/j.chiabu.2009.07.006

Milton, D. E. M. (2012) On the ontological status of autism: The 'double empathy problem'. *Disability & Society* 27(6), 883–887. https://doi.org/10.1080/09687599.2012.710008

Milton, D. E. M. (2017) *A Mismatch of Salience: Explorations of the Nature of Autism from Theory to Practice*. Shoreham-by-Sea: Pavilion Publishing and Media.

Morsanyi, K., van Bers, B. M. C. W., McCormack, T. and McGourty, J. (2018) The prevalence of specific learning disorder in mathematics and comorbidity with other developmental disorders in primary school-age children. *British Journal of Psychology* 109(4), 917–940. https://doi.org/10.1111/bjop.12322

Moseley, R. L., Druce, T. and Turner-Cobb, J. M. (2020) 'When my autism broke': A qualitative study spotlighting autistic voices on menopause. *Autism* 24(6), 1423–1437. https://doi.org/10.1177/1362361319901184

Mosley, D. V., Hargons, C. N., Meiller, C., Angyal, B., *et al.* (2021) Critical consciousness of anti-Black racism: A practical model to prevent and resist racial trauma. *Journal of Counseling Psychology* 68(1), 1–16. https://doi.org/10.1037/cou0000430

Mottron, L. and Burack, J. A. (2001) Enhanced Perceptual Functioning in the Development of Autism. In J. A. Burack, T. Charman, N. Yirmiya and P. R. Zelazo (eds) *The Development of Autism: Perspectives from Theory and Research* (pp.131–148). Mahwah, NJ: Lawrence Erlbaum Associates, Publishers.

Mottron, L., Dawson, M., Soulières, I., Hubert, B. and Burack, J. (2006) Enhanced perceptual functioning in autism: An update, and eight principles of autistic perception. *Journal of Autism and Developmental Disorders 36*(1), 27–43. https://doi.org/10.1007/s10803-005-0040-7

Mowlem, F. D., Rosenqvist, M. A., Martin, J., Lichtenstein, P., Asherson, P. and Larsson, H. (2019) Sex differences in predicting ADHD clinical diagnosis and pharmacological treatment. *European Child & Adolescent Psychiatry 28*(4), 481–489. https://doi.org/10.1007/s00787-018-1211-3

Mul, C., Stagg, S. D., Herbelin, B. and Aspell, J. E. (2018) The feeling of me feeling for you: Interoception, alexithymia and empathy in autism. *Journal of Autism and Developmental Disorders 48*(9), 2953–2967. https://doi.org/10.1007/s10803-018-3564-3

Mundy, K. (2022) Autistic masking and introducing autistic shielding. Aucademy webinar, 19 March. www.aucademy.co.uk

Murphy, D., Glaser, K., Hayward, H., Eklund, H., *et al.* (2018) Crossing the divide: A longitudinal study of effective treatments for people with autism and attention deficit hyperactivity disorder across the lifespan. *Programme Grants for Applied Research 6*(2), 1–240. https://doi.org/10.3310/pgfar06020

Murray, D. (2018) Monotropism – An Interest Based Account of Autism. In F. R. Volkmar (ed.) *Encyclopedia of Autism Spectrum Disorders* (pp. 1–3). New York: Springer New York. doi:10.1007/978-1-4614-6435-8_102269-1.

Murray, D., Lesser, M. and Lawson, W. (2005) Attention, monotropism and the diagnostic criteria for autism. *Autism 9*(2), 139–156. https://doi.org/10.1177/1362361305051398

Murray, M. L., Hsia, Y., Glaser, K., Simonoff, E., *et al.* (2014) Pharmacological treatments prescribed to people with autism spectrum disorder (ASD) in primary health care. *Psychopharmacology 231*(6), 1011–1021. https://doi.org/10.1007/s00213-013-3140-7

National Autistic Society and Mind (2021) *The Good Practice Guide for Mental Health Professionals*. www.autism.org.uk/what-we-do/news/adapt-mental-health-talking-therapies

Neumeier, S. M. (2018) 'To Siri with love' and the problem with neurodiversity lite. *Rewire News Group*, 9 February. Available at: https://rewire.news/article/2018/02/09/siri-love-problem-neurodiversity-lite, acessed on 12 July 2022.

Nicki, A. (2016) Borderline personality disorder, discrimination, and survivors of chronic childhood trauma. *International Journal of Feminist Approaches to Bioethics 9*(1), 218–245. https://www.jstor.org/stable/90011865

Nicolaidis, C., Milton, D., Sasson, N. J., Sheppard, E. and Yergeau, M. (2019) An expert discussion on autism and empathy. *Autism in Adulthood 1*(1), 4–11. https://doi.org/10.1089/aut.2018.29000.cjn

Nicolaidis, C., Raymaker, D. M., McDonald, K. E., Lund, E. M., *et al.* (2020) Creating accessible survey instruments for use with autistic adults and people with intellectual disability: Lessons learned and recommendations. *Autism in Adulthood 2*(1), 61–76. https://doi.org/10.1089/aut.2019.0074

Nicolaidis, C., Schnider, G., Lee, J., Raymaker, D. M., *et al.* (2021) Development and psychometric testing of the AASPIRE Adult Autism Healthcare Provider Self-Efficacy Scale. *Autism 25*(3), 767–773. https://doi.org/10.1177/1362361320949734

Nimmo-Smith, V., Heuvelman, H., Dalman, C., Lundberg, M., *et al.* (2020) Anxiety disorders in adults with autism spectrum disorder: A population-based study. *Journal of Autism and Developmental Disorders 50*(1), 308–318. https://doi.org/10.1007/s10803-019-04234-3

Nyrenius, J., Eberhard, J., Ghaziuddin, M., Gillberg, C. and Billstedt, E. (2022) Prevalence of Autism Spectrum Disorders in adult outpatient psychiatry. *Journal of Autism and Developmental Disorders*, 6 January. doi:10.1007/s10803-021-05411-z.

Oakley, B., Loth, E. and Murphy, D. G. (2021) Autism and mood disorders. *International Review of Psychiatry 33*(3), 280–299. https://doi.org/10.1080/09540261.2021.1872506

ONS (Office for National Statistics) (2020) Sexual orientation, UK: 2020. Experimental Statistics on sexual orientation in the UK in 2020 by region, sex, age, marital or legal partnership status, ethnic group and socio-economic classification, using data from the Annual Population Survey (APS). https://www.ons.gov.uk/peoplepopulationandcommunity/culturalidentity/sexuality/bulletins/sexualidentityuk/2020

Ostrolenk, A. and Bertone, A. (2016) Gender-specific differences in autism Spectrum cognitive profiles: Wechsler intelligence scales versus Raven's progressive matrices. *Clinical Psychiatry 66*(1), 3–8.

Ozonoff, S. (1997) Components of Executive Function in Autism and Other Disorders. In J. Russell (ed.) *Autism as an Executive Disorder* (pp.179–211). Oxford: Oxford University Press.

Palmqvist, M., Edman, G. and Bölte, S. (2014) Screening for substance use disorders in neurodevelopmental disorders: A clinical routine? *European Child & Adolescent Psychiatry 23*(5), 365–368. https://doi.org/10.1007/s00787-013-0459-x

Pearson, A. and Rose, K. (2021) A conceptual analysis of autistic masking: Understanding the narrative of stigma and the illusion of choice. *Autism in Adulthood* 3(1), 52–60. https://doi.org/10.1089/aut.2020.0043

Pearson, A., Rees, J. and Forster, S. (2022) 'This was just how this friendship worked': Experiences of interpersonal victimization among autistic adults. *Autism in Adulthood.* https://doi.org/10.1089/aut.2021.0035

Pecora, L. A., Mesibov, G. B. and Stokes, M. A. (2016) Sexuality in high-functioning autism: A systematic review and meta-analysis. *Journal of Autism and Developmental Disorders* 46(11), 3519–3556. https://doi.org/10.1007/s10803-016-2892-4

Pehlivanidis, A., Papanikolaou, K., Mantas, V., *et al.* (2020) Lifetime co-occurring psychiatric disorders in newly diagnosed adults with attention deficit hyperactivity disorder (ADHD) or/and autism spectrum disorder (ASD). *BMC Psychiatry 20,* 423. https://doi.org/10.1186/s12888-020-02828-1

Pellicano, E. and Burr, D. (2012) When the world becomes 'too real': A Bayesian explanation of autistic perception. *Trends in Cognitive Sciences* 16(10), 504–510. https://doi.org/10.1016/j.tics.2012.08.009

Polanczyk, G. V., Casella, C. and Jaffee, S. R. (2019) Commentary: ADHD lifetime trajectories and the relevance of the developmental perspective to psychiatry: reflections on Asherson and Agnew-Blais, (2019). *Journal of Child Psychology and Psychiatry* 60(4), 353–355. https://doi.org/10.1111/jcpp.13050

Poquérusse, J., Pastore, L., Dellantonio, S. and Esposito, G. (2018) Alexithymia and autism spectrum disorder: A complex relationship. *Frontiers in Psychology 9,* 1196. https://doi.org/10.3389/fpsyg.2018.01196

Postal, K. (2021) Comment on Cory, 2021: 'White privilege in clinical neuropsychology: an invisible "knapsack" in need of unpacking'. *The Clinical Neuropsychologist* 35(2), 224–226. https://doi.org/10.1080/13854046.2020.1844297

Purkis, Y. (2022) Why empathy is not as simple as it seems. Yenn Purkis Autism Page, 24 March. https://yennpurkis.home.blog/2022/03/24/why-empathy-is-not-as-simple-as-it-seems

Quirke, B., Heinen, M., Fitzpatrick, P., McKey, S., Malone, K. M. and Kelleher, C. (2020) Experience of discrimination and engagement with mental health and other services by Travellers in Ireland: Findings from the All Ireland Traveller Health Study (AITHS). *Irish Journal of Psychological Medicine*, 1–11. https://doi.org/10.1017/ipm.2020.90

Rainer, B., Barnett, A. L., Cairney, J., Green, D., *et al.* (2019) International clinical practice recommendations on the definition, diagnosis, assessment, intervention, and psychosocial aspects of developmental coordination disorder. *Developmental Neurology and Child Medicine, 61*(3), 242–285.

Rao, T. S. S. and Andrade, C. (2011) The MMR vaccine and autism: Sensation, refutation, retraction, and fraud. *Indian Journal of Psychiatry* 53(2), 95–96. doi:10.4103/0019-5545.82529.

Raznahan, A., Toro, R., Daly, E., Robertson, D., *et al.* (2010) Cortical anatomy in autism spectrum disorder: An in vivo MRI study on the effect of age. *Cerebral Cortex* 20(6), 1332–1340. https://doi.org/10.1093/cercor/bhp198

Reese, R. M., Jamison, T. R., Braun, M., Wendland, M., *et al.* (2015) Brief report: Use of interactive television in identifying autism in young children: Methodology and preliminary data. *Journal of Autism and Developmental Disorders* 45(5), 1474–1482. https://doi.org/10.1007/s10803-014-2269-5

Reuben, K. E., Stanzione, C. M. and Singleton, J. L. (2021) Interpersonal trauma and posttraumatic stress in autistic adults. *Autism in Adulthood* 3(3), 247–256. https://doi.org/10.1089/aut.2020.0073

Rødgaard, E.-M., Jensen, K., Miskowiak, K. W. and Mottron, L. (2021) Childhood diagnoses in individuals identified as autistics in adulthood. *Molecular Autism* 12(1), 73. https://doi.org/10.1186/s13229-021-00478-y

Roe, L., Galvin, M., Booi, L., Brandao, L., *et al.* (2020) To live and age as who we really are: Perspectives from older LGBT+ people in Ireland. *HRB Open Research 3,* 6. https://doi.org/10.12688/hrbopenres.12990.2

Roman-Urrestarazu, A., van Kessel, R., Allison, C., Matthews, F. E., Brayne, C. and Baron-Cohen, S. (2021) Association of race/ethnicity and social disadvantage with autism prevalence in 7 million school children in England. *JAMA Pediatrics* 175(6), e210054. https://doi.org/10.1001/jamapediatrics.2021.0054

Rose, J. (2009) *Identifying and Teaching Children and Young People with Dyslexia and Literacy Difficulties.* Nottingham: Department for Children, Schools and Families.

Rose, K. (2020) *How to Hide Your Autism.* Blackburn: Star Institute for Sensory Processing.

Rosenblum, S., Smits-Engelsman, B., Sugden, D., Wilson, P. and Vinçon, S. (2019) International clinical practice recommendations on the definition, diagnosis, assessment, intervention, and psychosocial aspects of developmental coordination disorder. *Developmental Neurology and Child Medicine* 61(3), 242–285. doi:10.1111/dmcn.14132.

Rubel, A. N. and Burleigh, T. J. (2020) Counting polyamorists who count: Prevalence and definitions of an under-researched form of consensual nonmonogamy. *Sexualities* 23(1–2), 3–27. https://doi.org/10.1177/1363460718779781

Rumball, F., Happé, F. and Grey, N. (2020) Experience of trauma and PTSD symptoms in autistic adults: Risk of PTSD development following DSM-5 and non-DSM-5 traumatic life events. *Autism Research* 13(12), 2122–2132. https://doi.org/10.1002/aur.2306

Russell, G., Stapley, S., Newlove-Delgado, T., Salmon, A., *et al.* (2021) Time trends in autism diagnosis over 20 years: A UK population-based cohort study. *Journal of Child Psychology and Psychiatry.* https://doi.org/10.1111/jcpp.13505

Rydzewska, E., Hughes-McCormack, L. A., Gillberg, C., Henderson, A., *et al.* (2019) Prevalence of sensory impairments, physical and intellectual disabilities, and mental health in children and young people with self/proxy-reported autism: Observational study of a whole country population. *Autism 23*(5), 1201–1209. https://doi.org/10.1177/1362361318791279

Sapey-Triomphe, L.-A. (2017) Perceptual Inference and Learning in Autism: A Behavioral and Neurophysiological Approach. PhD Thesis, Université de Lyon.

Sappok, T., Diefenbacher, A., Budczies, J., Schade, C., *et al.* (2013) Diagnosing autism in a clinical sample of adults with intellectual disabilities: How useful are the ADOS and the ADI-R? *Research in Developmental Disabilities 34*(5), 1642–1655. https://doi.org/10.1016/j.ridd.2013.01.028

Satterstrom, F. K., Kosmicki, J. A., Wang, J., Breen, M. S., *et al.* (2020) Large-scale exome sequencing study implicates both developmental and functional changes in the neurobiology of autism. *Cell 180*(3), 568–584.e23. doi:10.1016/j.cell.2019.12.036.

Sayal, K., Prasad, V., Daley, D., Ford, T. and Coghill, D. (2018) ADHD in children and young people: Prevalence, care pathways, and service provision. *The Lancet Psychiatry 5*(2), 175–186. https://doi.org/10.1016/S2215-0366(17)30167-0

Scantling, S. and Browder, S. (1993) *Ordinary Women, Extraordinary Sex: Every Woman's Guide to Pleasure and Beyond.* New York: Dutton Adult.

Schneebeli, M., Haker, H., Rüesch, A., Zahnd, N., *et al.* (2022) Disentangling 'Bayesian brain' theories of autism spectrum disorder [Preprint]. *Psychiatry and Clinical Psychology.* https://doi.org/10.1101/2022.02.07.22270242

Shaw, C. and Proctor, G. (2005) I. Women at the margins: A critique of the diagnosis of borderline personality disorder. *Feminism & Psychology 15*(4), 483–490. https://doi.org/10.1177/0959-353505057620

Shaywitz, S. E., Shaywitz, J. E. and Shaywitz, B. A. (2021) Dyslexia in the 21st century. *Current Opinion in Psychiatry 34*(2), 80–86. https://doi.org/10.1097/YCO.0000000000000670

Shumer, D. E., Reisner, S. L., Edwards-Leeper, L. and Tishelman, A. (2016) Evaluation of Asperger syndrome in youth presenting to a gender dysphoria clinic. *LGBT Health 3*(5), 387–390. https://doi.org/10.1089/lgbt.2015.0070

Silberman, S. (2016) *NeuroTribes: The Legacy of Autism and the Future of Neurodiversity.* New York: Avery Publishing.

Sinclair, J. (1993) Don't mourn for us. Our voice. *Autism Network International 1*(3). www.autreat.com/dont_mourn.html

Skokauskas, N. and Frodl, T. (2015) Overlap between autism spectrum disorder and bipolar affective disorder. *Psychopathology 48*(4), 209–216. https://doi.org/10.1159/000435787

Skokauskas, N. and Gallagher, L. (2010) Psychosis, affective disorders and anxiety in autistic spectrum disorder: Prevalence and nosological considerations. *Psychopathology 43*(1), 8–16. https://doi.org/10.1159/000255958

Smith, A. (2009) Emotional empathy in autism spectrum conditions: Weak, intact, or heightened? *Journal of Autism and Developmental Disorders 39*(12), 1747–1748. https://doi.org/10.1007/s10803-009-0799-z

Snapp, S. D., Watson, R. J., Russell, S. T., Diaz, R. M. and Ryan, C. (2015) Social support networks for LGBT young adults: Low cost strategies for positive adjustment. *Family Relations 64*(3), 420–430. https://doi.org/10.1111/fare.12124

Snouckaert, V. C. and Spek, A. A. (2020) The development of anorexia nervosa in people with an autism spectrum disorder: A qualitative, retrospective study. *Tijdschrift Voor Psychiatrie 62*(9), 760–767.

Snyder, H. R., Miyake, A. and Hankin, B. L. (2015) Advancing understanding of executive function impairments and psychopathology: Bridging the gap between clinical and cognitive approaches. *Frontiers in Psychology 6.* https://doi.org/10.3389/fpsyg.2015.00328

Soares, N. and Patel, D.R. (2015) Dyscalculia. *International Journal of Child and Adolescent Health 8*(1), 15–26.

Solbes-Canales, I., Valverde-Montesino, S. and Herranz-Hernández, P. (2020) Socialization of gender stereotypes related to attributes and professions among young Spanish school-aged children. *Frontiers in Psychology 11*, 609. https://doi.org/10.3389/fpsyg.2020.00609

Solomon, M., Miller, M., Taylor, S. L., Hinshaw, S. P. and Carter, C. S. (2012) Autism symptoms and internalizing psychopathology in girls and boys with autism spectrum disorders. *Journal of Autism and Developmental Disorders 42*(1), 48–59. https://doi.org/10.1007/s10803-011-1215-z

Solomon, S. D. and Davidson, J. R. (1997) Trauma: Prevalence, impairment, service use, and cost. *The Journal of Clinical Psychiatry 58*, Suppl. 9, 5–11.

South, M., Costa, A. P. and McMorris, C. (2021) Death by suicide among people with autism: Beyond Zebrafish. *JAMA Network Open 4*(1), e2034018. https://doi.org/10.1001/jamanetworkopen.2020.34018

Spielmann, V. (2021) *How to Deliver Neurodiversity Affirming Sensory Integration Therapy*. Blackburn: Star Institute.

Stack, A. and Lucyshyn, J. (2019) Autism spectrum disorder and the experience of traumatic events: Review of the current literature to inform modifications to a treatment model for children with autism. *Journal of Autism and Developmental Disorders 49*(4), 1613–1625. https://doi.org/10.1007/s10803-018-3854-9

Stewart, G. R., Corbett, A., Ballard, C., Creese, B., *et al.* (2022) Traumatic life experiences and post-traumatic stress symptoms in middle-aged and older adults with and without autistic traits. *International Journal of Geriatric Psychiatry 37*(2), gps.5669. https://doi.org/10.1002/gps.5669

Stoll, M. M., Bergamo, N. and Rossetti, K. G. (2021) Analyzing modes of assessment for children with autism spectrum disorder (ASD) using a culturally sensitive lens. *Advances in Neurodevelopmental Disorders 5*(3), 233–244. https://doi.org/10.1007/s41252-021-00210-0

Stone, W. S. and Chen, G. (2015) Comorbidity of autism spectrum and obsessive-compulsive disorders. *American Journal of Medicine and Science 8*(3), 109–112.

Straiton, D. and Sridhar, A. (2021) Short report: Call to action for autism clinicians in response to anti-Black racism. *Autism*. https://doi.org/10.1177/13623613211043643

Strang, J. F., Powers, M. D., Knauss, M., Sibarium, E., *et al.* (2018) 'They thought it was an obsession': Trajectories and perspectives of autistic transgender and gender-diverse adolescents. *Journal of Autism and Developmental Disorders 48*(12), 4039–4055. https://doi.org/10.1007/s10803-018-3723-6

Sullivan, P. F., Magnusson, C., Reichenberg, A., Boman, M., *et al.* (2012) Family history of schizophrenia and bipolar disorder as risk factors for autism. *Archives of General Psychiatry 69*(11). https://doi.org/10.1001/archgenpsychiatry.2012.730

Szalavitz, M. (2017) The hidden link between autism and addiction. *The Atlantic*, 2 March. www.theatlantic.com/health/archive/2017/03/autism-and-addiction/518289

Talcer, M. C., Duffy, O. and Pedlow, K. (2021) A qualitative exploration into the sensory experiences of autistic mothers. *Journal of Autism and Developmental Disorders*. https://doi.org/10.1007/s10803-021-05188-1

Taylor, S. (2004) The right not to work: Power and disability. *Monthly Review*, 1 March. www.monthlyreview.org/2004/03/01/the-right-not-to-work-power-and-disability

Tchanturia, K., Smith, K., Glennon, D. and Burhouse, A. (2020) Towards an improved understanding of the anorexia nervosa and autism spectrum comorbidity: PEACE pathway implementation. *Frontiers in Psychiatry 11*, 640. https://doi.org/10.3389/fpsyt.2020.00640

Testa, R. J., Habarth, J., Peta, J., Balsam, K. and Bockting, W. (2015) Development of the Gender Minority Stress and Resilience measure. *Psychology of Sexual Orientation and Gender Diversity 2*(1), 65–77. https://doi.org/10.1037/sgd0000081

Titman, N. (2018) The elephant in the room. Autscape, August. *Exploring Inclusion*, Tonbridge, Kent, England.

Tromans, S., Chester, V., Kiani, R., Alexander, R. and Brugha, T. (2018) The prevalence of autism spectrum disorders in adult psychiatric inpatients: A systematic review. *Clinical Practice & Epidemiology in Mental Health 14*, 177–187. https://doi.org/10.2174/1745017901814010177

Tromans, S., Chester, V., Gemegah, E., Roberts, K., *et al.* (2021) Autism identification across ethnic groups: A narrative review. *Advances in Autism 7*(3), 241–255. https://doi.org/10.1108/AIA-03-2020-0017

Tudge, J. R. H., Mokrova, I., Hatfield, B. E. and Karnik, R. B. (2009) Uses and misuses of Bronfenbrenner's bioecological theory of human development. *Journal of Family Theory & Review 1*(4), 198–210. https://doi.org/10.1111/j.1756-2589.2009.00026.x

United Nations (no date) What Is Domestic Abuse? www.un.org/en/coronavirus/what-is-domestic-abuse

van de Cruys, S., Evers, K., van der Hallen, R., van Eylen, L., *et al.* (2014) Precise minds in uncertain worlds: Predictive coding in autism. *Psychological Review 121*(4), 649–675. https://doi.org/10.1037/a0037665

van Dijke, A., Hopman, J. A. B. and Ford, J. D. (2018) Affect dysregulation, adult attachment problems, and dissociation mediate the relationship between childhood trauma and borderline personality disorder symptoms in adulthood. *European Journal of Trauma & Dissociation 2*(2), 91–99. https://doi.org/10.1016/j.ejtd.2017.11.002

van Leeuwen, T. M., Neufeld, J., Hughes, J. and Ward, J. (2020) Synaesthesia and autism: Different developmental outcomes from overlapping mechanisms? *Cognitive Neuropsychology 37*(7–8), 433–449. https://doi.org/10.1080/02643294.2020.1808455

Villani, J. and Barry, M. M. (2021) A qualitative study of the perceptions of mental health among the Traveller community in Ireland. *Health Promotion International 36*(5), 1450–1462. https://doi.org/10.1093/heapro/daab009

Walsh, R. J., Krabbendam, L., Dewinter, J. and Begeer, S. (2018) Brief report: Gender identity differences in autistic adults: Associations with perceptual and socio-cognitive profiles. *Journal of Autism and Developmental Disorders 48*(12), 4070–4078. https://doi.org/10.1007/s10803-018-3702-y

Ward, A. (2020). What is it like to have synesthesia? The Royal Institution, YouTube, 16 April. https://youtu.be/ZVC3E16FCrk

Ward, J. (2019) Individual differences in sensory sensitivity: A synthesizing framework and evidence from normal variation and developmental conditions. *Cognitive Neuroscience 10*(3), 139–157. https://doi.org/10.1080/17588928.2018.1557131

Ward, J., Brown, P., Sherwood, J. and Simner, J. (2018) An autistic-like profile of attention and perception in synaesthesia. *Cortex 107*, 121–130. https://doi.org/10.1016/j.cortex.2017.10.008

Ward, J., Hoadley, C., Hughes, J. E. A., Smith, P., *et al.* (2017) Atypical sensory sensitivity as a shared feature between synaesthesia and autism. *Scientific Reports 7*(1), 41155. https://doi.org/10.1038/srep41155

Warrier, V., Greenberg, D. M., Weir, E., Buckingham, C., *et al.* (2020) Elevated rates of autism, other neurodevelopmental and psychiatric diagnoses, and autistic traits in transgender and gender-diverse individuals. *Nature Communications 11*(1), 3959. https://doi.org/10.1038/s41467-020-17794-1

Wassell, C. and Burke, E. (2022) *Autism, Girls, & Keeping It All Inside*. Autistic Girls Network. https://autisticgirlsnetwork.org/keeping-it-all-inside.pdf

Weinberg, M. and Gil, S. (2016) Trauma as an objective or subjective experience: The association between types of traumatic events, personality traits, subjective experience of the event, and posttraumatic symptoms. *Journal of Loss and Trauma 21*(2), 137–146. https://doi.org/10.1080/15325024.2015.1011986

Weir, E., Allison, C. and Baron-Cohen, S. (2021a) Understanding the substance use of autistic adolescents and adults: A mixed-methods approach. *The Lancet Psychiatry 8*(8), 673–685. https://doi.org/10.1016/S2215-0366(21)00160-7

Weir, E., Allison, C. and Baron-Cohen, S. (2021b) The sexual health, orientation, and activity of autistic adolescents and adults. *Autism Research 14*(11), 2342–2354. https://doi.org/10.1002/aur.2604

Weiss, J. A. and Fardella, M. A. (2018) Victimization and perpetration experiences of adults with autism. *Frontiers in Psychiatry 9*, 203. https://doi.org/10.3389/fpsyt.2018.00203

WHO (World Health Organization) (2019) *International Classification of Diseases* (11th revision) (ICD-11). https://icd.who.int

Williams, D. (1996) *Autism, an Inside-Out Approach: An Innovative Look at the Mechanics of 'Autism' and its Developmental 'Cousins'*. London: Jessica Kingsley Publishers.

Wing, L. (1981) Asperger's syndrome: A clinical account. *Psychological Medicine 11*(1), 115–129. https://doi.org/10.1017/S0033291700053332

WrenAves (2022) Goodbye, You Will Not Be Missed: An Open Letter To NHS Mental Health Services. *Psychiatry is Driving Me Mad*. https://www.psychiatryisdrivingmemad.co.uk/post/goodbye-you-will-not-be-missed-an-open-letter-to-nhs-mental-health-services

Zablotsky, B., Bradshaw, C. P., Anderson, C. M. and Law, P. (2014) Risk factors for bullying among children with autism spectrum disorders. *Autism 18*(4), 419–427. https://doi.org/10.1177/1362361313477920

Zerbo, O., Massolo, M. L., Qian, Y. and Croen, L. A. (2015) A study of physician knowledge and experience with autism in adults in a large integrated healthcare system. *Journal of Autism and Developmental Disorders 45*(12), 4002–4014. https://doi.org/10.1007/s10803-015-2579-2

Zheng, L., Foley, K.-R., Grove, R., Elley, K., *et al.* (2021) The use of everyday and assistive technology in the lives of older autistic adults. *Autism*, 13623613211058585. https://doi.org/10.1177/13623613211058519

Ziegler, S., Bednasch, K., Baldofski, S. and Rummel-Kluge, C. (2021) Long durations from symptom onset to diagnosis and from diagnosis to treatment in obsessive-compulsive disorder: A retrospective self-report study. *PLoS ONE 16*(12), e0261169. https://doi.org/10.1371/journal.pone.0261169

Zisk, A. H. and Dalton, E. (2019) Augmentative and alternative communication for speaking autistic adults: Overview and recommendations. *Autism in Adulthood 1*(2), 93–100. https://doi.org/10.1089/aut.2018.0007

About the Authors

Davida Hartman is an Adjunct Professor in University College Dublin (UCD) School of Psychology and a Chartered Educational and Child Psychologist who has been working with Autistic children and adults for over 20 years. Having previously worked within the Irish health service in both disability and specialist services supporting Autistic children, in 2017 Davida co-founded The Children's Clinic, a multidisciplinary clinic in Dublin, Ireland, known for best practice, Neuro-Affirmative child autism assessments. In 2020, she founded The Adult Autism Practice, specialising in adult autism assessments, where she continues to be Clinical Director. Davida is also a lecturer and trainer, and has written five previous books with Jessica Kingsley Publishers.

Tara O'Donnell-Killen is an Autistic Coaching Psychologist, Integrative Therapist and founder of the non-profit Thriving Autistic, a global multidisciplinary team of neurodivergent practitioners who specialize in Neuro-Affirmative support for Autistic adults. Tara is also Support Lead for The Adult Autism Practice since its inception in 2020. She frequently lectures on Neuro-Affirmative Practice for universities and mental health charities across the UK and Ireland. Her current research projects include Neuro-Affirmative Parenting and therapeutic models of best practice for Neuro-Affirmative Support.

Jessica K. Doyle has a BA Honours in Psychology from Trinity College Dublin (TCD). She works as an Autistic Assistant Psychologist at The Adult Autism Practice, is a Director at Thriving Autistic, a Project Officer at TCD Sense, (2022) Chair of the Psychological Society of Ireland (PSI) Special Interest Group in Autism, and a Consultant and Researcher who is passionate about bridging the gaps between theory, researcher and practice. She is motivated to think outside the box, explore perceptions, develop understanding from below the surface, and reposition the lens away from changing the person or hiding their Authenticity to designing for diversity, fostering growth, self-awareness and empowerment, and committing to universal design.

Dr Maeve Kavanagh is a Chartered Clinical Psychologist who has worked on behalf of Autistic children and adults since 2008 in both the public and private healthcare sectors in Ireland. Maeve is a keen ally of the Autistic community and has a particular interest in gender identity and Autistic experiences. Maeve holds a BA in Psychology from University College Dublin (UCD) (2002), an MSc in Clinical Neuroscience from University College London (UCL) (2003) and a Doctorate in Clinical Psychology from Trinity College Dublin (TCD) (2008). Maeve is Principal Psychologist at The Adult Autism Practice, where she has worked since its foundation in 2020. She has worked with The Adult Autism Practice since its foundation in 2020, and is Co-Director of Childversity, specialising in Neuro-Affirmative autism assessments for children and adolescents.

Dr Anna Day is an Autistic Clinical Psychologist. Anna worked previously in the UK's National Health Service (NHS) and now works for The Adult Autism Practice, where she views the process of assessment as one of collaboratively exploring Autistic identity, and sees the discovery of one's autism as giving the potential for reviewing one's life through a new lens of understanding and reaching a perhaps unanticipated level of self-understanding and compassion. Anna has an Autistic daughter and is passionate about advocating for Autistic rights and Neuro-Affirmative approaches within mental healthcare and education.

Dr Juliana Azevedo is an experienced Senior Clinical Psychologist who obtained her undergraduate/Master's/Doctorate in Clinical Psychology from the Pontifical Catholic University of São Paulo (PUC-SP), Brazil and is a Chartered Member of the Psychological Society of Ireland (PSI). Working in Ireland for the past 18 years in lifespan public and private mental health services, she has developed a service identifying Autistic people referred to a psychology primary care service. Juliana has lectured in Trinity College Dublin (TCD) and University College Dublin (UCD), and holds additional qualifications in Cognitive Analytical Therapy. She also provides professional placements and clinical supervision to psychologists in training, both for the Doctorate Clinical Psychology course in TCD (where she holds an Honorary Tutor title) and for the Doctorate Educational Psychology course in UCD.

Subject Index

Author Index